江苏大学英文教材基金资助出版
江苏大学教改项目（2021JGZD011）资助出版
江苏大学留学本科生英文授课医学遗传学精品课程项目资助出版
来华留学生临床医学专业本科教育（英语授课）精品在线开放课程项目
（CEAIEJPK202101）资助出版

MEDICAL GENETICS

医学遗传学

主　编　邵根宝　金　洁　龚爱华
副主编　李明阳　杜凤移　纪立凯　张　徐
编　委　王浩然　张　颖　张柳平

江苏大学出版社
JIANGSU UNIVERSITY PRESS
镇 江

图书在版编目（CIP）数据

医学遗传学＝Medical Genetics：英文／邵根宝，金洁，龚爱华主编. -- 镇江：江苏大学出版社，2023.12
ISBN 978-7-5684-1777-8

Ⅰ.①医… Ⅱ.①邵… ②金… ③龚… Ⅲ.①医学遗传学 － 英文 Ⅳ.①R394

中国版本图书馆 CIP 数据核字（2021）第 281115 号

医学遗传学
Medical Genetics

主　　编／邵根宝　金　洁　龚爱华
责任编辑／宋燕敏
出版发行／江苏大学出版社
地　　址／江苏省镇江市京口区学府路 301 号（邮编：212013）
电　　话／0511-84446464（传真）
网　　址／http：//press.ujs.edu.cn
排　　版／镇江文苑制版印刷有限责任公司
印　　刷／江苏凤凰数码印务有限公司
开　　本／787 mm×1 092 mm　1/16
印　　张／17
字　　数／600 千字
版　　次／2023 年 12 月第 1 版
印　　次／2023 年 12 月第 1 次印刷
书　　号／ISBN 978-7-5684-1777-8
定　　价／95.00 元

如有印装质量问题请与本社营销部联系（电话：0511-84440882）

PREFACE

The genetic "revolution" that has occurred over the past 20 years has thrust clinical genetics into the mainstream of medical practice. Every component of health care delivery requires at least a working knowledge of core genetic principles. This fact is directly reflected in changes in medical school curricula. While the vast majority of medical students will not go on to specialize in medical genetics, all of them need to know much about genetic concepts and principles. Still, there truly is not a discipline in all of medicine that does not use genetic principles, genetic information, and genetic techniques in the practice of its field. Thus, a textbook in medical genetics must be broad and inclusive in the scope of material covered. There must be sufficient detail to guide the student to successful completion of the curriculum at his/her respective medical school. Most importantly, it should be a resource that students can use throughout their medical school years and beyond to refer to when questions arise during the times of residency and practice as a professional.

The compilation of this English textbook combines the overall requirements of the National Health and Family Planning Commission and the Ministry of Education, and adheres to the principles of "three basics, five characteristics, and three specifics". The presentation of basic theories and basic knowledge strives to be concise and easy to understand, while paying attention to ideological and scientific aspects. The textbook will reflect the timeliness and cutting-edge nature, keep up with the rapid development of biomedical research and application fields, and let MBBS students fully realize the mastery and application of the course "Medical Genetics", not just stay in the basic theory of this textbook. In terms of learning, it is a learning and application process that requires continuous follow-up of the times and scientific development. This textbook will play a great leading role in the study and practice of MBBS students in the field of clinical medicine in the future.

This textbook has made great efforts to update and rewrite the relevant knowledge and content of the common English textbooks on the market in a large area, with more emphasis, and a more concise and rigorous language. Taking genetic diseases as an example, the diseases discussed and involved in this textbook will be the most abundant and richest in domestic and foreign textbooks, which fully reflects the characteristics of MBBS students. The internal links of the textbook are set up reasonably, based on the characteristics of the readers, combined with the needs of the English textbook, adding modules such as this chapter review points, key terms, study questions, etc., to promote students' independent learning.

The overall framework of this textbook is divided into eleven chapters, with "genetic diseases" as the main line. Firstly, it briefly introduces the generation, development, tasks and prospects of medical genetics. Secondly, it introduces two key knowledge systems in detail, namely the human genome and Mendelian genetic diseases. Thirdly, it explores the structure of genes, gene mutations and related gene detection technologies from the micro level. From a macro perspective, using intracellular chromosomes and individuals, it reveals the inheritance patterns and influencing factors closely related to heredity. Finally, it ends with more complex core theoretical knowledge of tumor genetics, treatment and risk assessment of genetic diseases. The textbook goes from shallow to deep, from simple to complex, and from basic knowledge to practical application.

CONTENTS

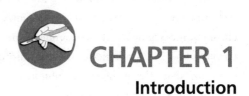

CHAPTER 1
Introduction

Purpose and Requirement:

In this chapter students should understand the fundamental and terminology of medical genetics, know the harm of genetic diseases and its status, and comprehend the researching category and characteristics.

1.1　The Birth and Development of Genetics and Genomics

Few areas of science and medicine are seeing advances at the pace we are experiencing in the related fields of genetics and genomics. It may appear surprising to many students today, then, to learn that an appreciation of the role of genetics in medicine dates back well over a century, to the recognition by the British physician Archibald Garrod and others that Mendel's laws of inheritance could explain the recurrence of certain clinical disorders in families. During the ensuing years, with developments in cellular and molecular biology, the field of **medical genetics** grew from a small clinical subspecialty concerned with a few rare hereditary disorders to a recognized medical specialty whose concepts and approaches are important components of the diagnosis and management of many disorders, both common and rare.

At the beginning of the 21st century, the **Human Genome Project** provided a virtually complete sequence of human DNA—our genome (the suffix-*ome* coming from the Greek for "all" or "complete")—which now serves as the foundation of efforts to catalogue all human genes, understand their structure and regulation, determine the extent of variation in these genes in different populations, and uncover how genetic variation contributes to disease. The human genome of any individual can now be studied in its entirety, rather than one gene at a time. These developments are making possible the field of **genomic medicine**, which seeks to apply a large-scale analysis of the human genome and its products, including the control of gene expression, human gene variation, and interactions between genes and the environment, to medical care.

1.2　Categories of Genetic Disease

Virtually any disease is the result of the combined action of genes and environment, but the relative role of the genetic component may be large or small. Among disorders caused wholly or partly by genetic factors, three main types are recognized: chromosome disorders, single-gene disorders, and multifactorial disorders.

In **chromosome disorders**, the defect is due not to a single mistake in the genetic blueprint but to an excess or a deficiency of the genes located on entire chromosomes or chromosome segments. For example, the presence of an extra copy of one chromosome, chromosome 21, underlies a specific disorder, Down syndrome, even though no individual gene on that chromosome is abnormal. Duplication or deletion of smaller segments of chromosomes, ranging in size from only a single gene up to a few percent of a chromosome's length, can cause complex birth defects like DiGeorge syndrome or even isolated autism without any obvious physical abnormalities. As a group, chromosome disorders are common, affecting approximately 7 per 1,000 liveborn infants and accounting for approximately half of all spontaneous abortions occurring in the first trimester of pregnancy. These types of disorders are discussed in Chapter 5.

Single-gene defects are caused by pathogenic mutations in individual genes. The mutation may be present on both chromosomes of a pair (one of paternal origin and one of maternal origin) or on only one chromosome of a pair (matched with a normal copy of that gene on the other copy of that chromosome). Single-gene defects often cause diseases that follow one of the classic inheritance patterns in families (autosomal recessive, autosomal dominant, or X-linked). In a few cases, the mutation is in the mitochondrial rather than in the nuclear genome. In any case, the cause is a critical error in the genetic information carried by a single gene. Single-gene disorders such as cystic fibrosis, sickle cell anemia, and Marfan syndrome usually exhibit obvious and characteristic pedigree patterns. Most such defects are rare, with a frequency that may be as high as 1 in 500 to 1,000 individuals but is usually much less. Although individually rare, single-gene disorders as a group are responsible for a significant proportion of disease and death. Overall, the incidence of serious single-gene disorders in the pediatric population has been estimated to be approximately 1 per 300 liveborn infants. Over an entire lifetime, the prevalence of single-gene disorders is 1 in 50. These disorders are discussed in Chapter 3.

Multifactorial disease with complex inheritance describes the majority of diseases in which there is a genetic contribution, as evidenced by increased risk for disease (compared to the general public) in identical twins or close relatives of affected individuals, and yet the family history does not fit the inheritance patterns seen typically in single-gene defects. Multifactorial diseases include congenital malformations such as Hirschsprung disease, cleft lip and palate, and congenital heart defects, as well as many common disorders of adult life, such as Alzheimer disease, diabetes, and coronary artery disease. There appears to be no single error in the genetic information in many of these conditions. Rather, the disease is the result of the combined impact of variant forms of many different genes; each variant may cause, protect from, or predispose to a serious defect, often in concert with or triggered by environmental factors. Estimates of the impact of multifactorial disease range from 5% in the pediatric population to more than 60% in the entire population. These disorders are the subject of Chapter 6.

1.3 Onward

During the 50-year professional life of today's professional and graduate students, extensive changes are likely to take place in the discovery, development, and use of genetic and genomic knowledge and tools in medicine. Judging from the quickening pace of discovery within only the past decade, it is virtually certain that we are just at the beginning of a revolution in integrating knowledge of genetics and the genome into public health and the practice of medicine. An introduction to the language and concepts of human and medical genetics and an appreciation of the genetic and genomic perspective on health and disease will form a framework for lifelong learning that is part of every health professional's career.

Review Points:

1. Medical genetics deals with the subset of human genetic variation that is of significance in the practice of medicine and in medical research.

2. Classification of genetic disorders:

(1) Single-gene disorders. (2) Chromosome disorders. (3) Multifactorial disorders.

3. Within human and medical genetics, there are many fields of interest: cytogenetic diseases involving chromosomal abnormalities, molecular and biochemical genetics involving the structure and function of individual genes, population genetics involving genetic variation in human populations and the factors that determine allele frequencies, clinical genetics involving the application of genetics to diagnosis and patient care, and genetic counseling which combines the provision of risk information while providing psychological and educational support.

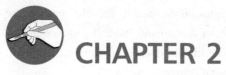

CHAPTER 2
Chromosomal Basis Heredity

Purpose and Requirement：

In this chapter students should understand the fundamental and terminology regarding to chromosome and mast the mitosis and meiosis.

Understanding the organization, variation, and transmission of the **human genome** is central to appreciating the role of genetics in medicine, as well as the emerging principles of genomic and personalized medicine. With the availability of the sequence of the human genome and a growing awareness of the role of genome variation in disease, it is now possible to begin to exploit the impact of that variation on human health on a broad scale. The comparison of individual genomes underscores the first major take-home lesson of this book—every individual has his or her own unique constitution of gene products, produced in response to the combined inputs of the genome sequence and one's particular set of environmental exposures and experiences. As pointed out in the previous chapter, this realization reflects what Garrod termed chemical individuality over a century ago and provides a conceptual foundation for the practice of genomic and personalized medicine.

Advances in genome technology and the resulting explosion in knowledge and information stemming from the Human Genome Project are thus playing an increasingly transformational role in integrating and applying concepts and discoveries in genetics to the practice of medicine.

2.1 The Human Genome and the Chromosomal Basis of Heredity

Appreciation of the importance of genetics to medicine requires an understanding of the nature of the hereditary material, how it is packaged into the human genome, and how it is transmitted from cell to cell during cell division and from generation to generation during reproduction. The human genome consists of large amounts of the chemical deoxyribonucleic acid (**DNA**) that contains within its structure the genetic information needed to specify all aspects of embryogenesis, development, growth, metabolism, and reproduction—essentially all aspects of what makes a human being a functional organism. Every nucleated cell in the body carries its own copy of the human genome, which contains, depending on how one defines the term, approximately 20,000 to 50,000 **genes**. Genes, which at this point we consider simply and most broadly as functional units of genetic information, are encoded in the DNA of the genome, organized into a number of rod-shaped organelles called **chromosomes** in the nucleus of each cell. The influence of genes and genetics on states of health and disease is profound, and its roots are found in the information encoded in the DNA that makes up the human genome.

Each species has a characteristic chromosome complement (**karyotype**) in terms of the number, morphology, and content of the chromosomes that make up its genome. The genes are in linear order along the chromosomes, each gene having a precise position or **locus**. A **gene map** is the map of the genomic location of the genes and is characteristic of each species and the individuals within a species.

The study of chromosomes, their structure, and their inheritance is called **cytogenetics**. The science of human cytogenetics dates from 1956, when it was first established that the normal human chromosome number is 46. Since that time, much has been learned about human chromosomes, their normal structure and composition, and the identity of the genes that they contain, as well as their numerous and varied abnormalities.

With the exception of cells that develop into gametes (**the germline**), all cells that contribute to one's body are called **somatic cells**. The genome contained in the nucleus of human somatic cells consists of 46 chromosomes, made up of 24 different types and arranged in 23 pairs (see Fig. 2-1). Of those 23 pairs, 22 are alike in males and females and are called **autosomes**, originally numbered in order of their apparent size from the largest to the smallest. The remaining pair comprises the two different types of **sex chromosomes**: an X and a Y chromosome in males and two X chromosomes in females. Central to the concept of the human genome, each chromosome carries a different subset of genes that are arranged linearly along its DNA. Members of a pair of chromosomes (referred to as **homologous chromosomes** or **homologues**) carry matching genetic information; that is, they typically have the same genes in the same order. At any specific locus, however, the homologues either may be identical or may vary slightly in sequence; these different forms of a gene are called **alleles**. One member of each pair of chromosomes is inherited from the father, the other from the mother. Normally, the members of a pair of autosomes are microscopically indistinguishable from each other. In females, the sex chromosomes, the two **X chromosomes**, are likewise largely indistinguishable. In males, however, the sex chromosomes differ. One is an X, identical to the Xs of the female, inherited by a male from his mother and transmitted to his daughters; the other, the **Y chromosome**, is inherited from his father and transmitted to his sons. In Chapter 5, as we explore the chromosomal and genomic basis of disease, we will look at some exceptions to the simple and almost universal rule that human females are XX and human males are XY.

In addition to the nuclear genome, a small but important part of the human genome resides in mitochondria in the cytoplasm (see Fig. 2-1). The mitochondrial chromosome has a number of unusual features that distinguish it from the rest of the human genome.

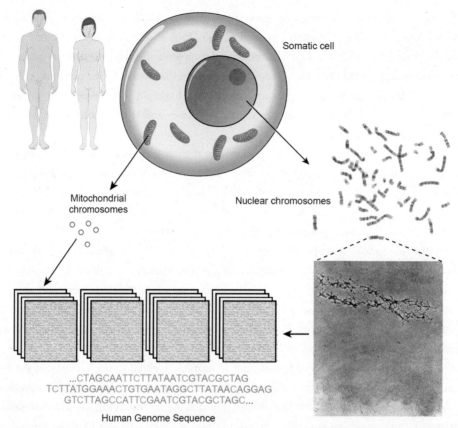

Figure 2-1 The human genome, encoded on both nuclear and mitochondrial chromosomes
(From PAULSON J R, LAEMMLI U K. The structure of histone-depleted metaphase chromosomes [J]. Cell, 1977,12(3):817-828.)

2.1.1 DNA Structure: A Brief Review

Before the organization of the human genome and its chromosomes is considered in detail, it is necessary to review the nature of the DNA that makes up the genome. DNA is a polymeric nucleic acid macromolecule composed of three types of units: a five-carbon sugar, deoxyribose; a nitrogen-containing base; and a phosphate group (see Fig. 2-2). The bases are of two types, **purines** and **pyrimidines**. In DNA, there are two purine bases, **adenine** (A) and **guanine** (G), and two pyrimidine bases, **thymine** (T) and **cytosine** (C). Nucleotides, each composed of a base, a phosphate, and a sugar moiety, polymerize into long polynucleotide chains held together by 5'-3' phosphodiester bonds formed between adjacent deoxyribose units (see Fig. 2-3A). In the human genome, these polynucleotide chains exist in the form of a double helix (see Fig. 2-3B) that can be hundreds of millions of nucleotides long in the case of the largest human chromosomes.

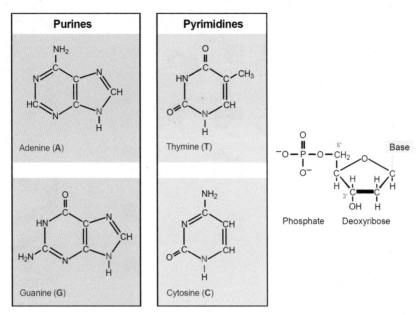

Figure 2-2   The four bases of DNA and the general structure of a nucleotide in DNA
Each of the four bases bonds with deoxyribose (through the nitrogen shown in *magenta*) and a phosphate group to form the corresponding nucleotides.

The anatomical structure of DNA carries the chemical information that allows the exact transmission of genetic information from one cell to its daughter cells and from one generation to the next. At the same time, the primary structure of DNA specifies the amino acid sequences of the polypeptide chains of proteins. DNA has elegant features that give it these properties. The native state of DNA, as elucidated by James Watson and Francis Crick in 1953, is a double helix (see Fig. 2-3B). The helical structure resembles a right-handed spiral staircase in which its two polynucleotide chains run in opposite directions, held together by hydrogen bonds between pairs of bases: T of one chain paired with A of the other, and G with C. The specific nature of the genetic information encoded in the human genome lies in the sequence of C's, A's, G's, and T's on the two strands of the double helix along each of the chromosomes, both in the nucleus and in mitochondria (see Fig. 2-1). Because of the complementary nature of the two strands of DNA, knowledge of the sequence of nucleotide bases on one strand automatically allows one to determine the sequence of bases on the other strand. The double-stranded structure of DNA molecules allows them to replicate precisely by separation of the two strands, followed by synthesis of two new complementary strands, in accordance with the sequence of the original template strands (see Fig. 2-4). Similarly, when necessary, the base complementarity allows efficient and correct repair of damaged DNA molecules.

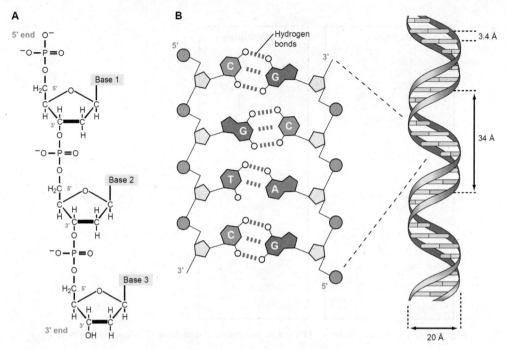

Figure 2-3　The structure of DNA

(A) A portion of a DNA polynucleotide chain, showing the 3′-5′ phosphodiester bonds that link adjacent nucleotides. (B) The double-helix model of DNA, as proposed by Watson and Crick. The horizontal "rungs" represent the paired bases. The helix is said to be right-handed because the strand going from lower left to upper right crosses over the opposite strand. The detailed portion of the figure illustrates the two complementary strands of DNA, showing the AT and GC base pairs. Note that the orientation of the two strands is antiparallel.

(From WATSON J D, CRICK F H C. Molecular structure of nucleic acids: a structure for deoxyribose nucleic acid[J]. Nature, 1953,171(4356):737-738.)

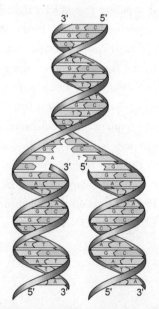

Figure 2-4　The replication of DNA

Replication of a DNA double helix, resulting in two identical daughter molecules, each composed of one parental strand and one newly synthesized strand.

2.1.2 Structure of Human Chromosomes

The composition of genes in the human genome, as well as the determinants of their expression, is specified in the DNA of the 46 human chromosomes in the nucleus plus the mitochondrial chromosome. Each human chromosome consists of a single, continuous DNA double helix; that is, each chromosome is one long, double-stranded DNA molecule, and the nuclear genome consists, therefore, of 46 linear DNA molecules, totaling more than 6 billion nucleotide pairs (see Fig. 2-1).

Chromosomes are not naked DNA double helices, however. Within each cell, the genome is packaged as **chromatin**, in which genomic DNA is complexed with several classes of specialized proteins. Except during cell division, chromatin is distributed throughout the nucleus and is relatively homogeneous in appearance under the microscope. When a cell divides, however, its genome condenses to appear as microscopically visible chromosomes. Chromosomes are thus visible as discrete structures only in dividing cells, although they retain their integrity between cell divisions.

The DNA molecule of a chromosome exists in chromatin as a complex with a family of basic chromosomal proteins called **histones**. This fundamental unit interacts with a heterogeneous group of nonhistone proteins, which are involved in establishing a proper spatial and functional environment to ensure normal chromosome behavior and appropriate gene expression.

Five major types of histones play a critical role in the proper packaging of chromatin. Two copies each of the four core histones H2A, H2B, H3, and H4 constitute an octamer, around which a segment of DNA double helix winds, like thread around a spool (see Fig. 2-5). Approximately 140 base pairs (bp) of DNA are associated with each histone core, making just under two turns around the octamer. After a short (20- to 60-bp) "spacer" segment of DNA, the next core DNA complex forms, and so on, giving chromatin the appearance of beads on a string. Each complex of DNA with core histones is called a **nucleosome** (see Fig. 2-5), which is the basic structural unit of chromatin, and each of the 46 human chromosomes contains several hundred thousand to well over a million nucleosomes. A fifth histone, H1, appears to bind to DNA at the edge of each nucleosome, in the internucleosomal spacer region. The amount of DNA associated with a core nucleosome, together with the spacer region, is approximately 200 bp.

In addition to the major histone types, a number of specialized histones can substitute for H3 or H2A and confer specific characteristics on the genomic DNA at that location. Histones can also be modified by chemical changes, and these modifications can change the properties of nucleosomes that contain them. The pattern of major and specialized histone types and their modifications can vary from cell type to cell type and is thought to specify how DNA is packaged and how accessible it is to regulatory molecules that determine gene expression or other genome functions.

During the cell cycle, chromosomes pass through orderly stages of condensation and decondensation. However, even when chromosomes are in their most decondensed state, in a stage of the cell cycle called **interphase**, DNA packaged in chromatin is substantially more condensed than it would be as a native, protein-free, double helix. Further, the long strings of nucleosomes are themselves compacted into a secondary helical structure, a cylindrical "solenoid" fiber that appears to be the fundamental unit of chromatin organization (see Fig. 2-5). The solenoids are themselves packed into **loops** or domains attached at intervals of approximately 100,000 bp (equivalent to 100 kilobase pairs [kb], because 1 kb = 1,000 bp) to a protein **scaffold** within the nucleus. It has been speculated that these loops are the functional units of the genome and that the attachment points of each loop are specified along the chromosomal DNA. As we shall see, one level of control of gene expression depends on how DNA and genes are packaged into chromosomes and on their association with chromatin proteins in the packaging process.

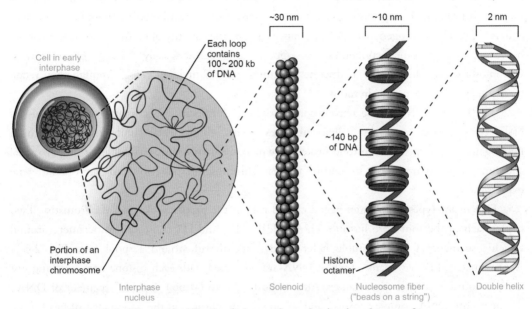

Figure 2-5 Hierarchical levels of chromatin packaging in a human chromosome

The enormous amount of genomic DNA packaged into a chromosome can be appreciated when chromosomes are treated to release the DNA from the underlying protein scaffold (see Fig. 2-1). When DNA is released in this manner, long loops of DNA can be visualized, and the residual scaffolding can be seen to reproduce the outline of a typical chromosome.

(1) The Mitochondrial Chromosome

As mentioned earlier, a small but important subset of genes encoded in the human genome resides in the cytoplasm in the mitochondria (see Fig. 2-1). Mitochondrial genes exhibit exclusively maternal inheritance. Human cells can have hundreds to thousands of mitochondria, each containing a number of copies of a small circular molecule, the mitochondrial chromosome. The mitochondrial DNA molecule is only 16 kb in length (just a tiny fraction of the length of even the smallest nuclear chromosome) and encodes only 37 genes. The products of these genes function in mitochondria, although the vast majority of proteins within the mitochondria are, in fact, the products of nuclear genes. Mutations in mitochondrial genes have been demonstrated in several maternally inherited as well as sporadic disorders.

(2) The Human Genome Sequence

With a general understanding of the structure and clinical importance of chromosomes and the genes they carry, scientists turned attention to the identification of specific genes and their location in the human genome. From this broad effort emerged the **Human Genome Project**, an international consortium of hundreds of laboratories around the world, formed to determine and assemble the sequence of the 3.3 billion base pairs of DNA located among the 24 types of human chromosome.

Over the course of a decade and a half, powered by major developments in DNA-sequencing technology, large sequencing centers collaborated to assemble sequences of each chromosome. The genomes actually being sequenced came from several different individuals, and the consensus sequence that resulted at the conclusion of the Human Genome Project was reported in 2003 as a "reference" sequence assembly, to be used as a basis for later comparison with sequences of individual genomes. This reference sequence is maintained in publicly accessible databases to facilitate scientific discovery and its translation into useful advances for medicine. Genome sequences are typically presented in a 5′ to 3′ direction on just one of the two strands of the double helix, because—owing to the complementary nature of DNA structure described earlier—if one knows the sequence of one strand, one can infer the sequence of the other strand (see Fig. 2-6).

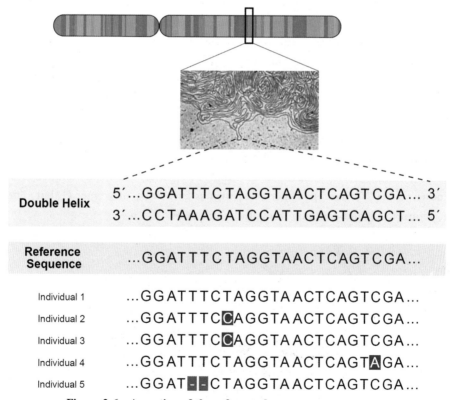

Figure 2-6   A portion of the reference human genome sequence

By convention, sequences are presented from one strand of DNA only, because the sequence of the complementary strand can be inferred from the double-stranded nature of DNA (shown above the reference sequence). The sequence of DNA from a group of individuals is similar but not identical to the reference, with single nucleotide changes in some individuals and a small deletion of two bases in another.

2.2 Transmission of the Genome

The chromosomal basis of heredity lies in the copying of the genome and its transmission from a cell to its progeny during typical cell division and from one generation to the next during reproduction, when single copies of the genome from each parent come together in a new embryo.

To achieve these related but distinct forms of genome inheritance, there are two kinds of cell division, mitosis and meiosis. **Mitosis** is ordinary somatic cell division by which the body grows, differentiates, and effects tissue regeneration. Mitotic division normally results in two daughter cells, each with chromosomes and genes identical to those of the parent cell. There may be dozens or even hundreds of successive mitoses in a lineage of somatic cells. In contrast, **meiosis** occurs only in cells of the germline. Meiosis results in the formation of reproductive cells (**gametes**), each of which has only 23 chromosomes—one of each kind of autosome and either an X or a Y. Thus, whereas somatic cells have the **diploid** or the 2n chromosome complement (i. e., 46 chromosomes), gametes have the **haploid** or the n complement (i. e., 23 chromosomes). Abnormalities of chromosome number or structure, which are usually clinically significant, can arise either in somatic cells or in cells of the germline by errors in cell division.

2.2.1 The Cell Cycle

A human being begins life as a fertilized ovum (**zygote**), a diploid cell from which all the cells of the body (estimated to be approximately 100 trillion in number) are derived by a series of dozens or even hundreds of mitoses. Mitosis is obviously crucial for growth and differentiation, but it takes up only a small part of the life cycle of a cell. The period between two successive mitoses is called **interphase**, the state in which most of the life of a cell is spent.

Immediately after mitosis, the cell enters a phase, called G_1, in which there is no DNA synthesis (see Fig. 2-7). Some cells pass through this stage in hours; others spend a long time, days or years, in G_1. In fact, some cell types, such as neurons and red blood cells, do not divide at all once they are fully differentiated; rather, they are permanently arrested in a distinct phase known as G_0("G zero"). Other cells, such as liver cells, may enter G_0 but, after organ damage, return to G_1 and continue through the cell cycle.

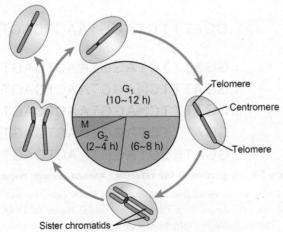

Figure 2-7 A typical mitotic cell cycle

The telomeres, the centromere, and sister chromatids are indicated.

The cell cycle is governed by a series of **checkpoints** that determine the timing of each step in mitosis. In addition, checkpoints monitor and control the accuracy of DNA synthesis as well as the assembly and attachment of an elaborate network of microtubules that facilitate chromosome movement. If damage to the genome is detected, these mitotic checkpoints halt cell cycle progression until repairs are made or, if the damage is excessive, until the cell is instructed to die by programmed cell death (a process called **apoptosis**).

During G_1, each cell contains one diploid copy of the genome. As the process of cell division begins, the cell enters **S phase**, the stage of programmed DNA synthesis, ultimately leading to the precise replication of each chromosome's DNA. During this stage, each chromosome, which in G_1 has been a single DNA molecule, is duplicated and consists of **two sister chromatids** (see Fig. 2-7), each of which contains an identical copy of the original linear DNA double helix. The two sister chromatids are held together physically at the **centromere**, a region of DNA that associates with a number of specific proteins to form the **kinetochore**. This complex structure serves to attach each chromosome to the microtubules of the **mitotic spindle** and to govern chromosome movement during mitosis. DNA synthesis during S phase is not synchronous throughout all chromosomes or even within a single chromosome; rather, along each chromosome, it begins at hundreds to thousands of sites, called **origins of DNA replication**. Individual chromosome segments have their own characteristic time of replication during the 6- to 8-hour S phase. The ends of each chromosome (or chromatid) are marked by **telomeres**, which consist of specialized repetitive DNA sequences that ensure the integrity of the chromosome during cell division. Correct maintenance of the ends of chromosomes requires a special enzyme called **telomerase**, which ensures that the very ends of each chromosome are replicated.

The essential nature of these structural elements of chromosomes and their role in ensuring genome integrity is illustrated by a range of clinical conditions that result from defects in elements of the telomere or kinetochore or cell cycle machinery or from inaccurate replication of even small portions of the genome.

By the end of S phase, the DNA content of the cell has doubled, and each cell now contains two copies of the diploid genome. After S phase, the cell enters a brief stage called G_2. Throughout the whole cell cycle, the cell gradually enlarges, eventually doubling its total mass before the next mitosis. G_2 is ended by mitosis, which begins when individual chromosomes begin to condense and become visible under the microscope as thin, extended threads, a process that is considered in greater detail in the following section.

The G1, S, and G2 phases together constitute interphase. In typical dividing human cells, the three phases take a total of 16 to 24 hours, whereas mitosis lasts only 1 to 2 hours (see Fig. 2-7). There is great variation, however, in the length of the cell cycle, which ranges from a few hours in rapidly dividing cells, such as those of the dermis of the skin or the intestinal mucosa, to months in other cell types.

2.2.2 Mitosis

During the mitotic phase of the cell cycle, an elaborate apparatus ensures that each of the two daughter cells receives a complete set of genetic information. This result is achieved by a mechanism that distributes one chromatid of each chromosome to each daughter cell (see

Fig. 2-8). The process of distributing a copy of each chromosome to each daughter cell is called **chromosome segregation**. The importance of this process for normal cell growth is illustrated by the observation that many tumors are invariably characterized by a state of genetic imbalance resulting from mitotic errors in the distribution of chromosomes to daughter cells.

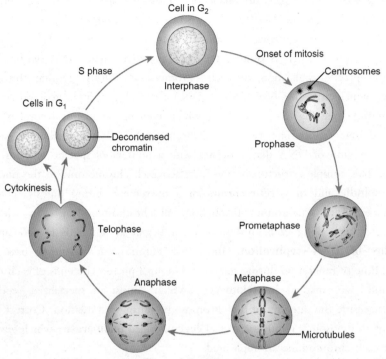

Figure 2-8   Mitosis

Only two chromosome pairs are shown.

The process of mitosis is continuous, but five stages, illustrated in Figure 2-8, are distinguished: prophase, prometaphase, metaphase, anaphase, and telophase.

- **Prophase.** This stage is marked by gradual condensation of the chromosomes, formation of the mitotic spindle, and formation of a pair of **centrosomes**, from which microtubules radiate and eventually take up positions at the poles of the cell.

- **Prometaphase.** Here, the nuclear membrane dissolves, allowing the chromosomes to disperse within the cell and to attach, by their kinetochores, to microtubules of the mitotic spindle.

- **Metaphase.** At this stage, the chromosomes are maximally condensed and line up at the equatorial plane of the cell.

- **Anaphase.** The chromosomes separate at the centromere, and the sister chromatids of each chromosome now become independent **daughter chromosomes**, which move to opposite poles of the cell.

- **Telophase.** Now, the chromosomes begin to decondense from their highly contracted state, and a nuclear membrane begins to re-form around each of the two daughter nuclei, which resume their interphase appearance. To complete the process of cell division, the cytoplasm cleaves by a process known as cytokinesis.

There is an important difference between a cell entering mitosis and one that has just completed the process. A cell in G_2 has a fully replicated genome (i.e., a 4n complement of DNA), and each chromosome consists of a pair of sister chromatids. In contrast, after mitosis, the chromosomes of each daughter cell have only one copy of the genome. This copy will not be duplicated until a daughter cell in its turn reaches the S phase of the next cell cycle (see Fig. 2-7). The entire process of mitosis thus ensures the orderly duplication and distribution of the genome through successive cell divisions.

2.2.3　Meiosis

Meiosis, the process by which diploid cells give rise to haploid gametes, involves a type of cell division that is unique to germ cells. In contrast to mitosis, meiosis consists of one round of DNA replication followed by two rounds of chromosome segregation and cell division (see meiosis Ⅰ and meiosis Ⅱ in Fig. 2-9). As outlined here and illustrated in Figure 2-10, the overall sequence of events in male and female meiosis is the same. However, the timing of gametogenesis is very different in the two sexes.

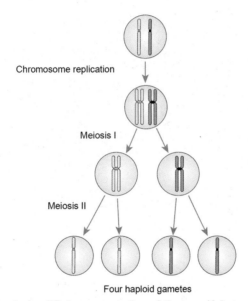

Chromosome replication

Meiosis I

Meiosis II

Four haploid gametes

Figure 2-9　A simplified representation of the essential steps in meiosis

Meiosis consists of one round of DNA replication followed by two rounds of chromosome segregation, meiosis Ⅰ and meiosis Ⅱ.

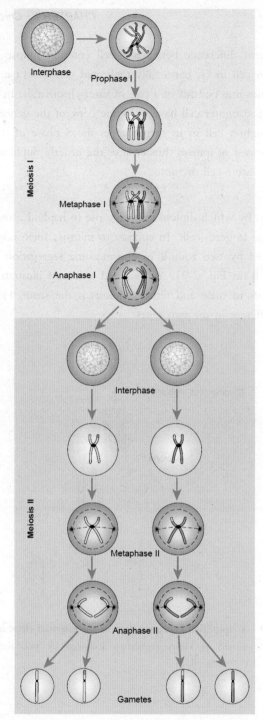

Figure 2-10　Meiosis and its consequences

A single chromosome pair and a single crossover are shown, leading to formation of four distinct gametes. The chromosomes replicate during interphase and begin to condense as the cell enters prophase of meiosis Ⅰ. In meiosis Ⅰ, the chromosomes synapse and recombine. A crossover is visible as the homologues align at metaphase Ⅰ, with the centromeres oriented toward opposite poles. In anaphase Ⅰ, the exchange of DNA between the homologues is apparent as the chromosomes are pulled to opposite poles. After completion of meiosis Ⅰ and cytokinesis, meiosis Ⅱ proceeds with a mitosis-like division. The sister kinetochores separate and move to opposite poles in anaphase Ⅱ, yielding four haploid products.

Meiosis Ⅰ is also known as the **reduction division** because it is the division in which the chromosome number is reduced by half through the pairing of homologues in prophase and by their segregation to different cells at anaphase of meiosis Ⅰ. Meiosis Ⅰ is also notable because it is the stage at which genetic **recombination** (also called **meiotic crossing over**) occurs. In this process, as shown for one pair of chromosomes in Figure 2-10, homologous segments of DNA are exchanged between nonsister chromatids of each pair of homologous chromosomes, thus ensuring that none of the gametes produced by meiosis will be identical to another.

Prophase of meiosis Ⅰ differs in a number of ways from mitotic prophase, with important genetic consequences, because homologous chromosomes need to pair and exchange genetic information. The most critical early stage is called **zygotene**, when homologous chromosomes begin to align along their entire length. The process of meiotic pairing—called **synapsis**—is normally precise, bringing corresponding DNA sequences into alignment along the length of the entire chromosome pair. The paired homologues—now called **bivalents**—are held together by a ribbon-like proteinaceous structure called the **synaptonemal complex**, which is essential to the process of recombination. After synapsis is complete, meiotic crossing over takes place during **pachytene**, after which the synaptonemal complex breaks down.

Metaphase Ⅰ begins, as in mitosis, when the nuclear membrane disappears. A spindle forms, and the paired chromosomes align themselves on the equatorial plane with their centromeres oriented toward different poles (see Fig. 2-10).

Anaphase of meiosis Ⅰ again differs substantially from the corresponding stage of mitosis. Here, it is the two members of each bivalent that move apart, not the sister chromatids (contrast Fig. 2-10 with Fig. 2-8). The homologous centromeres (with their attached sister chromatids) are drawn to opposite poles of the cell, a process termed **disjunction**. Thus the chromosome number is halved, and each cellular product of meiosis Ⅰ has the haploid chromosome number. The 23 pairs of homologous chromosomes assort independently of one another, and as a result, the original paternal and maternal chromosome sets are sorted into random combinations. The possible number of combinations of the 23 chromosome pairs that can be present in the gametes is 2^{23} (more than 8 million). Owing to the process of crossing over, however, the variation in the genetic material that is transmitted from parent to child is actually much greater than this. As a result, each chromatid typically contains segments derived from each member of the original parental chromosome pair, as illustrated schematically in Figure 2-10. For example, at this stage, a typical large human chromosome would be composed of three to five segments, alternately paternal and maternal in origin, as inferred from DNA sequence variants that distinguish the respective parental genomes (see Fig. 2-11).

After telophase of meiosis Ⅰ, the two haploid daughter cells enter meiotic interphase. In contrast to mitosis, this interphase is brief, and meiosis Ⅱ begins. The notable point that distinguishes meiotic and mitotic interphase is that there is no S phase (i.e., no DNA synthesis and duplication of the genome) between the first and second meiotic divisions.

Meiosis Ⅱ is similar to an ordinary mitosis, except that the chromosome number is 23 instead of 46; the chromatids of each of the 23 chromosomes separate, and one chromatid of each chromosome passes to each daughter cell (see Fig. 2-10). However, as mentioned earlier, because of crossing over in meiosis Ⅰ, the chromosomes of the resulting gametes are not identical (see Fig. 2-11).

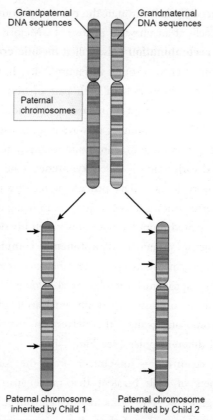

Figure 2-11　The effect of homologous recombination in meiosis

In this example, representing the inheritance of sequences on a typical large chromosome, an individual has distinctive homologues, one containing sequences inherited from his father (*blue*) and one containing homologous sequences from his mother (*purple*). After meiosis in spermatogenesis, he transmits a single complete copy of that chromosome to his two offspring. However, as a result of crossing over (*arrows*), the copy he transmits to each child consists of alternating segments of the two grandparental sequences. Child 1 inherits a copy after two crossovers, whereas child 2 inherits a copy with three crossovers.

2.3　Human Gametogenesis and Fertilization

　　The cells in the germline that undergo meiosis, primary spermatocytes or primary oocytes, are derived from the zygote by a long series of mitoses before the onset of meiosis. Male and female gametes have different histories, marked by different patterns of gene expression that reflect their developmental origin as an XY or XX embryo. The human primordial germ cells are recognizable by the fourth week of development outside the embryo proper, in the endoderm of the yolk sac. From there, they migrate during the sixth week to the genital ridges and associate with somatic cells to form the primitive gonads, which soon differentiate into testes or ovaries, depending on the cells' sex chromosome constitution (XY or XX). Both spermatogenesis and oogenesis require meiosis but have important differences in detail and timing that may have clinical and genetic consequences for the offspring. Female meiosis is initiated once, early during fetal life, in a limited number of cells. In contrast, male meiosis is initiated continuously in many cells from a dividing cell population throughout the adult life of a male.

In the female, successive stages of meiosis take place over several decades—in the fetal ovary before the female in question is even born, in the oocyte near the time of ovulation in the sexually mature female, and after fertilization of the egg that can become that female's offspring. Although postfertilization stages can be studied in vitro, access to the earlier stages is limited. Testicular material for the study of male meiosis is less difficult to obtain, inasmuch as testicular biopsy is included in the assessment of many men attending infertility clinics. Much remains to be learned about the cytogenetic, biochemical, and molecular mechanisms involved in normal meiosis and about the causes and consequences of meiotic irregularities.

2.3.1 Spermatogenesis

The stages of spermatogenesis are shown in Figure 2-12. The seminiferous tubules of the testes are lined with **spermatogonia**, which develop from the primordial germ cells by a long series of mitoses and which are in different stages of differentiation. **Sperm** (spermatozoa) are formed only after sexual maturity is reached. The last cell type in the developmental sequence is the **primary spermatocyte**, a diploid germ cell that undergoes meiosis I to form two haploid **secondary spermatocytes**. Secondary spermatocytes rapidly enter meiosis II, each forming two **spermatids**, which differentiate without further division into sperm. In humans, the entire process takes approximately 64 days. The enormous number of sperm produced, typically approximately 200 million per ejaculate and an estimated 10^{12} in a lifetime, requires several hundred successive mitoses.

As discussed earlier, normal meiosis requires pairing of homologous chromosomes followed by recombination. The autosomes and the X chromosomes in females present no unusual difficulties in this regard; but what of the X and Y chromosomes during spermatogenesis? Although the X and Y chromosomes are different and are not homologues in a strict sense, they do have relatively short identical segments at the ends of their respective short arms (Xp and Yp) and long arms (Xq and Yq). Pairing and crossing over occurs in both regions during meiosis I. These homologous segments are called **pseudoautosomal** to reflect their autosome-like pairing and recombination behavior, despite being on different sex chromosomes.

2.3.2 Oogenesis

Whereas spermatogenesis is initiated only at the time of puberty, oogenesis begins during a female's development as a fetus (see Fig. 2-13). The **ova** develop from **oogonia**, cells in the ovarian cortex that have descended from the primordial germ cells by a series of approximately 20 mitoses. Each oogonium is the central cell in a developing follicle. By approximately the third month of fetal development, the oogonia of the embryo have begun to develop into **primary oocytes**, most of which have already entered prophase of meiosis I. The process of oogenesis is not synchronized, and both early and late stages coexist in the fetal ovary. Although there are several million oocytes at the time of birth, most of these degenerate; the others remain arrested in prophase I (see Fig. 2-10) for decades. Only approximately 400 eventually mature and are ovulated as part of a woman's menstrual cycle.

After a woman reaches sexual maturity, individual follicles begin to grow and mature, and a few (on average one per month) are ovulated. Just before ovulation, the oocyte rapidly completes meiosis Ⅰ, dividing in such a way that one cell becomes the secondary oocyte (an egg or **ovum**), containing most of the cytoplasm with its organelles; the other cell becomes the first polar body (see Fig. 2-13). Meiosis Ⅱ begins promptly and proceeds to the metaphase stage during ovulation, where it halts again, only to be completed if fertilization occurs.

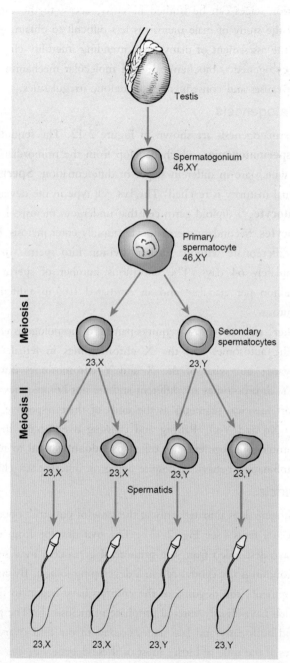

Figure 2-12　Human spermatogenesis in relation to the two meiotic divisions

The sequence of events begins at puberty and takes approximately 64 days to be completed. The chromosome number (46 or 23) and the sex chromosome constitution (X or Y) of each cell are shown. (From MOORE K L, PERSAUD T V N. The developing human: clinically oriented embryology [M]. 6th ed. Philadelphia: W.B. Saunders, 1998.)

2.3.3 Fertilization

Fertilization of the egg usually takes place in the fallopian tube within a day or so of ovulation. Although many sperm may be present, the penetration of a single sperm into the ovum sets up a series of biochemical events that usually prevent the entry of other sperms.

Fertilization is followed by the completion of meiosis Ⅱ, with the formation of the second polar body (see Fig. 2-13). The chromosomes of the now-fertilized egg and sperm form **pronuclei**,

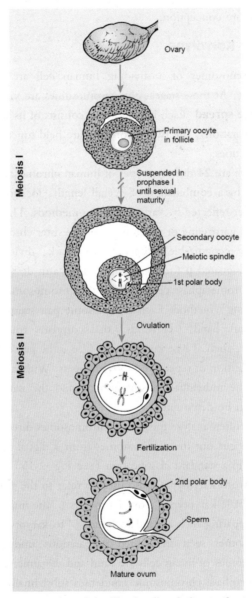

Figure 2-13 Human oogenesis and fertilization in relation to the two meiotic divisions

The primary oocytes are formed prenatally and remain suspended in prophase of meiosis Ⅰ for years until the onset of puberty. An oocyte completes meiosis Ⅰ as its follicle matures, resulting in a secondary oocyte and the first polar body. After ovulation, each oocyte continues to metaphase of meiosis Ⅱ. Meiosis Ⅱ is completed only if fertilization occurs, resulting in a fertilized mature ovum and the second polar body.

each surrounded by its own nuclear membrane. It is only upon replication of the parental genomes after fertilization that the two haploid genomes become one diploid genome within a shared nucleus. The diploid **zygote** divides by mitosis to form two diploid daughter cells, the first in the series of cell divisions that initiate the process of embryonic development.

Although the development begins at the time of conception, with the formation of the zygote, in clinical medicine the stage and duration of pregnancy are usually measured as the "menstrual age", dating from the beginning of the mother's last menstrual period, typically approximately 14 days before conception.

2.4　The Human Karyotype

The condensed chromosomes of a dividing human cell are most readily analyzed at metaphase or prometaphase. At these stages, the chromosomes are visible under the microscope as a so-called **chromosome spread**. Each chromosome consists of its sister chromatids, although in most chromosome preparations, the two chromatids are held together so tightly that they are rarely visible as separate entities.

As stated earlier, there are 24 different types of human chromosome, each of which can be distinguished cytologically by a combination of overall length, location of the centromere, and sequence content, the latter reflected by various staining methods. The centromere is apparent as a **primary constriction**, a narrowing or pinching-in of the sister chromatids due to formation of the kinetochore. This is a recognizable cytogenetic landmark, dividing the chromosome into two **arms**, a short arm designated **p** (for *petit*) and a long arm designated **q**.

Figure 2-14 shows a prometaphase cell in which the chromosomes have been stained by the Giemsa-staining (**G-banding**) method. Each chromosome pair stains in a characteristic pattern of alternating light and dark bands (G bands) that correlates roughly with features of the underlying DNA sequence, such as base composition (i.e., the percentage of base pairs that are GC or AT) and the distribution of repetitive DNA elements. With such banding techniques, all of the chromosomes can be individually distinguished, and the nature of many structural or numerical abnormalities can be determined.

Although experts can often analyze metaphase chromosomes directly under the microscope, a common procedure is to cut out the chromosomes from a digital image or photomicrograph and arrange them in pairs in a standard classification (see Fig. 2-15). The completed picture is called a **karyotype**. The word karyotype is also used to refer to the standard chromosome set of an individual ("a normal male karyotype") or of a species ("the human karyotype") and, as a verb, to the process of preparing such a standard figure ("to karyotype").

Unlike the chromosomes seen in stained preparations under the microscope or in photographs, the chromosomes of living cells are fluid and dynamic structures. During mitosis, the chromatin of each interphase chromosome condenses substantially (see Fig. 2-16). When maximally condensed at metaphase, DNA in chromosomes is approximately $1/10,000$ of its fully extended state. When chromosomes are prepared to reveal bands (as in Figs. 2-14 and 2-15), as many as $1,000$ or more bands can be recognized in stained preparations of all the chromosomes. Each cytogenetic band therefore contains as many as 50 or more genes, although the density of genes in the genome, as mentioned previously, is variable.

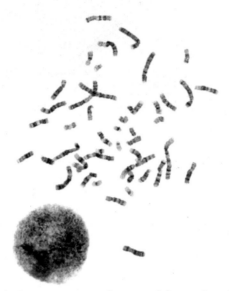

Figure 2-14   A chromosome spread prepared from a lymphocyte culture

The darkly stained nucleus adjacent to the chromosomes is from a different cell in interphase, when chromosomal material is diffuse throughout the nucleus.

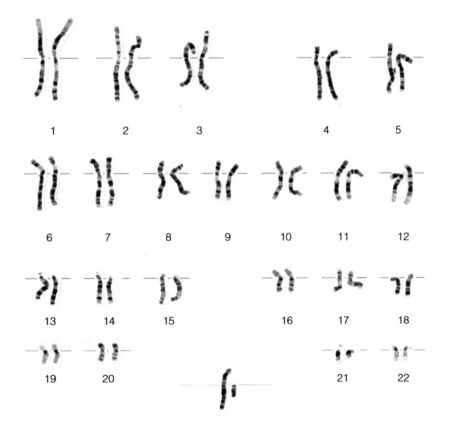

SEX CHROMOSOMES

Figure 2-15   A human male karyotype

The chromosomes are at the prometaphase stage of mitosis and are arranged in a standard classification, numbered 1 to 22 in order of length, with the X and Y chromosomes shown separately.

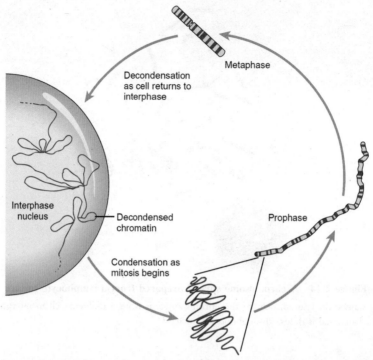

Figure 2-16 Cycle of condensation and decondensation as a chromosome proceeds through the cell cycle

2.5 Medical Relevance of Mitosis and Meiosis

The biological significance of mitosis and meiosis lies in ensuring the constancy of chromosome number—and thus the integrity of the genome—from one cell to its progeny and from one generation to the next. The medical relevance of these processes lies in errors of one or the other mechanism of cell division, leading to the formation of an individual or of a cell lineage with an abnormal number of chromosomes and thus an abnormal dosage of genomic material.

Meiotic nondisjunction, particularly in oogenesis, is the most common mutational mechanism in our species, responsible for chromosomally abnormal fetuses in at least several percent of all recognized pregnancies. Among pregnancies that survive to term, chromosome abnormalities are a leading cause of developmental defects, failure to thrive in the newborn period, and intellectual disability.

Mitotic nondisjunction in somatic cells also contributes to genetic disease. Nondisjunction soon after fertilization, either in the developing embryo or in extraembryonic tissues like the placenta, leads to chromosomal mosaicism that can underlie some medical conditions, such as a proportion of patients with Down syndrome. Further, abnormal chromosome segregation in rapidly dividing tissues, such as in cells of the colon, is frequently a step in the development of chromosomally abnormal tumors, and thus evaluation of chromosome and genome balance is an important diagnostic and prognostic test in many cancers.

Review Points:

1. Structure of human chromosomes: DNA double helix; Nucleosome; 30-nm-diameter fiber; loop of chromatin.

2. Mitosis: The process of mitosis is continuous, but five stages are distinguished: prophase, prometaphase, metaphase, anaphase, and telophase.

3. Meiosis: Meiosis is the type of cell division by which the diploid cell of the germ line give rise to haploid gametes. Meiosis consists of one round of DNA synthesis followed by rounds of chromosome segregation and cell division. The two successive meiotic divisions are called meiosis I and meiosis II. Meiosis I is also known as the reduction division because it is the division in which the chromosome number is reduced from diploid to haploid by the pairing of homologs in prophase and by their segregation to different cells at anaphase of meiosis I. Meiosis II follows meiosis I without an intervening step of DNA replication. As in ordinary mitosis, the chromatids separate, and one chromatid of each chromosome passes to each daughter cell.

Study Questions:

1. At a certain locus, a person has two alleles, A and a.

a. What alleles will be present in this person's gametes?

b. When do A and a segregate (1) if there is no crossing over between the locus and the centromere of the chromosome? (2) if there is a single crossing over between the locus and the centromere?

2. What is the main cause of numerical chromosome abnormalities in humans?

3. Disregarding crossing over, which increases the amount of genetic variability, estimate the probability that all your chromosomes have come to you from your father's mother and your mother's mother. Would you be male or female?

4. A chromosome entering meiosis is composed of two sister chromatids, each of which is a single DNA molecule.

a. In our species, at the end of meiosis I, how many chromosomes are there per cell? How many chromatids?

b. At the end of meiosis II, how many chromosomes are there per cell? How many chromatids?

c. When is the diploid chromosome number restored? When is the two-chromatid structure of a typical metaphase chromosome restored?

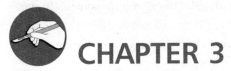

CHAPTER 3
Patterns of Single-Gene Inheritance

Purpose and Requirement:

In this chapter students should understand the typical patterns of transmission of single-gene disorders are discussed and mast heterogeneity, penetrance, expressivity, pleiotropy, and germline mosaicism.

In Chapter 1, we introduced and briefly characterized the three main categories of genetic disorders—single-gene, chromosomal, and complex. In this chapter, the typical patterns of transmission of single-gene disorders are discussed in detail, building on the mechanisms of gene and genome transmission presented generally in Chapters 2; the emphasis here is on the various inheritance patterns of genetic disease in families. Later, in Chapter 6, we will examine more complex patterns of inheritance, including multifactorial disorders that result from the interaction between variants at one or more genes, as well as environmental factors.

3.1 Overview and Concepts

➢ Genotype and Phenotype

For autosomal loci (and X-linked loci in females), the **genotype** of a person at a locus consists of both of the alleles occupying that locus on the two homologous chromosomes (see Fig. 3-1). Genotype should not be confused with **haplotype**, which refers to the set of alleles at two or more neighboring loci on one of the two homologous chromosomes. More broadly, the term genotype can refer to all of the allele pairs that collectively make up an individual's genetic constitution across the entire genome. **Phenotype** is the expression of genotype as a morphological, clinical, cellular, or biochemical trait, which may be clinically observable or may only be detected by blood or tissue testing. The phenotype can be discrete—such as the presence or absence of a disease—or can be a measured quantity, such as body mass index or blood glucose levels. A phenotype may, of course, be either normal or abnormal in a given individual, but in this book, which emphasizes disorders of medical significance, the focus is on disease phenotypes—that is, genetic disorders.

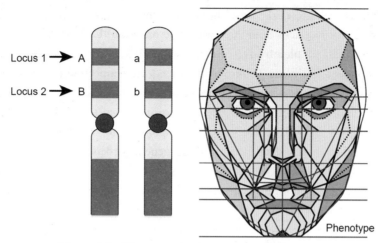

Figure 3-1   The concepts of genotype and phenotype

(*Left*) The genotype refers to information encoded in the genome. Diagram of one pair of homologous chromosomes and two loci on that chromosome, Locus 1 and Locus 2, in an individual who is heterozygous at both loci. He has alleles A and a at locus 1 and alleles B and b at locus 2. The locus 1 genotype is Aa, while the locus 2 genotype is Bb. The two haplotypes on these homologous chromosomes are A-B and a-b. (*Right*) The phenotype is the physical, clinical, cellular, or biochemical manifestation of the genotype, as illustrated here by morphometric aspects of an individual's face.

When a person has a pair of identical alleles at a locus encoded in nuclear DNA, he or she is said to be **homozygous**, or a **homozygote**. When the alleles are different and one of the alleles is the wild-type allele, he or she is **heterozygous**, or a **heterozygote**. The term **compound heterozygote** is used to describe a genotype in which two different mutant alleles of a gene are present, rather than one wild-type and one mutant allele. These terms (*homozygous, heterozygous, and compound heterozygous*) can be applied either to a person or to a genotype. In the special case in which a male has an abnormal allele for a gene located on the X chromosome and there is no other copy of the gene, he is neither homozygous nor heterozygous but is referred to as **hemizygous**. Mitochondrial DNA is still another special case. In contrast to the two copies of each gene per diploid cell, mitochondrial DNA molecules, and the genes encoded by the mitochondrial genome, are present in tens to thousands of copies per cell. For this reason, the terms *homozygous, heterozygous, and hemizygous* are not used to describe genotypes at mitochondrial loci.

A **single-gene disorder** is one that is determined primarily by the alleles at a single locus. The disease follows one of the classic inheritance patterns in families (autosomal recessive, autosomal dominant, X-linked) and is therefore referred to as **mendelian** because, like the characteristics of the garden peas Gregor Mendel studied, they occur on average in fixed and predictable proportions among the offspring of specific types of matings.

A single abnormal gene or gene pair often produces multiple diverse phenotypic effects in multiple organ systems, with a variety of signs and symptoms occurring at different points during the life span. To cite just one example, individuals with a mutation in the *VHL* gene can have hemangioblastomas of the brain, spinal cord, and retina; renal cysts; pancreatic cysts; renal cell carcinoma; pheochromocytoma; and endolymphatic tumors of the inner ear; as well as tumors of the epididymis in males or of the broad ligament of the uterus in females—even though all of these disease manifestations stem from the same single mutation. Under these circumstances, the disorder is said to exhibit **pleiotropy**, and the expression of the gene defect is said to be **pleiotropic**. At present, for many pleiotropic disorders, the connection between the gene defect and the various manifestations is neither obvious nor well understood.

Single-gene disorders affect children disproportionately, but not exclusively. Serious single-gene disorders affect 1 in 300 neonates and are responsible for an estimated 7% of pediatric hospitalizations. Although less than 10% of single-gene disorders manifest after puberty, and only 1% occur after the end of the reproductive period, mendelian disorders are nonetheless important to consider in adult medicine. There are nearly 200 mendelian disorders whose phenotypes include common adult illnesses such as heart disease, stroke, cancer, and diabetes. Although mendelian disorders are by no means the major contributory factor in causing these common diseases in the population at large, they are important in individual patients because of their significance for the health of other family members and because of the availability of genetic testing and detailed management options for many of them.

Penetrance and Expressivity

For some genetic conditions, a disease-causing genotype is always fully expressed at birth as an abnormal phenotype. Clinical experience, however, teaches that other disorders are not expressed at all or may vary substantially in their signs and symptoms, clinical severity, or age of onset, even among members of a family who all share the same disease-causing genotype. Geneticists use distinct terms to describe such differences in clinical expression.

Penetrance is the probability that a mutant allele or alleles will have any phenotypic expression at all. When the frequency of expression of a phenotype is less than 100%—that is, when some of those who have the relevant genotype completely fail to express it—the disorder is said to show **reduced** or **incomplete penetrance**. Penetrance is all or nothing. It is the percentage of people at any given age with a predisposing genotype who are affected, regardless of the severity.

Penetrance of some disorders is age dependent; that is, it may occur any time, from early in intrauterine development all the way to the postreproductive years. Some disorders are lethal prenatally, whereas others can be recognized prenatally (e.g., by ultrasonography) but are consistent with a liveborn infant; still others may be recognized only at birth (**congenital**). Other disorders have their onset typically or exclusively in childhood or in adulthood. Even in these, however, and sometimes even in the same family, two individuals carrying the same disease-causing genotype may develop the disease at very different ages.

In contrast to penetrance, **expressivity** refers not to the presence or absence of a phenotype, but to the severity of expression of that phenotype among individuals with the same disease-causing genotype. When the severity of disease differs in people who have the same genotype, the phenotype is said to show **variable expressivity**. Even in the same family, two individuals carrying the same mutant genes may have some signs and symptoms in common, whereas their other disease manifestations may be quite different, depending on which tissues or organs happen to be affected. The challenge to the clinician caring for these families is to not miss very subtle signs of a disorder in a family member and, as a result, either mistake mild expressivity for lack of penetrance or infer that the individual does not have the disease-causing genotype.

3.2 Pedigrees

Single-gene disorders are characterized by their patterns of transmission in families. To establish the pattern of transmission, a usual first step is to obtain information about the family history of the patient and to summarize the details in the form of a **pedigree**, a graphical representation of the family tree, with use of standard symbols (see Fig. 3-2). The extended family depicted in such pedigrees is a **kindred** (see Fig. 3-3). An affected individual through whom a family with a genetic disorder is first brought to the attention of the geneticist (i.e., is ascertained) is the **proband, propositus**, or **index case**. The person who brings the family to attention by consulting a geneticist is referred to as the **consultand**; the consultand may be an affected individual or an unaffected relative of a proband. A family may have more than one proband, if they are ascertained through more than one source. Brothers and sisters are called **sibs** or **siblings**, and a family of sibs forms a **sibship**. Relatives are classified as **first degree** (parents, sibs, and offspring of the proband), **second degree** (grandparents and grandchildren, uncles and aunts, nephews and nieces, and half-sibs), or **third degree** (e.g., first cousins), and so forth, depending on the number of steps in the pedigree between the two relatives. Couples who have one or more ancestors in common are **consanguineous**. If the proband is the only affected member in a family, he or she is an **isolated** case (see Fig. 3-3). If an isolated case is proven to be due to new mutation in the proband, it is referred to as a **sporadic** case. When there is a definitive diagnosis based on comparisons to other patients, well-established patterns of inheritance in other families with the same disorder can often be used as a basis for counseling, even if the patient is an isolated case in the family. Thus, even when a patient has no similarly affected relatives, it may still be possible to recognize that the disorder is genetic and determine the risk to other family members.

Examining a pedigree is an essential first step in determining the inheritance pattern of a genetic disorder in a family. There are, however, a number of situations that may make the inheritance pattern of an individual pedigree difficult to discern. The inheritance pattern in a family with a lethal disorder affecting a fetus early in pregnancy may be obscure because all that one observes are multiple miscarriages or reduced fertility. Conversely, for phenotypes with variable age of onset, an affected individual may have unaffected family members who have not yet reached the age at which the mutant gene reveals itself. In addition to reduced penetrance or variable expressivity that may mask the existence of relatives carrying the mutant genotype, the geneticist may lack accurate information about the presence of the disorder in relatives or about family relationships. Finally, with the small family size typical of most developed countries today, the patient may by chance alone be the only affected family member, making determination of any inheritance pattern very difficult.

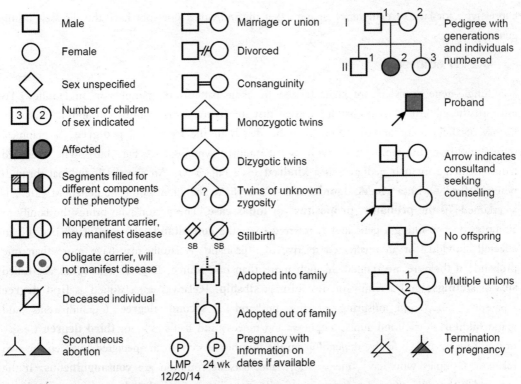

Figure 3-2 Symbols commonly used in pedigree charts

Although there is no uniform system of pedigree notation, the symbols used here are according to recent recommendations made by professionals in the field of genetic counseling.

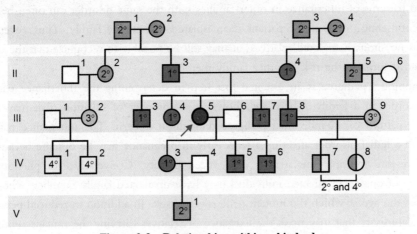

Figure 3-3 Relationships within a kindred

The proband, III-5 (*arrow*), represents an isolated case of a genetic disorder. She has four siblings, III-3, III-4, III-7, and III-8. Her partner/spouse is III-6, and they have three children (their F1 progeny). The proband has nine first-degree relatives (her parents, siblings, and offspring), nine second-degree relatives (grandparents, uncles and aunts, nieces and nephews, and grandchildren), two third-degree relatives (first cousins), and four fourth-degree relatives (first cousins once removed). IV-3, IV-5, and IV-6 are second cousins of IV-1 and IV-2. IV-7 and IV-8, whose parents are consanguineous, are doubly related to the proband: second-degree relatives through their father and fourth-degree relatives through their mother.

3.3   Mendelian Inheritance

The patterns of inheritance shown by single-gene disorders in families depend chiefly on two factors:

- Whether the chromosomal location of the gene locus is on an autosome (chromosomes 1 to 22), on a sex chromosome (X and Y chromosomes), or in the mitochondrial genome.
- Whether the phenotype is **dominant** (expressed when only one chromosome carries the mutant allele) or **recessive** (expressed only when both chromosomes of a pair carry mutant alleles at a locus).

3.3.1   Autosomal, X-Linked, and Mitochondrial Inheritance

The different patterns of transmission of the autosomes, sex chromosomes, and mitochondria during meiosis result in distinctive inheritance patterns of mutant alleles on these different types of chromosome. Because only one of the two copies of each autosome passes into a single gamete during meiosis, males and females heterozygous for a mutant allele on an autosome have a 50% chance of passing that allele on to any offspring, regardless of the child's sex. Mutant alleles on an X chromosome, however, are not distributed equally to sons and daughters. Males pass their Y chromosome to their sons and their X to their daughters. They therefore cannot pass an allele on the X chromosome to their sons and always pass the allele to their daughters. Because mitochondria are inherited from the mother only, regardless of the sex of the offspring, mutations in the mitochondrial genome are not inherited according to a mendelian pattern. Autosomal, X-linked, and mitochondrial inheritance will be discussed in the rest of the chapter that follows.

3.3.2   Dominant and Recessive Traits

(1) Autosomal Loci

As classically defined, a phenotype is **recessive** if it is expressed only in homozygotes, hemizygotes, or compound heterozygotes, all of whom lack a wild-type allele, and never in heterozygotes, who do have a wild-type allele. In contrast, a **dominant** inheritance pattern occurs when a phenotype is expressed in heterozygotes as well as in homozygotes (or compound heterozygotes). For the vast majority of inherited dominant diseases, homozygotes or compound heterozygotes for mutant alleles at autosomal loci are more severely affected than are heterozygotes, an inheritance pattern known as **incompletely dominant** (or **semidominant**). Very few diseases are known in which homozygotes (or compound heterozygotes) show the same phenotype as heterozygotes. In such cases, the disorder is referred to as a **pure dominant** disease. Finally, if phenotypic expression of both alleles at a locus occurs in a compound heterozygote, inheritance is termed **codominant**.

ABO Blood Group

One medically important trait that demonstrates codominant expression is the ABO blood group system important in blood transfusion and tissue transplantation. The *A*, *B*, and *O* alleles at the *ABO* locus form a three-allele system in which two alleles (*A* and *B*) govern expression of either the A or B carbohydrate antigen on the surface of red cells as a codominant trait; a third allele (O) results in expression of neither the A nor the B antigen and is recessive. The difference between the A and B antigen is which of two different sugar molecules makes up the terminal sugar on a cell surface glycoprotein called H. Whether the A or B form of the glycoprotein is made is specified by an enzyme encoded by the *ABO* gene that adds one or the other sugar molecule to the H antigen depending on which version of the enzyme is encoded by alleles at the *ABO* locus. There are therefore four phenotypes possible: O, A, B, and AB (see Table 3-1). Type A individuals have antigen A on their red blood cells, type B individuals have antigen B, type AB individuals have both antigens, and type O individuals have neither.

Table 3-1 ABO Genotypes and Serum Reactivity

Genotype	Phenotype in RBCs	Reaction with Anti-A	Reaction with Anti-B	Antibodies in Serum
OO	O	−	−	Anti-A, anti-B
AA or *AO*	A	+	−	Anti-B
BB or *BO*	B	−	+	Anti-A
AB	AB	+	+	Neither

Note: − Represents no reaction; + represents reaction. RBC, red blood cell.

A feature of the ABO groups not shared by other blood group systems is the reciprocal relationship, in an individual, between the antigens present on the red blood cells and the antibodies in the serum (see Table 3-1). When the red blood cells lack antigen A, the serum contains anti-A antibodies; when the cells lack antigen B, the serum contains anti-B. Formation of anti-A and anti-B antibodies in the absence of prior blood transfusion is believed to be a response to the natural occurrence of A-like and B-like antigens in the environment (e.g., in bacteria).

(2) X-Linked Loci

For X-linked disorders, a condition expressed only in hemizygotes and never in heterozygotes has traditionally been referred to as an X-linked recessive, whereas a phenotype that is always expressed in heterozygotes as well as in hemizygotes has been called X-linked dominant. Because of epigenetic regulation of X-linked gene expression in carrier females due to X chromosome inactivation, it can be difficult to determine phenotypically if a disease with an X-linked inheritance pattern is dominant or recessive, and some geneticists have therefore chosen not to use these terms when describing the inheritance of X-linked disease.

Strictly speaking, the terms *dominant* and *recessive* refer to the inheritance pattern of a phenotype rather than to the alleles responsible for that phenotype. Similarly, a gene is not dominant or recessive; it is the phenotype produced by a particular mutant allele in that gene that shows dominant or recessive inheritance.

3.4 Autosomal Patterns of Mendelian Inheritance

3.4.1 Autosomal Recessive Inheritance

Autosomal recessive disease occurs only in individuals with two mutant alleles and no wild-type allele. Such homozygotes must have inherited a mutant allele from each parent, each of whom is (barring rare exceptions that we will consider later) a heterozygote for that allele.

When a disorder shows recessive inheritance, the mutant allele responsible generally reduces or eliminates the function of the gene product, a so-called **loss-of-function** mutation. For example, many recessive diseases are caused by mutations that impair or eliminate the function of an enzyme. The remaining normal gene copy in a heterozygote is able to compensate for the mutant allele and prevent the disease from occurring. However, when no normal allele is present, as in homozygotes or compound heterozygotes, disease occurs.

Three types of matings can lead to homozygous offspring affected with an autosomal recessive disease. The most common mating by far is between two unaffected heterozygotes, who are often referred to as **carriers**. However, any mating in which each parent has at least one recessive allele can produce homozygous affected offspring. The transmission of a recessive condition can be followed if we symbolize the mutant recessive allele as *r* and its normal dominant allele as *R*.

Table 3-2   Autosomal Recessive Inheritance

Carrier by Carrier		Parent 2 Genotype R/r Gametes		Risk for Disease
		R	r	
Parent 1 Genotype R/r	R	R/R	R/r	¼ Unaffected (R/R) ½ Unaffected carriers (R/r) ¼ Affected (r/r)
Gametes	r	R/r	r/r	

Carrier by Affected		Parent 2 Genotype r/r Gametes		Risk for Disease
		r	r	
Parent 1 Genotype R/r	R	R/r	R/r	½ Unaffected carriers (R/r) ½ Affected (r/r)
Gametes	r	r/r	r/r	

Affected by Affected		Parent 2 Genotype r/r Gametes		Risk for Disease
		r	r	
Parent 1 Genotype r/r	r	r/r	r/r	All affected (r/r)
Gametes	r	r/r	r/r	

Note: The wild-type allele is denoted by uppercase R, a mutant allele by lowercase r.

As seen in the Table 3-2, when both parents of an affected person are carriers, their children's risk for receiving a recessive allele is 50% from each parent. The chance of inheriting two recessive alleles and therefore being affected is thus $1/2 \times 1/2$ or 1 in 4 with each pregnancy. The 25% chance for two heterozygotes to have a child with an autosomal recessive disorder is independent of how many previous children there are who are either affected or unaffected. The proband may be the only affected family member, but if any others are affected, they are usually in the same sibship and not elsewhere in the kindred (see Fig. 3-4).

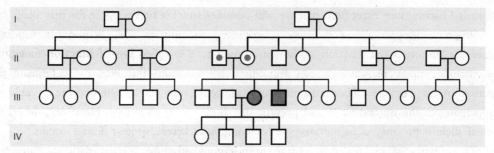

Figure 3-4　Typical pedigree showing autosomal recessive inheritance

(1) Sex-Influenced Autosomal Recessive Disorders

Because males and females both have the same complement of autosomes, autosomal recessive disorders generally show the same frequency and severity in males and females. There are, however, exceptions. Some autosomal recessive diseases demonstrate a **sex-influenced phenotype**, that is, the disorder is expressed in both sexes but with different frequencies or severity. For example, **hereditary hemochromatosis** is an autosomal recessive phenotype that is 5 to 10 times more common in males than in females. Affected individuals have enhanced absorption of dietary iron that can lead to iron overload and serious damage to the heart, liver, and pancreas. The lower incidence of the clinical disorder in homozygous females is believed to be due to their lower dietary iron intake, lower alcohol usage, and increased iron loss through menstruation.

(2) Gene Frequency and Carrier Frequency

Mutant alleles responsible for a recessive disorder are generally rare, and so most people will not have even one copy of the mutant allele. Because an autosomal recessive disorder must be inherited from both parents, the risk that any carrier will have an affected child depends partly on the chance that his or her mate is also a carrier of a mutant allele for the condition. Thus knowledge of the carrier frequency of a disease is clinically important for genetic counseling.

The most common autosomal recessive disorder in white children is **cystic fibrosis** (CF), caused by mutations in the *CFTR* gene. Among white populations, approximately 1 child in 2,000 has two mutant CFTR alleles and has the disease, from which we can infer that 1 in 23 individuals is a silent carrier who has no disease. Mutant alleles may be handed down from carrier to carrier for numerous generations without ever appearing in the homozygous state and causing overt disease. The presence of such hidden recessive genes is not revealed unless the carrier happens to mate with someone who also carries a mutant allele at the same locus and the two deleterious alleles are both inherited by a child.

Estimates of the number of deleterious alleles in each of our genomes range from 50 to 200 based on examining an individual's complete exome or genome sequence for clearly deleterious mutations in the coding regions of the genome. This estimate is imprecise, however. It may be an underestimate, because it does not include mutant alleles whose deleterious effect is not obvious from a simple examination of the DNA sequence. It may also, however, be an overestimate, because it includes mutations in many genes that are not known to cause disease.

(3) Consanguinity

Because most mutant alleles are generally uncommon in the population, people with rare autosomal recessive disorders are typically **compound heterozygotes** rather than true homozygotes. One well-recognized exception to this rule occurs when an affected individual inherits the exact same mutant allele from both parents because the parents are consanguineous (i.e., they are related and carry the identical mutant allele inherited from a common ancestor). Finding consanguinity in the parents of a patient with a genetic disorder is strong evidence (although not proof) for the autosomal recessive inheritance of that condition. For example, the disorder in the pedigree in Figure 3-5 is likely to be an autosomal recessive trait, even though other information in the pedigree may seem insufficient to establish this inheritance pattern.

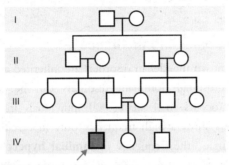

Figure 3-5   Pedigree in which parental consanguinity suggests autosomal recessive inheritance
Note: *Arrow* indicates the proband.

Consanguinity is more frequently found in the background of patients with very rare conditions than in those with more common recessive conditions. This is because it is less likely that two individuals mating at random in the population will both be carriers of a very rare disorder by chance alone than it is that they would both be carriers because they inherited the same mutant allele from a single common ancestor. For example, in **xeroderma pigmentosum**, a very rare autosomal recessive condition of DNA repair, more than 20% of cases occur among the offspring of marriages between first cousins. In contrast, in more common recessive conditions, most cases of the disorder result from matings between *unrelated* persons, each of whom happens by chance to be a carrier. Thus most affected persons with a relatively common disorder, such as CF, are not the result of consanguinity, because the mutant allele is so common in the general population.

The genetic risk to the offspring of marriages between related people is not as great as is sometimes imagined. For marriages between first cousins, the absolute risks of abnormal offspring, including not only known autosomal recessive diseases but also stillbirth, neonatal death, and congenital malformation, is 3% to 5%, approximately double the overall background risk of 2% to 3% for offspring born to any unrelated couple. Consanguinity at the level of third cousins or more remote relationships is not considered to be genetically significant, and the increased risk for abnormal offspring is negligible in such cases.

The incidence of first-cousin marriage is low (≈ 1 to 10 per 1,000 marriages) in many populations in western societies today. However, it remains relatively common in some ethnic groups, for example, in families from rural areas of the Indian subcontinent, in other parts of Asia, and in the Middle East, where between 20% and 60% of all marriages are between cousins.

Characteristics of Autosomal Recessive Inheritance

- An autosomal recessive phenotype, if not isolated, is typically seen only in the sibship of the proband, and not in parents, offspring, or other relatives.
- For most autosomal recessive diseases, males and females are equally likely to be affected.
- Parents of an affected child are asymptomatic carriers of mutant alleles.
- The parents of the affected person may in some cases be consanguineous. This is especially likely if the gene responsible for the condition is rare in the population.
- The recurrence risk for each sib of the proband is 1 in 4 (25%).

3.4.2 Autosomal Dominant Inheritance

More than half of all known mendelian disorders are inherited as autosomal dominant traits. The incidence of some autosomal dominant disorders can be high. For example, adult **polycystic kidney disease** occurs in 1 in 1,000 individuals in the United States. Other autosomal dominant disorders show a high frequency only in certain populations from specific geographical areas: for example, the frequency of **familial hypercholesterolemia** is 1 in 100 for Afrikaner populations in South Africa and of **myotonic dystrophy** is 1 in 550 in the Charlevoix and Saguenay-Lac Saint Jean regions of northeastern Quebec. The burden of autosomal dominant disorders is further increased because of their hereditary nature. When they are transmitted through families, they raise medical and even social problems not only for individuals but also for whole kindreds, often through many generations.

The risk and severity of dominantly inherited disease in the offspring depend on whether one or both parents are affected and whether the trait is a pure dominant or is incompletely dominant. There are a number of different ways that one mutant allele can cause a dominantly inherited trait to occur in a heterozygote despite the presence of a normal allele.

Denoting D as the mutant allele and d as the wild-type allele, matings that produce children with an autosomal dominant disease can be between two heterozygotes (D/d) for the mutation or, more frequently, between a heterozygote for the mutation (D/d) and a homozygote for a normal allele (d/d).

As seen in the Table 3-3, each child of a D/d by d/d mating has a 50% chance of receiving the affected parent's abnormal allele D and a 50% chance of receiving the normal allele d. In the population as a whole, then, the offspring of D/d by d/d parents are approximately 50% D/d and 50% d/d. Of course, each pregnancy is an independent event, not governed by the outcome of previous pregnancies. Thus, within a family, the distribution of affected and unaffected children may be quite different from the theoretical expected ratio of 1 : 1, especially if the sibship is small. Typical autosomal dominant inheritance can be seen in the pedigree of a family with a dominantly inherited form of hereditary deafness (see Fig. 3-6).

Table 3-3 Autosomal Dominant Inheritance

Affected by Unaffected		Parent 2 Genotype d/d Gametes		Risk for Disease
		d	d	
Parent 1 Genotype D/d Gametes	D	D/d	D/d	½ Affected (D/d) ½ Unaffected (d/d)
	d	d/d	d/d	

Affected by Affected		Parent 2 Genotype D/d Gametes		Risk for Disease
		D	d	
Parent 1 Genotype D/d Gametes	D	D/D	D/d	Strictly dominant ¾ Affected (D/D and D/d) ¼ Unaffected (d/d)
	d	D/d	d/d	Incompletely dominant ¼ Severely affected (D/D) ½ Affected (D/d) ¼ Unaffected (d/d)

Note: The mutant allele causing dominantly inherited disease is denoted by uppercase D; the normal or wild-type allele is denoted by lowercase d.

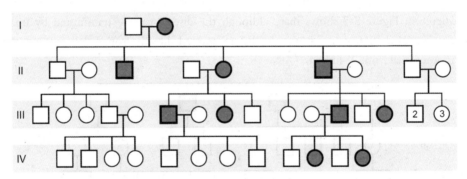

Figure 3-6 Typical inheritance of a form of adult-onset progressive sensorineural deafness (DFNA1) inherited as an autosomal dominant trait

In medical practice, homozygotes for dominant phenotypes are not often seen because matings that could produce homozygous offspring are rare. Again denoting the abnormal allele as D and the wild-type allele as d, the matings that can produce a D/D homozygote might theoretically be D/d by D/d, D/D by D/d, or D/D by D/D. In the case of two heterozygotes mating, three fourths of the offspring of a D/d by D/d mating will be affected to some extent and one fourth unaffected.

(1) Pure Dominant Inheritance

As mentioned earlier, very few human disorders demonstrate a purely dominant pattern of inheritance. Even **Huntington disease**, which is frequently considered to be a pure dominant because the disease is generally similar in the nature and severity of symptoms in heterozygotes and homozygotes, appears to have a somewhat accelerated time course from the onset of disease to death in homozygous individuals compared with heterozygotes.

(2) Incompletely Dominant Inheritance

Achondroplasia is an incompletely dominant skeletal disorder of short-limbed dwarfism and large head caused by certain mutations in the fibroblast growth factor receptor 3 gene (*FGFR3*). Most achondroplasia patients have normal intelligence and lead normal lives within their physical capabilities. Marriages between two patients with achondroplasia are not uncommon. A pedigree of a mating between two individuals heterozygous for the most common mutation that causes achondroplasia is shown in Figure 3-6B. The deceased child, individual III-3, was a homozygote for the condition and had a disorder far more severe than in either parent, resulting in death soon after birth.

(3) Sex-Limited Phenotype in Autosomal Dominant Disease

As discussed earlier for the autosomal recessive condition hemochromatosis, autosomal dominant phenotypes may also demonstrate a sex ratio that differs significantly from 1 : 1. Extreme divergence of the sex ratio is seen in sex-limited phenotypes, in which the defect is autosomally transmitted but expressed in only one sex. An example is **male-limited precocious puberty**, an autosomal dominant disorder in which affected boys develop secondary sexual characteristics and undergo an adolescent growth spurt at approximately 4 years of age. In some families, the defect has been traced to mutations in the *LCGR* gene, which encodes the receptor for luteinizing hormone. These mutations constitutively activate the receptor's signaling action, even in the absence of its hormone. The defect shows no effect in heterozygous females. The pedigree in Figure 3-7 shows that, although the disease can be transmitted by unaffected (nonpenetrant carrier) females, it can also be transmitted directly from father to son, showing that it is autosomal, not X-linked.

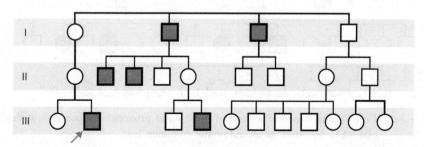

Figure 3-7 Part of a large pedigree of male-limited precocious puberty in one family
This autosomal dominant disorder can be transmitted by affected males or by unaffected carrier females. Male-to-male transmission shows that inheritance is autosomal, not X-linked. Transmission of the trait through carrier females shows that inheritance cannot be Y-linked. *Arrow* indicates proband.

Characteristics of Autosomal Dominant Inheritance

• The phenotype usually appears in every generation, each affected person having an affected parent. Exceptions or apparent exceptions to this rule in clinical genetics are (1) cases originating from fresh mutations in a gamete of a phenotypically normal parent and (2) cases in which the disorder is not expressed (nonpenetrant) or is expressed only subtly in a person who has inherited the responsible mutant allele.

- Any child of an affected parent has a 50% risk for inheriting the trait. This is true for most families, in which the other parent is phenotypically normal. Because statistically each family member is the result of an "independent event", wide deviation from the expected 1 : 1 ratio may occur by chance in a single family.

- Phenotypically normal family members do not transmit the phenotype to their children. Failure of penetrance or subtle expression of a condition may lead to apparent exceptions to this rule.

- Males and females are equally likely to transmit the phenotype, to children of either sex. In particular, male-to-male transmission can occur, and males can have unaffected daughters.

- A significant proportion of isolated cases are sporadic cases due to new mutation.

(4) Effect of Incomplete Penetrance, Variable Expressivity, and New Mutations on Autosomal Dominant Inheritance Patterns

Some of the difficulties raised by incomplete penetrance in fully understanding the inheritance of a disease phenotype are demonstrated by the **split-hand/foot malformation**, a type of ectrodactyly. The split-hand malformation originates in the sixth or seventh week of development, when the hands and feet are forming. Failure of penetrance in pedigrees of split-hand malformation can lead to apparent skipping of generations, and this complicates genetic counseling because an at-risk person with normal hands may nevertheless carry the mutation for the condition and thus be capable of having children who are affected.

Figure 3-8 is a pedigree of split-hand deformity in which the unaffected sister of an affected man sought genetic counseling. Her mother is a nonpenetrant carrier of the split-hand mutation. The literature on split-hand deformity suggests that there is reduced penetrance of approximately 70% (i.e., only 70% of the people who have the mutation exhibit the clinical defect). Using this pedigree information to calculate conditional probabilities, one can calculate that the risk that the consultand might herself be a nonpenetrant carrier is 23% and her chance of having a child with the abnormality is therefore approximately 8% (carrier risk×the risk for transmission× penetrance, or 23% ×50% ×70%).

An autosomal dominant inheritance pattern may also be obscured by variable expressivity. **Neurofibromatosis 1 (NF1)**, a common disorder of the nervous system, demonstrates both age-dependent penetrance and variable expressivity in a single family. Some adults may have only multiple flat, irregular pigmented skin lesions, known as café au lait spots, and small benign tumors (hamartomas) called Lisch nodules on the iris of the eye. Other family members can have these signs as well as multiple benign fleshy tumors (neurofibromas) in the skin. And, still others may have a much more severe phenotype, with intellectual disability, diffuse plexiform neurofibromas, or malignant tumors of nervous system or muscle in addition to the café au lait spots, Lisch nodules, and neurofibromas. Unless one looks specifically for mild manifestations of the disease in the relatives of the proband, heterozygous carriers may be incorrectly classified as unaffected, noncarriers.

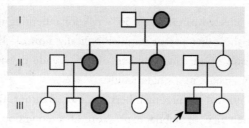

Figure 3-8　Pedigree of split-hand deformity

This pedigree demonstrates failure of penetrance in the mother of the proband (*arrow*) and his sister, the consultand. Reduced penetrance must be taken into account in genetic counseling.

Furthermore, the signs of NF1 may require many years to develop. For example, in the newborn period, less than half of all affected newborns show even the most subtle sign of the disease, an increased incidence of café au lait spots. Eventually, however, multiple café au lait spots and Lisch nodules do appear so that, by adulthood, heterozygotes always demonstrate some sign of the disease.

Finally, in classic autosomal dominant inheritance, every affected person in a pedigree has an affected parent, who also has an affected parent, and so on, as far back as the disorder can be traced. In fact, however, many dominant conditions of medical importance occur because of a spontaneous, de novo mutation in a gamete inherited from a noncarrier parent (see Fig. 3-6). An individual with an autosomal dominant disorder caused by new mutation will look like an isolated case, and his or her parents, aunts and uncles, and cousins will all be unaffected noncarriers. He or she will still be at risk for passing the mutation down to his or her own children, however. Once a new mutation has arisen, it will be transmitted to future generations following standard principles of inheritance, and, as we discuss in the next section, its survival in the population depends on the fitness of persons carrying it.

3.5　X-Linked Inheritance

In contrast to genes on the autosomes, genes on the X and Y chromosomes are distributed unequally to males and females in families. The patrilineal inheritance of the Y chromosome is straightforward. However, there are very few strictly Y-linked genes, almost all of which are involved in primary sex determination or the development of secondary male characteristics, and they will not be considered here. Approximately 800 protein-coding and 300 noncoding RNA genes have been identified on the X chromosome to date, of which over 300 genes are presently known to be associated with X-linked disease phenotypes. Phenotypes determined by genes on the X have a characteristic sex distribution and a pattern of inheritance that is usually easy to identify and easy to distinguish from the patterns of autosomal inheritance we just explored.

Because males have one X chromosome but females have two, there are only two possible genotypes in males and four in females with respect to mutant alleles at an X-linked locus. A male with a mutant allele at an X-linked locus is **hemizygous** for that allele, whereas females may be a homozygote for the wild-type allele, a homozygote for a mutant allele, a compound heterozygote for two different mutant alleles, or a heterozygous carrier of a mutant allele. For example, if X_H is the wild-type allele for an X-linked disease gene and a mutant allele, X_h, is the disease allele, the genotypes expected in males and females are as follows:

Table 3-4 Genotypes and Phenotypes in X-linked Disease

Sex	Genotypes	Phenotypes
Males	Hemizygous X_H Hemizygous X_h	Unaffected affected
Females	Homozygous X_H/X_H Heterozygous X_H/X_h Homozygous X_h/X_h	Unaffected Carrier (may or may not be affected) affected

3.5.1 X Inactivation, Dosage Compensation, and the Expression of X-Linked Genes

X inactivation is a normal physiological process in which most of the genes on one of the two X chromosomes in normal females, but not the genes on the single X chromosome in males, are inactivated in somatic cells, thus equalizing the expression of most X-linked genes in the two sexes. The clinical relevance of X inactivation in X-linked diseases is profound. It leads to females having two cell populations, which express alleles of X-linked genes on one or the other of the two X chromosomes. These two cell populations are thus genetically identical but functionally distinct, and both cell populations in human females can be readily detected for some disorders. For example, in **Duchenne muscular dystrophy**, female carriers exhibit typical mosaic expression of their dystrophin immunostaining (see Fig. 3-9). Depending on the pattern of random X inactivation of the two X chromosomes, two female heterozygotes for an X-linked disease may have very different clinical presentations because they differ in the proportion of cells that have the mutant allele on the active X in a relevant tissue (as seen in **manifesting heterozygotes**).

3.5.2 Recessive and Dominant Inheritance of X-Linked Disorders

As mentioned earlier in this chapter, the use of the terms *dominant* and *recessive* is somewhat different in X-linked conditions than we just saw for autosomal disorders. So-called X-linked dominant and recessive patterns of inheritance are typically distinguished on the basis of the phenotype in heterozygous females. Some X-linked phenotypes are consistently apparent clinically, at least to some degree, in carriers and are thus referred to as dominant, whereas others typically are not and are considered to be recessive. The difficulty in classifying an X-linked disorder as dominant or recessive arises because females who are heterozygous for the same mutant allele in a family may or may not demonstrate the disease, depending on the pattern of random X inactivation and the proportion of the cells in pertinent tissues that have the mutant allele on the active or inactive X.

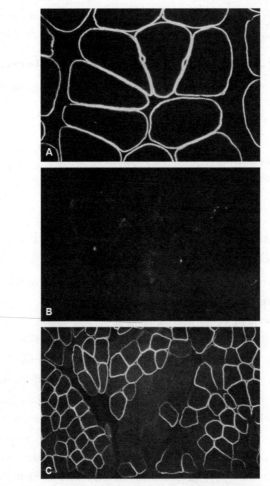

Figure 3-9　Immunostaining for dystrophin in muscle specimens

（A）A normal female（×480）.（B）A male with Duchenne muscular dystrophy（DMD）（×480）.
（C）A carrier female（×240）. Staining creates the bright signals seen here encircling individual muscle
fibers. Muscle from DMD patients lacks dystrophin staining. Muscle from DMD carriers exhibits both
positive and negative patches of dystrophin immunostaining, representing fibers with either the normal
or mutant allele on the active X.

　　Nearly a third of X-linked disorders are penetrant in some but not all female heterozygotes
and cannot be classified as either dominant or recessive. Even for disorders that can be so
classified, they show incomplete penetrance that varies as a function of X inactivation patterns,
not inheritance patterns. Because clinical expression of an X-linked condition does not depend
strictly on the particular gene involved or even the particular mutation in the same family, some
geneticists have recommended dispensing altogether with the terms *recessive* and *dominant* for
X-linked disorders. Be that as it may, the terms are widely applied to X-linked disorders, and
we will continue to use them, recognizing that they describe extremes of a continuum of
penetrance and expressivity in female carriers of X-linked diseases.

（1）X-Linked Recessive Inheritance

　　The inheritance of X-linked recessive phenotypes follows a well-defined and easily
recognized pattern（see Fig. 3-10）. An X-linked recessive mutation is expressed phenotypically

in all males who receive it, and, consequently, X-linked recessive disorders are generally restricted to males.

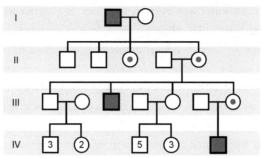

Figure 3-10   Pedigree pattern demonstrating an X-linked recessive disorder such as hemophilia A, transmitted from an affected male through females to an affected grandson and great-grandson

Hemophilia A is a classic X-linked recessive disorder in which the blood fails to clot normally because of a deficiency of factor VIII, a protein in the clotting cascade. The hereditary nature of hemophilia and even its pattern of transmission have been recognized since ancient times, and the condition became known as the "royal hemophilia" because of its occurrence among descendants of Britain's Queen Victoria, who was a carrier.

As in the earlier discussion, suppose X_h represents the mutant factor VIII allele causing hemophilia A, and X_H represents the normal allele. If a male with hemophilia mates with a normal female, all the sons receive their father's Y chromosome and a maternal X and are unaffected, but all the daughters receive the paternal X chromosome with its hemophilia allele and are obligate carriers. If a daughter of the affected male mates with an unaffected male, four genotypes are possible in the progeny, with equal probabilities (see Table 3-5).

Table 3-5   X-Linked Recessive Inheritance

Affected Male by Noncarrier Female		Female Genotype X_H/X_H Gametes		Risk for Disease
		X_H	X_H	
Male Genotype X_h/Y	X_h	X_H/X_h	X_H/X_h	All female carriers (X_H/X_h)
Gametes	Y	X_H/Y	X_H/Y	All males unaffected (X_H/Y)

Unaffected Male by Carrier Female		Female Genotype X_H/X_h Gametes		Risk for Disease
		X_H	X_h	
Male Genotype X_H/Y	X_H	X_H/X_H	X_H/X_h	¼ Noncarrier female (X_H/X_H) ¼ Carrier female (X_H/X_h)
Gametes	Y	X_H/Y	X_h/Y	¼ Normal male (X_H/Y) ¼ Affected male (X_h/Y)

Note: The wild-type allele at the X-linked hemophilia locus is denoted as X_H with an uppercase H, and the mutant allele is denoted as X_h with a lowercase h.

The hemophilia of an affected grandfather, which did not appear in any of his own children, has a 50% chance of appearing in each son of his daughters. It will not reappear among the descendants of his sons, however. A daughter of a carrier has a 50% chance of being a carrier herself (see Fig. 3-10). By chance, an X-linked recessive allele may be transmitted undetected through a series of female carriers before it is expressed in a male descendant.

Characteristics of X-Linked Recessive Inheritance

- The incidence of the trait is much higher in males than in females.
- Heterozygous females are usually unaffected, but some may express the condition with variable severity as determined by the pattern of X inactivation.
- The gene responsible for the condition is transmitted from an affected man through all his daughters. Any of his daughters' sons has a 50% chance of inheriting it.
- The mutant allele is never transmitted directly from father to son, but it is transmitted by an affected male to all his daughters.
- The mutant allele may be transmitted through a series of carrier females; if so, the affected males in a kindred are related through females.
- A significant proportion of isolated cases are due to new mutation.

(2) Affected Females in X-linked Recessive Disease

Although X-linked conditions are classically seen only in males, they can be observed in females under two circumstances. In one, such a female can be homozygous for the relevant disease allele, although most X-linked diseases are so rare that this scenario is highly unlikely unless her parents are consanguineous. However, a few X-linked conditions, such as X-linked color blindness, are sufficiently common that such homozygotes are seen in female offspring of an affected father and a carrier mother.

More commonly, an affected female represents a carrier of a recessive X-linked allele who shows phenotypic expression of the disease and is referred to as a **manifesting heterozygote**. Whether a female carrier will be a manifesting heterozygote depends on a number of features of X inactivation. First, the choice of which X chromosome is to become inactive is a random one, but it occurs when there is a relatively small number of cells in the developing female embryo. By chance alone, therefore, the fraction of cells in various tissues of carrier females in which the normal or mutant allele happens to remain active may deviate substantially from the expected 50%, resulting in **unbalanced** or "**skewed**" **X inactivation**. A female carrier may have signs and symptoms of an X-linked disorder if the skewed inactivation is unfavorable (i.e., a large majority of the active X chromosomes in pertinent tissues happen to contain the deleterious allele).

Favorably unbalanced or skewed inactivation, in which the mutant allele is found preferentially on the inactive X in some or all tissues of an unaffected heterozygous female, also occurs. Such skewed inactivation may simply be due to chance alone, as we just saw (albeit in the opposite direction). However, there are certain X-linked conditions in which there is reduced cell survival or a proliferative disadvantage for those cells that originally had the mutant allele on the active X early in development, resulting in a pattern of highly skewed inactivation that favors cells with the normal allele on the active X in relevant tissues. For example, highly skewed X inactivation is the rule in female carriers of certain **X-linked immunodeficiencies**, in whom only those early progenitor cells that happen to carry the normal allele on their active X chromosome can populate certain lineages in the immune system.

(3) X-Linked Dominant Inheritance

As discussed earlier, an X-linked phenotype can be described as dominant if it is regularly expressed in heterozygotes. X-linked dominant inheritance can readily be distinguished from autosomal dominant inheritance by the lack of **male-to-male transmission**, which is impossible for X-linked inheritance because males transmit the Y chromosome, not the X, to their sons (see Table 3-6).

Table 3-6   X-Linked Dominant Inheritance

Unaffected Male by Affected Female		Female Genotype X_D/X_d Gametes		Risk for Disease
		X_D	X_d	
Male Genotype X_d/Y	X_d	X_D/X_d	X_d/X_d	¼ Affected females (X_D/X_d)
				¼ Unaffected females (X_d/X_d)
Gametes	Y	X_D/Y	X_d/Y	¼ Affected males (X_D/Y)
				¼ Unaffected males (X_d/Y)
Affected Male by Noncarrier Female		Female Genotype X_d/X_d Gametes		Risk for Disease
		X_d	X_d	
Male Genotype X_D/Y	X_D	X_D/X_d	X_D/X_d	All females affected (X_D/X_d)
Gametes	Y	X_d/Y	X_d/Y	All males unaffected (X_d/Y)

Note: The wild-type allele at the hypophosphatemic rickets locus is denoted as X_d, and the mutant allele is denoted as X_D.

Thus the distinguishing feature of a fully penetrant X-linked dominant pedigree (see Fig. 3-11) is that all the daughters and none of the sons of affected males are affected. If any daughter is unaffected or any son is affected, the inheritance must be autosomal, not X-linked. The pattern of inheritance through females is no different from the autosomal dominant pattern. Because females have a pair of X chromosomes just as they have pairs of autosomes, each child of an affected female has a 50% chance of inheriting the trait, regardless of sex. Across multiple families with an X-linked dominant disease, the expression is usually milder in heterozygous females, because the mutant allele is located on the inactive X chromosome in a proportion of their cells. Thus most X-linked dominant disorders are incompletely dominant, as is the case with most autosomal dominant disorders.

Characteristics of X-Linked Dominant Inheritance

- Affected males with normal mates have no affected sons and no normal daughters.
- Both male and female offspring of female carriers have a 50% risk for inheriting the phenotype. The pedigree pattern is similar to that seen with autosomal dominant inheritance.
- Affected females are approximately twice as common as affected males, but affected females typically have milder (although variable) expression of the phenotype.
- One example of an X-linked dominant disorder is X-linked **hypophosphatemic rickets** (also known as vitamin D-resistant rickets), in which the ability of the kidney tubules to reabsorb filtered phosphate is impaired. This disorder fits the criterion of an X-linked dominant disorder in that both sexes are affected, although the serum phosphate level is less depressed and the rickets less severe in heterozygous females than in affected males.

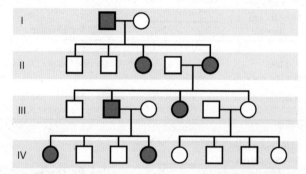

Figure 3-11　Pedigree pattern demonstrating X-linked dominant inheritance

(4) X-Linked Dominant Disorders with Male Lethality

Although most X-linked conditions are typically apparent only in males, a few rare X-linked defects are expressed exclusively or almost exclusively in females. These X-linked dominant conditions are lethal in males before birth (see Fig. 3-12). Typical pedigrees of these conditions show transmission by affected females, who produce affected daughters, normal daughters, and normal sons in equal proportions (1 : 1 : 1); affected males are not seen.

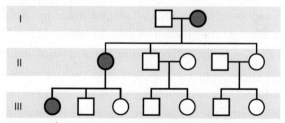

Figure 3-12　Pedigree pattern demonstrating X-linked dominant inheritance of a disorder that is lethal in males during the prenatal period

Rett syndrome is a striking disorder that occurs nearly exclusively in females and meets all criteria for being an X-linked dominant disorder that is usually lethal in hemizygous males. The syndrome is characterized by normal prenatal and neonatal growth and development, followed by the rapid onset of neurological symptoms in affected girls. The disease mechanism is thought to reflect abnormalities in the regulation of a set of genes in the developing brain. The cause of male lethality is unknown but presumably reflects a requirement during early development for at least one functional copy of the *MECP2* gene on the X chromosome that is mutated in this syndrome.

(5) X-Linked Dominant Disorders with Male Sparing

Other disorders are manifest only in carrier females because hemizygous males are largely spared the consequences of the mutation they carry. One such disorder is female-limited, X-linked **epilepsy and cognitive impairment**. Affected females are asymptomatic at birth and appear to be developing normally but then develop seizures, generally in the second year of life, after which development begins to regress. Most affected females go on to be developmentally delayed, which can vary from mild to severe. In contrast, male hemizygotes in the same families are completely unaffected (see Fig. 3-13). The disorder is due to loss-of-function mutations in the protocadherin gene 19, an X-linked gene that encodes a cell surface molecule expressed on neurons in the central nervous system.

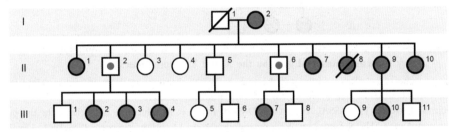

Figure 3-13 Pedigree pattern of familial female epilepsy and cognitive impairment

The explanation for this unusual pattern of inheritance is not clear. It is hypothesized that the epilepsy occurs in females because mosaicism for expression of protocadherin 19, resulting from random X inactivation in the brain, disrupts communication between groups of neurons with and without the cell surface protein. Neurons in males uniformly lack the cell surface molecule, but their brains are apparently spared cell-cell miscommunication by a different, compensating protocadherin.

3.6 Pseudoautosomal Inheritance

As we first saw in Chapter 2, meiotic recombination between X-linked loci only occurs between the two homologous X chromosomes and is therefore restricted to females. X-linked loci do not participate in meiotic recombination in males, who have a Y chromosome and only one X chromosome. There are, however, a small number of contiguous loci located at the tips of the p and q arms of the sex chromosomes that are homologous between the X and Y and do recombine between them in male meiosis. As a consequence, during spermatogenesis, a mutant allele at one of these loci on the X chromosome can be transferred onto the Y chromosome and passed on to male offspring, thereby demonstrating the male-to-male transmission characteristic of autosomal inheritance. Because these unusual loci on the X and Y demonstrate autosomal inheritance but are not located on an autosome, they are referred to as **pseudoautosomal** loci, and the segments of the X and Y chromosomes where they are located are referred to as the **pseudoautosomal regions**.

One example of a disease caused by a mutation at a pseudoautosomal locus is **dyschondrosteosis**, a dominantly inherited skeletal dysplasia with disproportionate short stature and deformity of the forearms. Although a greater prevalence of the disease in females as compared with males initially suggested an X-linked dominant disorder, the presence of male-to-male transmission clearly ruled out strict X-linked inheritance (see Fig. 3-14). Mutations in the *SHOX* gene, located in the pseudoautosomal region on Xp and Yp, have been found responsible for this condition.

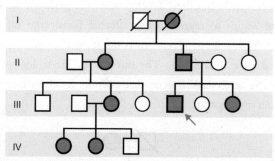

Figure 3-14   Pedigree showing inheritance of dyschondrosteosis due to mutations in *SHOX*, a pseudoautosomal gene on the X and Y chromosomes

The *arrow* shows a male who inherited the trait on his Y chromosome from his father. His father, however, inherited the trait on his X chromosome from his mother.

(From SHEARS D J, VASSAL H J, GOODMAN F R, et al. Mutation and deletion of the pseudoautosomal gene SHOX cause Leri-Weill dyschondrosteosis[J]. Nature genetics, 1998,19(1):70−73.)

3.7   Mosaicism

Although we are used to thinking of ourselves as being composed of cells that all carry exactly the same complement of genes and chromosomes, this is in reality an oversimplified view. Mosaicism is the presence in an individual or a tissue of at least two cell lineages that differ genetically but are derived from a single zygote. Mutations that occur after conception in a single cell in either prenatal or postnatal life can give rise to clones of cells genetically different from the original zygote because, given the nature of DNA replication, the mutation will persist in all the clonal descendants of that cell (see Fig. 3-15). Mosaicism for numerical or structural abnormalities of chromosomes is a clinically important phenomenon, and somatic mutation is recognized as the major contributor to most types of cancer.

Mosaicism can affect any cells or tissue within a developing embryo or at any point after conception to adulthood, and it can be a diagnostic dilemma to determine just how widespread the mosaic pattern is. For example, the population of cells that carry a mutation in a mosaic pregnancy might be found only in extraembryonic tissue and not in the embryo proper (**confined placental mosaicism**), might be present in some tissues of the embryo but not in the gametes (pure **somatic mosaicism**), might be restricted to the gamete lineage only and nowhere else (pure **germline mosaicism**), or might be present in both somatic lineages and the germline—all depending on whether the mutation occurred before or after the separation of the inner cell mass, the germline cells, and the somatic cells during embryogenesis. Because there are approximately 30 mitotic divisions in the cells of the germline before meiosis in the female and several hundred in the male, there is ample opportunity for mutations to occur in germline cells after the separation from somatic cells, resulting in pure gonadal mosaicism.

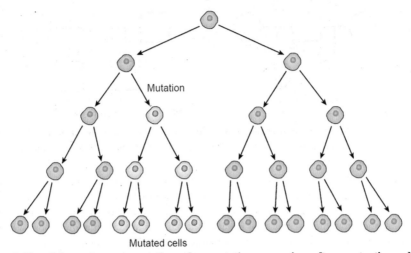

Figure 3-15   Schematic representation of a mutation occurring after conception, during mitotic cell divisions

Such a mutation can lead to a proportion of cells carrying the mutation—that is, to either somatic or germline mosaicism, depending on at what stage of embryonic or postnatal development the mutation occurred.

Determining whether mosaicism for a mutation is present only in the germline or only in somatic tissues may be difficult because failure to find a mutation in a subset of cells from a readily accessible somatic tissue (e.g., peripheral white blood cells, skin, or buccal cells) does not ensure that the mutation is not present elsewhere in the body, including the germline.

3.7.1 Segmental Mosaicism

A mutation affecting morphogenesis and occurring during embryonic development might be manifested as a segmental or patchy abnormality, depending on the stage at which the mutation occurred and the lineage of the somatic cell in which it originated. For example, **neurofibromatosis 1 (NF1)** is sometimes segmental, affecting only one part of the body. Segmental NF1 is caused by somatic mosaicism for a mutation that occurred after conception. Although the parents of such a patient would be unaffected and considered not at risk for transmitting the mutant gene, a patient with segmental NF1 could be at risk for having an affected child, whose phenotype would be typical for NF1, that is, not segmental. Whether the patient is at risk for transmitting the defect will depend on whether the mutation occurred before separation of germline cells from the somatic cell line that carries the mutation.

3.7.2 Germline Mosaicism

In pedigrees with germline mosaicism, unaffected individuals with no evidence of a disease-causing mutation in their genome (as evidenced by the failure to find the mutation in DNA extracted from their peripheral white blood cells) may still be at risk for having more than one child who inherited the mutation from them (see Fig. 3-16). The existence of germline mosaicism means that geneticists and genetic counselors must be aware of the potential inaccuracy of assuming that normal examination results and normal gene test results of the parents of a child with an autosomal dominant or X-linked phenotype means the child must be a new mutation.

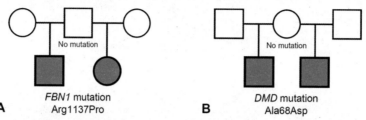

A   FBN1 mutation   B   DMD mutation
           Arg1137Pro   Ala68Asp

Figure 3-16   Pedigrees demonstrating two affected siblings with the autosomal dominant disorder Marfan syndrome (Family A) and the X-linked condition Becker muscular dystrophy (Family B)

In Family A, the affected children have the same point mutation inherited from their father, who is unaffected and does not carry the mutation in DNA from examined somatic tissues. He must have been a mosaic for the *FBN1* mutation in his germline. In Family B, the affected children have the same point mutation inherited from their mother who is unaffected and does not carry the mutation in DNA from examined somatic tissues. She must have been a mosaic for the *DMD* mutation in her germline.

3.8   Parent-of-Origin Effects on Inheritance Patterns

➤ Unusual Inheritance Patterns due to Genomic Imprinting

According to Mendel's laws of heredity, a mutant allele of an autosomal gene is equally likely to be transmitted from a parent of either sex to an offspring of either sex. Similarly, a female is equally likely to transmit a mutated X-linked gene to a child of either sex. Originally, little attention was paid to whether the sex of the parent had any effect on the expression of the genes each parent transmits. However, in some genetic disorders, such as **Prader-Willi syndrome** and **Angelman syndrome**, the expression of the disease phenotype depends on whether the mutant allele has been inherited from the father or from the mother, a phenomenon known as **genomic imprinting**. The hallmark of genomic imprinting is that the sex of the parent who transmits the abnormality determines whether there is expression of the disorder in a child. This is very different from sex-limited inheritance, in which expression of the disease depends on the sex of the child who inherits the abnormality.

Imprinting can cause unusual inheritance patterns in pedigrees, in that a disorder can appear to be inherited in a dominant manner when transmitted from one parent, but not the other. For example, the **hereditary paragangliomas** (PGLs) are a group of autosomal dominant disorders in which multiple tumors develop in sympathetic and parasympathetic ganglia of the autonomic nervous system. Patients with paraganglioma can also develop a catecholamine-producing tumor known as a pheochromocytoma, either in the adrenal medulla or in sympathetic ganglia along the vertebral column. A pedigree of one type of PGL family is shown in Figure 3-17. The striking observation is that, although both males and females can be affected, this is only if they inherited the mutation from their father and not from their mother. A male heterozygote who has inherited his mutation from his mother will remain unaffected throughout life but is still at a 50% risk for transmitting the mutation to each of his children, who are then at high risk for developing the disease.

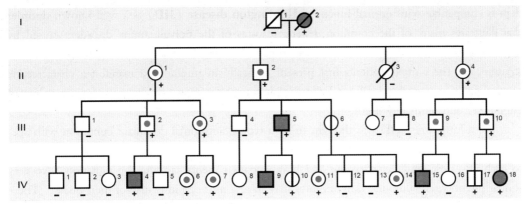

Figure 3-17 Pedigree of a family with paraganglioma syndrome 1 caused by a mutation in the SDHD gene
Individuals II-1, II-2, II-4, III-2, III-3, III-9, III-10, IV-6, IV-7, IV-11, and IV-14 each inherited the mutation from their mothers but are unaffected. However, when the males in this group pass on the mutation, those children can be affected. In addition to the imprinting, the family also demonstrates the effect of reduced and age-dependent penetrance in the children (III-6, IV-10, IV-17) of heterozygous fathers. The + and − symbols refer to the presence or absence of the *SDHD* mutation in this family.

3.9 Dynamic Mutations: Unstable Repeat Expansions

In all of the types of inheritance presented thus far in this chapter, the responsible mutation, once it occurs, is stable when it is transmitted from one generation to the next. That is, all affected members of a family share the identical inherited mutation. In contrast, an entirely different class of genetic disease has been recognized, diseases due to **dynamic mutations** that change from generation to generation. These conditions are characterized by an unstable expansion within the affected gene of a segment of DNA consisting of repeating units of three or more nucleotides that occur in tandem. Many such repeat units consist of three nucleotides, such as CAG or CCG, and the repeat will therefore be CAGCAGCAGCAG or CCGCCGCCGCCG. In general, genes associated with these diseases all have wild-type alleles that are polymorphic. That is, there is a variable number of repeat units in the normal population. As the gene is passed from generation to generation, however, the number of repeats can increase and undergo **expansion**, far beyond the normal polymorphic range, leading to abnormalities in gene expression and function. The discovery of this unusual group of conditions has dispelled the orthodox notions of germline stability and provided a biological basis for peculiarities of familial transmission, that previously had no known mechanistic explanation.

More than a dozen diseases are known to result from unstable repeat expansions of this type. All of these conditions are primarily neurological. Here, we will review the inheritance patterns of two different unstable expansion diseases that illustrate the effects that different dynamic mutations can have on patterns of inheritance.

3.9.1 Polyglutamine Disorders

Several different neurological diseases share the property that the protein encoded by the gene mutated in each condition is characterized by a variable string of consecutive glutamine residues, the codon for which is the trinucleotide CAG. These so-called **polyglutamine disorders** result when an expansion of the CAG repeat leads to a protein with more glutamines than is compatible with normal function. **Huntington disease (HD)** is a well-known disorder that illustrates many of the common genetic features of the polyglutamine disorders caused by expansion of an unstable repeat. The neuropathology is dominated by degeneration of the striatum and the cortex. Patients first present clinically in midlife and manifest a characteristic phenotype of motor abnormalities (chorea, dystonia), personality changes, a gradual loss of cognition, and ultimately death.

For a long time, HD was thought to be a typical autosomal dominant condition with age-dependent penetrance. The disease is transmitted from generation to generation with a 50% risk to each offspring, and heterozygous and homozygous patients carrying the mutation have very similar phenotypes, although homozygotes may have a more rapid course of their disease. There are, however, obvious peculiarities in its inheritance that cannot be explained by simple autosomal dominant inheritance. Firstly, the disease appears to develop at an earlier and earlier age as it is transmitted through the pedigree, a phenomenon referred to as **anticipation**. Secondly, anticipation seems to occur only when the mutant allele is transmitted by an affected father and not by an affected mother, a situation known as **parental transmission bias**.

The peculiarities of inheritance of HD are now readily explained by the discovery that the mutation is composed of an abnormally long CAG expansion in the coding region of the *HD* gene. Normal individuals carry alleles with between 9 and 35 CAG repeats in their *HD* gene, with the average being 18 or 19. Individuals affected with HD, however, have 40 or more repeats, with the average being around 46. Repeat numbers in the range of 40 to 50 usually result in disease later in life, which explains the age-dependent penetrance that is a hallmark of this condition. A borderline repeat number of 36 to 39, although usually associated with HD, can be found in a few individuals who show no signs of the disease even at a fairly advanced age. The age of onset varies with how many CAG repeats are present (see Fig. 3-18).

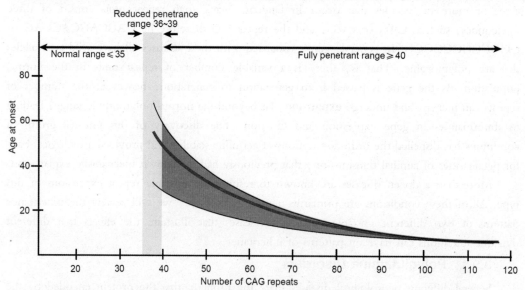

Figure 3-18   Graph correlating approximate age of onset of Huntington disease with the number of CAG repeats found in the HD gene

The *solid line* is the average age of onset, and the *shaded area* shows the range of age of onset for any given number of repeats.

How, then, does an individual come to have an expanded CAG repeat in his or her *HD* gene? Firstly, he or she may inherit it from a parent who already has an expanded repeat beyond the normal range but has not yet developed the disease. Secondly, he or she may inherit an expanded repeat from a parent with repeat length of 35 to 40, which may or may not cause disease in the parent's lifetime but may expand on transmission, resulting in earlier-onset disease in later generations (and thus explaining anticipation). For example, in the pedigree shown in Figure 3-19, individual I-1, now deceased, was diagnosed with HD at the age of 64 years and was heterozygous for an expanded allele with 37 CAG repeats and a normal, stable allele with 25 repeats. Four of his children inherited the unstable allele, with CAG repeat lengths ranging from 42 to more than 100 repeats. Finally, unaffected individuals may carry alleles with repeat lengths at the upper limit of the normal range (29 to 35 CAG repeats) that can expand during meiosis to 40 or more repeats. CAG repeat alleles at the upper limits of normal that do not cause disease but are capable of expanding into the disease-causing range are known as **premutations**.

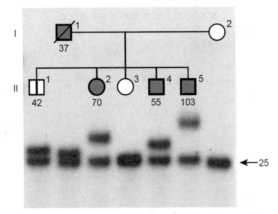

Figure 3-19   Pedigree of family with Huntington disease

Shown beneath the pedigree is a Southern blot analysis for CAG repeat expansions in the HD gene. In addition to a normal allele containing 25 CAG repeats, individual I-1 and his children, II-1, II-2, II-4, and II-5, are all heterozygous for expanded alleles, each containing a different number of CAG repeats. The repeat number is indicated below each individual. II-2, II-4, and II-5 are all affected; individual II-1 is unaffected at the age of 50 years but will develop the disease later in life.

Expansion in HD shows a paternal transmission bias and occurs most frequently during male gametogenesis, which is why the severe early-onset juvenile form of the disease, seen with the largest expansions (70 to 121 repeats), is always paternally inherited.

3.9.2   Fragile X Syndrome

The **fragile X syndrome** is the most common heritable form of moderate intellectual disability, one of many conditions now considered to be among the autism spectrum disorders. The name fragile X refers to a cytogenetic marker on the X chromosome at Xq27.3, a so-called **fragile site** induced in cultured cells in which the chromatin fails to condense properly during mitosis. The syndrome is inherited as an X-linked disorder with penetrance in females in the 50% to 60% range. The fragile X syndrome has a frequency of 1 in 3,000 to 4,000 male births and is so common that it requires consideration in the differential diagnosis of intellectual disability or autism in both males and females. Testing for the fragile X syndrome is among the most frequent indications for genome analysis, genetic counseling, and prenatal diagnosis.

Like HD, fragile X syndrome is caused by an unstable repeat expansion. However, in this case, a massive expansion of a different triplet repeat, CGG, occurs in the 5' untranslated region of a gene called *FMR1* (see Fig. 3-20). The normal number of repeats is up to 55, whereas more than 200 (and even up to several thousand) repeats are found in patients with the "full" fragile X syndrome mutation. The syndrome is due to a lack of expression of the *FMR1* gene and failure to produce the encoded protein. The expanded repeat leads to excessive methylation of cytosines in the promoter of *FMR1*; DNA methylation at CpG islands prevents normal promoter function and leads to gene silencing.

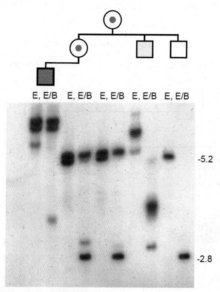

Figure 3-20   Southern blot DNA from the members of a family in which fragile X syndrome is segregating

In the family shown at the top, DNA samples were digested either with the endonuclease EcoRI alone (E) or with the combination of EcoRI and BssH2 (B), an endonuclease that will not cut when the cytosines in its recognition sequence are methylated. EcoRI digestion normally yields a 5. 2-kb fragment containing the region of the repeat, but the size of the fragment increases proportionately to the expansion of the triplet repeat. Digestion with BssH2 along with EcoRI (E/B) will reduce the 5.2-kb fragment generated by EcoRI to a 2.8-kb fragment containing the repeats if the CGG repeats are unmethylated, as is the case on the active X chromosome in a female, or if the repeats are not expanded into the full mutation range (>200 repeats). BssH2 cannot cut the 5.2-kb fragment coming from an inactive X or a fully expanded *FMR1* allele. The affected individual has a large EcoRI fragment, much greater than 5.2 kb, that contains the expanded CGG repeat and is resistant to BssH2 digestion because it is mostly methylated. His mother has two fragments after EcoRI digestion, one normal in size and the other a few hundred base pairs larger, indicating she is a premutation carrier, as is her mother, the proband's grandmother. Upon double digestion, two fragments are seen, the normal at 2.8 kb and a premutation allele that is a few hundred base pairs larger. The proband has two uncles, one (shown in light blue) who appears mildly affected and has an expanded allele (based on EcoRI digestion) that is only partially methylated (based on BssH2 digestion). The other uncle is a normal male with a normal sized, unmethylated allele.

Triplet repeat numbers between 56 and 200 constitute an intermediate premutation stage of the fragile X syndrome. Expansions in this range are unstable when they are transmitted from mother to child and have an increasing tendency to undergo full expansion to more than 200 copies of the repeat during gametogenesis in the female (but almost never in the male), with the risk for expansion increasing dramatically with increasing premutation size (see Fig. 3-21). The overall premutation frequency in females in the population is estimated to be greater than 1 in 200.

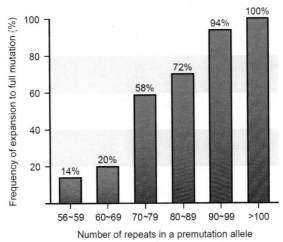

Figure 3-21   Frequency of expansion of a premutation triplet repeat in FMR1 to a full mutation in oogenesis as a function of the length of the premutation allele carried by a heterozygous female

The risk for fragile X syndrome to her sons is approximately half this frequency, because there is a 50% chance a son will inherit the expanded allele. The risk for fragile X syndrome to her daughters is approximately one-fourth this frequency, because there is a 50% chance a daughter would inherit the full mutation, and penetrance of the full mutation in a female is approximately 50%.
(From NOLIN S L, LEWIS F A 3rd, YE L L, et al. Familial transmission of the FMR1 CGG repeat [J]. American journal of human genetics, 1996,59(6):1252-1261.)

3.9.3   Similarities and Differences in Huntington Disease and Fragile X Pedigrees

A comparison of HD with the fragile X syndrome reveals some similarities but also many differences that illustrate many of the features of disorders due to dynamic mutations:

- Premutation expansions causing an increased risk for passing on full mutations are the rule in both of these disorders, and anticipation is commonly seen in both.
- However, the number of repeats in premutation alleles in HD is 29 to 35, far less than the 55 to 200 repeats in fragile X syndrome premutations.
- Premutation carriers for fragile X syndrome are at risk for adult-onset ataxia (in males) and ovarian failure (in females). But premutation carriers in HD are, by definition, disease-free.
- The expansion of premutation alleles occurs primarily in the female germline in fragile X syndrome. In contrast, the largest expansions causing juvenile-onset HD occur in the male germline.

3.10   Correlating Genotype and Phenotype

An important component of medical genetics is identifying and characterizing the genotypes responsible for particular disease phenotypes. In doing so, it is important not to adhere to an overly simplistic view that each disease phenotype is caused uniquely by one particular mutation in a specific gene or that mutations in a particular gene always cause the same phenotype. In fact, there is often substantial heterogeneity in the complex relationship(s) among disease phenotypes, the genes that are mutated in those diseases, and the nature of the mutations found in those genes. Here, we introduce them and outline their distinguishing features.

- **Allelic heterogeneity**, in which different mutations in a gene may produce the same phenotype.
- **Locus heterogeneity**, in which mutations in different genes may cause the same phenotype.
- **Clinical or phenotypic heterogeneity**, in which different mutations in a gene may result in different phenotypes.

3.10.1 Allelic Heterogeneity

Many loci possess more than one mutant allele. In fact, at a given locus, there may be several or many mutations in the population. Allelic heterogeneity may be responsible for differences in the severity or degree of pleiotropy demonstrated for a particular condition. As one example, more than 1,000 different mutations have been found worldwide in the cystic fibrosis transmembrane conductance regulator gene (*CFTR*) among patients with CF. Sometimes these different mutations result in clinically indistinguishable disorders. In other cases, different mutant alleles at the same locus produce a similar phenotype but along a continuum of severity. In autosomal recessive disorders, in particular, the fact that many patients are compound heterozygotes for two different alleles further adds to phenotypic variability of a disorder. For example, homozygotes or compound heterozygotes for many *CFTR* mutations have classic CF with pancreatic insufficiency, severe progressive lung disease, and congenital absence of the vas deferens in males, whereas other patients with combinations of other mutant alleles may have lung disease but normal pancreatic function, and still others will have only the abnormality of the male reproductive tract.

Allelic heterogeneity may also be manifest in the pattern of inheritance demonstrated for a particular condition. For example, in **retinitis pigmentosa**, a common cause of hereditary visual impairment due to photoreceptor degeneration, some mutations in the *ORP1* gene, encoding an oxygen-regulated photoreceptor protein, cause an autosomal recessive form of the disease, whereas others in the same gene result in an autosomal dominant form.

3.10.2 Locus Heterogeneity

Locus heterogeneity describes the situation in which clinically similar and even indistinguishable disorders may arise from mutations in different loci in different patients. For some phenotypes, pedigree analysis alone has been sufficient to demonstrate locus heterogeneity. Taking retinitis pigmentosa again as an example, it was recognized many years ago that the disease occurs in both autosomal and X-linked forms. Now, pedigree analysis combined with gene mapping has demonstrated that this single clinical entity can be caused by mutations in at least 56 different genes, 54 of which are autosomal and 2 of which are X-linked.

3.10.3　Clinical Heterogeneity

Different mutations in the same gene may produce very dissimilar phenotypes in different families, a phenomenon known as **clinical** or **phenotypic heterogeneity**. This situation occurs with mutations in the *LMNA* gene, which encodes a nuclear membrane protein. Different *LMNA* mutations have been associated with at least a half dozen phenotypically distinct disorders, including a form of muscular dystrophy, one form of hereditary dilated cardiomyopathy, one form of the Charcot-Marie-Tooth peripheral neuropathy, a disorder of adipose tissue called lipodystrophy, and the premature aging syndrome known as Hutchinson-Gilford progeria.

3.11　Importance of the Family History in Medical Practice

Among medical specialties, medical genetics is distinctive in that it focuses not only on the patient but also on the entire family. A comprehensive family history is an important first step in the analysis of any disorder, whether or not the disorder is known to be genetic. As the late Barton Childs stated succinctly: "To fail to take a good family history is bad medicine." Despite the sophisticated cytogenetic, molecular, and genome testing now available to geneticists, an accurate family history (including the family pedigree) still remains a fundamental tool for all physicians and genetic counselors to use for determining the pattern of inheritance of a disorder in the family, forming a differential diagnosis, determining what genetic testing might be needed, and designing an individualized management and treatment plan for their patients. Furthermore, recognizing a familial component to a medical disorder allows the risk in other family members to be estimated so that proper management, prevention, and counseling can be offered to the patient and the family, as we will discuss in many of the chapters to follow.

Review Points:

1. Allelic heterogeneity is an important cause of clinical variation. Many loci possess more than one mutant allele. In fact, at a given locus there may be several of many mutations. Sometimes, these different mutations result in clinically indistinguishable or closely similar disorders. But the inheritants of these mutants may be different. It may be AD or AR. For example, sickle cell disease, the mutants of β-globin may be AD or AR.

2. For many phenotypes, pedigree analysis alone has been sufficient to demonstrate genetic heterogeneity. For example, congenital deafness, has long been known to occur in autosomal dominant, autosomal recessive, and X-linked forms. In recent years, pedigree analysis combined with gene mapping has demonstrated that there are at least two dozen loci responsible for 4 X-linked forms, 41 autosomal dominant forms, and 6 autosomal recessive forms.

3. The measurement of consanguinity is relevant in medical genetics because the risk of a child's being homozygous for a rare recessive allele is proportional to how related the parents are. The coefficient of inbreeding (F) is the probability that a homozygote has received both alleles at a locus from the same ancestral source. It is also the proportion of loci at which a person is homozygous or identical by descent.

4. Penetrance is the probability that a gene will have any phenotypic expression at all.

5. Expressivity is the severity of expression of the phenotype.

6. When a single abnormal gene or gene pair produces diverse phenotypic effects, such as which organ system are involved and which particular signs and symptoms occur, its expression is said to be pleiotropic.

7. Mosaicism is defined as the presence in an individual or a tissue of at least two cell lines that differ genetically but are derived from a single zygote. A mutation occuring during cell proliferation, in either somatic cells or during gametogenesis, leads to a proportion of cells carrying the mutation. That is, to either somatic or germline mosaicism.

Study Questions:

1. Cathy is pregnant for the second time. Her first child, Donald, has cystic fibrosis (CF). Cathy has two brothers, Charles and Colin, and a sister, Cindy. Colin and Cindy are unmarried. Charles is married to an unrelated woman, Carolyn, and has a 2-year-old daughter, Debbie. Cathy's parents are Bob and Betty. Betty's sister Barbara is the mother of Cathy's husband, Calvin, who is 25. There is no previous family history of CF.
   a. Sketch the pedigree, using standard symbols.
   b. What is the pattern of transmission of CF, and what is the risk for CF for Cathy's next child?
   c. Which people in this pedigree are obligate heterozygotes?

2. George and Grace, who have normal hearing, have eight children; two of their five daughters and two of their three sons are congenitally deaf. Another couple, Harry and Helen, both with normal hearing, also have eight children; two of their six daughters and one of their two sons are deaf. A third couple, Gilbert and Gisele, who are congenitally deaf, have four children, also deaf. Their daughter Hedy marries Horace, a deaf son of George and Grace, and Hedy and Horace in turn have four deaf children. Their eldest son Isaac marries Ingrid, a daughter of Harry and Helen; although both Isaac and Ingrid are deaf, their six sons all have normal hearing. Sketch the pedigree and answer the following questions. (Hint: How many different types of congenital deafness are segregating in this pedigree?)
   a. State the probable genotypes of the children in the last generation.
   b. Why are all the children of Gilbert and Gisele and of Hedy and Horace deaf?

3. Don and his maternal grandfather Barry both have hemophilia A. Don's partner Diane is his maternal aunt's daughter. Don and Diane have one son, Edward, and two daughters, Elise and Emily, all of whom have hemophilia A. They also have an unaffected daughter, Enid.
   a. Draw the pedigree.
   b. Why are Elise and Emily affected?
   c. What is the probability that a son of Elise would be hemophilic? What is the probability that her daughter would be hemophilic?
   d. What is the probability that a son of Enid would be hemophilic? A daughter?

4. A boy is born with a number of malformations but does not have a recognized syndrome. The parents are unrelated, and there is no family history of a similar condition. Which of the following conditions could explain this situation? Which are unlikely? Why?

   a. Autosomal dominant inheritance with new mutation.

   b. Autosomal dominant inheritance with reduced penetrance.

   c. Autosomal dominant inheritance with variable expressivity.

   d. Autosomal recessive inheritance.

   e. X-linked recessive inheritance.

   f. Autosomal dominant inheritance, misattributed paternity.

   g. Maternal ingestion of a teratogenic drug at a sensitive stage of embryonic development.

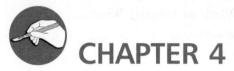

CHAPTER 4
Principle of Clinical Cytogenetics

Purpose and Requirement:

In this chapter students should understand the general principles of clinical cytogenetics and the various types of numerical and structural abnormalities observed in human karyotypes.

Clinical cytogenetics is the study of chromosomes, their structure, and their inheritance, as applied to the practice of medicine. It has been apparent for over 50 years that chromosome abnormalities—microscopically visible changes in the number or structure of chromosomes—could account for a number of clinical conditions that are thus referred to as **chromosome disorders**. With their focus on the complete set of genetic material, cytogeneticists were the first to bring a genome-wide perspective to the practice of medicine. Today, chromosome analysis—with increasing resolution and precision at both the cytological and genomic levels—is an important diagnostic procedure in numerous areas of clinical medicine. Current genome analyses that use approaches to be explored in this chapter, including **chromosomal microarrays** and **whole-genome sequencing**, represent impressive improvements in capacity and resolution, but ones that are conceptually similar to microscopic methods focusing on chromosomes (see Fig. 4-1).

Chromosome disorders form a major category of genetic disease. They account for a large proportion of all reproductive wastage, congenital malformations, and intellectual disability and play an important role in the pathogenesis of cancer. Specific cytogenetic disorders are responsible for hundreds of distinct syndromes that collectively are more common than all the single-gene diseases together. Cytogenetic abnormalities are present in nearly 1% of live births, in approximately 2% of pregnancies in women older than 35 years who undergo prenatal diagnosis, and in fully half of all spontaneous, first-trimester abortions.

The spectrum of analysis from microscopically visible changes in chromosome number and structure to anomalies of genome structure and sequence detectable at the level of whole-genome sequencing encompasses literally the entire field of medical genetics (see Fig. 4-1). In this chapter, we present the general principles of chromosome and genome analysis and focus on the **chromosome mutations** and **regional mutations**. We restrict our discussion to disorders due to genomic imbalance—either for the hundreds to thousands of genes found on individual chromosomes or for smaller numbers of genes located within a particular chromosome region. Application of these principles to some of the most common and best-known chromosomal disorders will then be presented in Chapter 5.

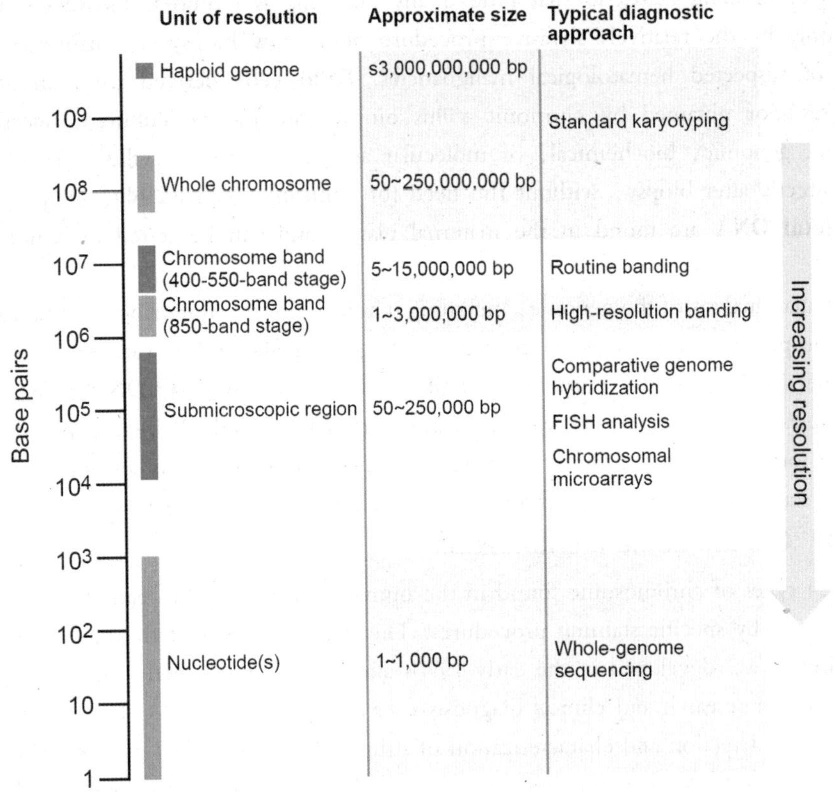

Unit of resolution	Approximate size	Typical diagnostic approach
■ Haploid genome	s3,000,000,000 bp	
10^9		Standard karyotyping
10^8 Whole chromosome	50~250,000,000 bp	
10^7 Chromosome band (400-550-band stage)	5~15,000,000 bp	Routine banding
Chromosome band (850-band stage)	1~3,000,000 bp	High-resolution banding
10^6		
10^5 Submicroscopic region	50~250,000 bp	Comparative genome hybridization
		FISH analysis
10^4		Chromosomal microarrays
10^3		
10^2		
	Nucleotide(s)	1~1,000 bp Whole-genome sequencing
10		
1		

Base pairs (vertical axis label)

Increasing resolution (vertical label)

Figure 4-1   Spectrum of resolution in chromosome and genome analysis

The typical resolution and range of effectiveness are given for various diagnostic approaches used routinely in chromosome and genome analysis. FISH, Fluorescence in situ hybridization.

4.1 Introduction to Cytogenetics and Genome Analysis

To be examined by chromosome analysis for clinical purposes, cells must be capable of proliferation in culture. The most accessible cells that meet this requirement are white blood cells, specifically T lymphocytes. To prepare a short-term culture that is suitable for cytogenetic analysis of these cells, a sample of peripheral blood is obtained, and the white blood cells are collected, placed in tissue culture medium, and stimulated to divide. After a few days, the dividing cells are arrested in **metaphase** with chemicals that inhibit the mitotic spindle. Cells are treated with a hypotonic solution to release the chromosomes, which are then fixed, spread on slides, and stained by one of several techniques, depending on the particular diagnostic procedure being performed. They are then ready for analysis.

Although ideal for rapid clinical analysis, cell cultures prepared from peripheral blood have the disadvantage of being short-lived (3 to 4 days). Long-term cultures suitable for permanent storage or further studies can be derived from a variety of other tissues. Skin biopsy, a minor surgical procedure, can provide samples of tissue that in culture produce **fibroblasts**, which can be used for a variety of biochemical and molecular studies as well as for chromosome and genome analysis. White blood cells can also be transformed in culture to form **lymphoblastoid** cell lines that are potentially immortal. **Bone marrow** has the advantage of containing a high proportion of dividing cells, so that little if any culturing is required. However, it can be obtained only by the relatively invasive procedure of marrow biopsy. Its main use is in the diagnosis of suspected hematological malignancies. **Fetal cells** derived from amniotic fluid (amniocytes) or obtained by chorionic villus biopsy can also be cultured successfully for cytogenetic, genomic, biochemical, or molecular analysis. Chorionic villus cells can also be analyzed directly after biopsy, without the need for culturing. Remarkably, small amounts of **cell-free fetal DNA** are found in the maternal plasma and can be tested by whole-genome sequencing.

Molecular analysis of the genome, including whole-genome sequencing, can be carried out on any appropriate clinical material, provided that good-quality DNA can be obtained. Cells need not be dividing for this purpose, and thus it is possible to study DNA from tissue and tumor samples, for example, as well as from peripheral blood. Which approach is most appropriate for a particular diagnostic or research purpose is a rapidly evolving area as the resolution, sensitivity, and ease of chromosome and genome analysis increase.

4.1.1 Chromosome Identification

The 24 types of chromosome found in the human genome can be readily identified at the cytological level by specific staining procedures. The most common of these, Giemsa banding (**G banding**), was developed in the early 1970s and was the first widely used whole-genome analytical tool for research and clinical diagnosis (see Figs. 2-1 and 2-14). It has been the gold standard for the detection and characterization of structural and numerical genomic abnormalities in clinical diagnostic settings for both constitutional (postnatal or prenatal) and acquired (cancer) disorders.

G-banding and other staining procedures can be used to describe individual chromosomes and their variants or abnormalities, using an internationally accepted system of chromosome classification. Figure 4-2 is an ideogram of the banding pattern of a set of normal human chromosomes at metaphase, illustrating the alternating pattern of light and dark bands used for chromosome identification. The pattern of bands on each chromosome is numbered on each arm from the centromere to the telomere, as shown in detail in Figure 4-3 for several chromosomes. The identity of any particular band (and thus the DNA sequences and genes within it) can be described precisely and unambiguously by use of this regionally based and hierarchical numbering system.

Human chromosomes are often classified into three types that can be easily distinguished at metaphase by the position of the **centromere**, the primary constriction visible at metaphase (see Fig. 4-2): **metacentric** chromosomes, with a more or less central centromere and arms of approximately equal length; **submetacentric** chromosomes, with an off-center centromere and arms of clearly different lengths; and **acrocentric** chromosomes, with the centromere near one end. A potential fourth type of chromosome, **telocentric**, with the centromere at one end and only a single arm, does not occur in the normal human karyotype, but it is occasionally observed in chromosome rearrangements. The human acrocentric chromosomes (chromosomes 13, 14, 15, 21, and 22) have small, distinctive masses of chromatin known as **satellites** attached to their short arms by narrow stalks (called secondary constrictions). The stalks of these five chromosome pairs contain hundreds of copies of genes for ribosomal RNA (the major component of ribosomes) as well as a variety of repetitive sequences.

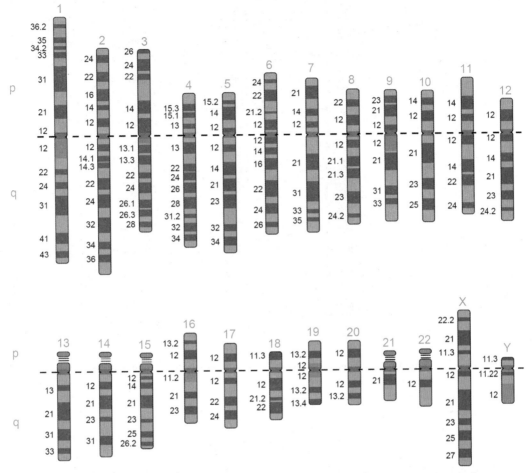

Figure 4-2 Ideogram showing G-banding patterns for human chromosomes at metaphase, with approximately 400 bands per haploid karyotype

As drawn, chromosomes are typically represented with the sister chromatids so closely aligned that they are not recognized as distinct entities. Centromeres are indicated by the primary constriction and narrow *dark gray* regions separating the p and q arms. For convenience and clarity, only the G-dark bands are numbered. For examples of full numbering scheme, see Figure 4-3.

In addition to changes in banding pattern, nonstaining gaps—called **fragile sites**—are occasionally observed at particular sites on several chromosomes that are prone to regional genomic instability. Over 80 common fragile sites are known, many of which are heritable variants. A small proportion of fragile sites are associated with specific clinical disorders. The fragile site most clearly shown to be clinically significant is seen near the end of the long arm of the X chromosome in males with a specific and common form of X-linked intellectual disability, **fragile X syndrome**, as well as in some female carriers of the same genetic defect.

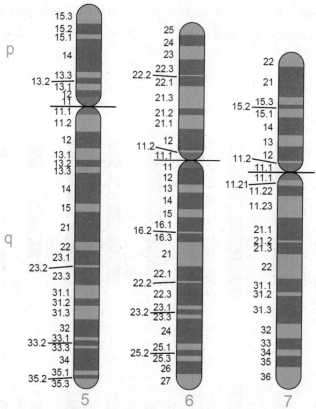

Figure 4-3 Examples of G-banding patterns for chromosomes 5, 6, and 7 at the 550-band stage of condensation

Band numbers permit unambiguous identification of each G-dark or G-light band, for example, chromosome 5p15.2 or chromosome 7q21.2.

4.1.2　High-Resolution Chromosome Analysis

The standard G-banded karyotype at a 400- to 550-band stage of resolution, as seen in a typical metaphase preparation, allows detection of deletions and duplications of greater than approximately 5 to 10 Mb anywhere in the genome (see Fig. 4-1). However, the sensitivity of G-banding at this resolution may be lower in regions of the genome in which the banding patterns are less specific.

To increase the sensitivity of chromosome analysis, high-resolution banding (also called **prometaphase banding**) can be achieved by staining chromosomes that have been obtained at an early stage of mitosis (prophase or prometaphase), when they are still in a relatively uncondensed state. High-resolution banding is especially useful when a subtle structural abnormality of a chromosome is suspected. Staining of prometaphase chromosomes can reveal up to 850 bands or even more in a haploid set, although this method is frequently replaced now by microarray analysis. A comparison of the banding patterns at three different stages of resolution is shown for one chromosome in Figure 4-4, demonstrating the increase in diagnostic precision that one obtains with these longer chromosomes. Development of high-resolution chromosome analysis in the early 1980s allowed the discovery of a number of new so-called **microdeletion syndromes** caused by smaller genomic deletions or duplications in the 2- to 3-Mb size range (see Fig. 4-1). However, the time-consuming and technically difficult nature of this method precludes its routine use for whole-genome analysis.

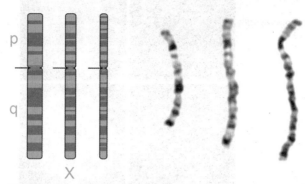

Figure 4-4　The X chromosome: ideograms and photomicrographs at metaphase, prometaphase, and prophase (*left to right*)

4.1.3　Fluorescence in Situ Hybridization

Targeted high-resolution chromosome banding was largely replaced in the early 1990s by **fluorescence in situ hybridization (FISH)**, a method for detecting the presence or absence of a particular DNA sequence or for evaluating the number or organization of a chromosome or chromosomal region in situ (literally, "in place") in the cell. This convergence of genomic and cytogenetic approaches—variously termed *molecular cytogenetics*, *cytogenomics*, or *chromonomics*—dramatically expanded both the scope and precision of chromosome analysis in routine clinical practice.

FISH technology takes advantage of the availability of ordered collections of recombinant DNA clones containing DNA from around the entire genome, generated originally as part of the Human Genome Project. Clones containing specific human DNA sequences can be used as probes to detect the corresponding region of the genome in chromosome preparations or in interphase nuclei for a variety of research and diagnostic purposes, as illustrated in Figure 4-5:

- DNA probes specific for individual chromosomes, chromosomal regions, or genes can be labeled with different fluorochromes and used to identify particular chromosomal rearrangements or to rapidly diagnose the existence of an abnormal chromosome number in clinical material.
- Repetitive DNA probes allow detection of satellite DNA or other repeated DNA elements localized to specific chromosomal regions. Satellite DNA probes, especially those belonging to the α-satellite family of centromere repeats, are widely used for determining the number of copies of a particular chromosome.

Although FISH technology provides much higher resolution and specificity than G-banded chromosome analysis, it does not allow for efficient analysis of the entire genome, and thus its use is limited by the need to target a specific genomic region based on a clinical diagnosis or suspicion.

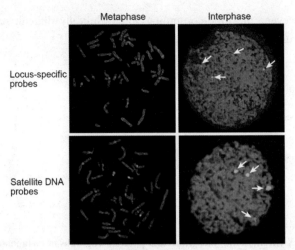

Figure 4-5   Fluorescence in situ hybridization to human chromosomes at metaphase and interphase, with different types of DNA probe

Top, Single-copy DNA probes specific for sequences within bands 4q12 (*red* fluorescence) and 4q31.1 (*green* fluorescence). *Bottom*, Repetitive α-satellite DNA probes specific for the centromeres of chromosomes 18 (*aqua*), X (*green*), and Y (*red*).

4.1.4 Genome Analysis Using Microarrays

Although the G-banded karyotype remains the front-line diagnostic test for most clinical applications, it has been complemented or even replaced by genome-wide approaches for detecting copy number imbalances at higher resolution (see Fig. 4-1), extending the concept of targeted FISH analysis to test the entire genome. Instead of examining cells and chromosomes in situ one probe at a time, chromosomal microarray techniques simultaneously query the whole genome represented as an ordered array of genomic segments on a microscope slide containing overlapping or regularly spaced DNA segments that represent the entire genome. In one approach based on **comparative genome hybridization (CGH)**, one detects relative copy number gains and losses in a genome-wide manner by hybridizing two samples—one a control genome and one from a patient—to such microarrays. An excess of sequences from one or the other genome indicates an overrepresentation or underrepresentation of those sequences in the patient genome relative to the control (see Fig. 4-6). An alternative approach uses "single nucleotide polymorphism (SNP) arrays" that contain versions of sequences corresponding to the two alleles of various SNPs around the genome. In this case, the relative representation and intensity of alleles in different regions of the genome indicate if a chromosome or chromosomal region is present at the appropriate dosage (see Fig. 4-6).

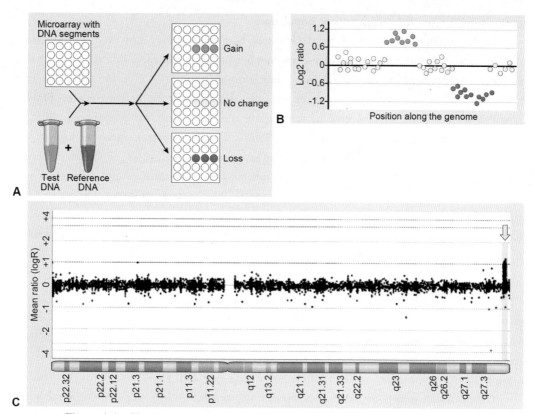

Figure 4-6   Chromosomal microarray to detect chromosome and genomic dosage
(A) Schematic of an array assay based on comparative genome hybridization (CGH), where a patient's genome (denoted in *green*) is cohybridized to the array with a control reference genome (denoted in *red*). The probes are mixed and allowed to hybridize to their complementary sequences on the array. Relative intensities of hybridization of the two probes are measured, indicating equivalent dosage between the two genomes (*yellow*) or a relative gain (*green*) or loss (*red*) in the patient sample. (B) A typical output plots the logarithm of the fluorescence ratios as a function of the position along the genome. (C) Array CGH result for a patient with Rett syndrome, indicating a duplication of approximately 800 kb in band Xq28 containing the *MECP2* gene. LogR of fluorescence ratios are plotted along the length of the X chromosome. Each dot represents the ratio for an individual sequence on the array. Sequences corresponding to the *MECP2* gene and its surrounding region are duplicated in the patient's genome, leading to an increased ratio, indicated by the *green arrow* and *shaded box* in that region of the chromosome.

For routine clinical testing of suspected chromosome disorders, probe spacing on the array provides a resolution as high as 250 kb over the entire unique portion of the human genome. A higher density of probes can be used to achieve even higher resolution (<25 ~ 50 kb) over regions of particular clinical interest, such as those associated with known developmental disorders or congenital anomalies (see Fig. 4-6). This approach, which is being used in an increasing number of clinical laboratories, complements conventional karyotyping and provides a much more sensitive, high-resolution assessment of the genome. Microarrays have been used successfully to identify chromosome and genome abnormalities in children with unexplained developmental delay, intellectual disability, or birth defects, revealing a number of pathogenic genomic alterations that were not detectable by conventional G banding. Based on this significantly increased yield, genome-wide arrays are replacing the G-banded karyotype as the routine frontline test for certain patient populations.

Two important limitations of this technology bear mentioning, however. Firstly, array-based methods measure only the relative copy number of DNA sequences but not whether they have been translocated or rearranged from their normal position (s) in the genome. Thus confirmation of suspected chromosome or genome abnormalities by karyotyping or FISH is important to determine the nature of an abnormality and thus its risk for recurrence, either for the individual or for other family members. Secondly, high-resolution genome analysis can reveal variants, in particular small differences in copy number, that are of uncertain clinical significance. An increasing number of such variants are being documented and catalogued even within the general population. Many are likely to be benign **copy number variants**. Their existence underscores the unique nature of each individual's genome and emphasizes the diagnostic challenge of assessing what is considered a "normal" karyotype and what is likely to be pathogenic.

4.1.5　Genome Analysis by Whole-Genome Sequencing

At the extreme end but on the same spectrum as cytogenetic analysis and microarray analysis, the ultimate resolution for clinical tests to detect chromosomal and genomic disorders would be to sequence patient genomes in their entirety. Indeed, as the efficiency of whole-genome sequencing has increased and its costs have fallen, it is becoming increasingly practical to consider sequencing patient samples in a clinical setting (see Fig. 4-1).

The principles underlying such an approach are straightforward, because the number and composition of any particular segment of an individual's genome will be reflected in the DNA sequences generated from that genome. Although the sequences routinely obtained with today's technology are generally short (approximately 50 to 500 bp) compared to the size of a chromosome or even a single gene, a genome with an abnormally low or high representation of those sequences from a particular chromosome or segment of a chromosome is likely to have a numerical or structural abnormality of that chromosome. To detect numerical abnormalities of an entire chromosome, it is generally not necessary to sequence a genome to completion. Even a limited number of sequences that align to a particular chromosome of interest should reveal whether those sequences are found in the expected number (e.g., equivalent to two copies per diploid genome for an autosome) or whether they are significantly overrepresented or underrepresented (see Fig. 4-7). This concept is now being applied to the prenatal diagnosis of fetal chromosome imbalance.

To detect balanced rearrangements of the genome, however, in which no DNA in the genome is either gained or lost, a more complete genome sequence is required. Here, instead of sequences that align perfectly to the reference human genome sequence, one finds rare sequences that align to two different and normally noncontiguous regions in the reference sequence (whether on the same chromosome or on different chromosomes) (see Fig. 4-7). This approach has been used to identify the specific genes involved in some cancers, and in children with various congenital defects due to translocations, involving the juxtaposition of sequences that are normally located on different chromosomes.

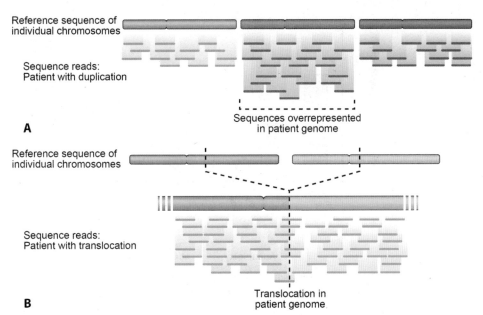

Figure 4-7   **Strategies for detection of numerical and structural chromosome abnormalities by whole-genome sequence analysis**

Although only a small number of reads are illustrated schematically here, in practice many millions of sequence reads are analyzed and aligned to the reference genome to obtain statistically significant support for a diagnosis of aneuploidy or a structural chromosome abnormality. (A) Alignment of sequence reads from a patient's genome to the reference sequence of three individual chromosomes. Overrepresentation of sequences from the *red* chromosome indicates that the patient is aneuploid for this chromosome. (B) Alignment of sequence reads from a patient's genome to the reference sequence of two chromosomes reveals a number of reads that contain contiguous sequences from both chromosomes. This indicates a translocation in the patient's genome involving the *blue* and *orange* chromosomes at the positions designated by the *dotted lines*.

4.2   Chromosome Abnormalities

Abnormalities of chromosomes may be either numerical or structural and may involve one or more autosomes, sex chromosomes, or both simultaneously. The overall incidence of chromosome abnormalities is approximately 1 in 154 live births (see Fig. 4-8), and their impact is therefore substantial, both in clinical medicine and for society. By far the most common type of clinically significant chromosome abnormality is **aneuploidy**, an abnormal chromosome number due to an extra or missing chromosome. An aneuploid karyotype is always associated with physical or mental abnormalities or both. **Structural abnormalities** (rearrangements involving one or more chromosomes) are also relatively common (see Fig. 4-8). Depending on whether or not a structural rearrangement leads to an imbalance of genomic content, these may or may not have a phenotypic effect. However, as explained later in this chapter, even balanced chromosome abnormalities may be at an increased risk for abnormal offspring in the subsequent generation.

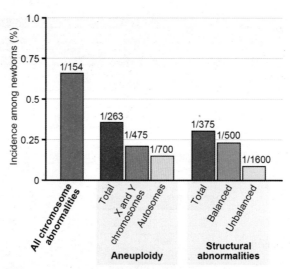

Figure 4-8   Incidence of chromosome abnormalities in newborn surveys, based on chromosome analysis of over 68,000 newborns

Chromosome abnormalities are described by a standard set of abbreviations and nomenclature that indicate the nature of the abnormality and (in the case of analyses performed by FISH or microarrays) the technology used. Some of the more common abbreviations and examples of abnormal karyotypes and abnormalities are listed in Table 4-1.

Table 4-1   Some Abbreviations Used for Description of Chromosomes and Their Abnormalities (With Representative Examples)

Abbreviation	Meaning	Example	Condition
		46,XX	Normal female karyotype
		46,XY	Normal male karyotype
cen	Centromere		
del	Deletion	46, XX, del (5) (q13)	Female with terminal deletion of one chromosome 5 distal to band 5q13
der	Derivative chromosome	der(1)	Translocation chromosome derived from chromosome 1 and containing the centromere of chromosome 1
dic	Dicentric chromosome	dic(X;Y)	Translocation chromosome containing the centromeres of both the X and Y chromosomes
dup	Duplication		
inv	Inversion	inv(3)(p25q21)	Pericentric inversion of chromosome 3
mar	Marker chromosome	47,XX, +mar	Female with an extra, unidentified chromosome
mat	Maternal origin	47,XY, +der (1) mat	Male with an extra der (1) chromosome inherited from his mother
p	Short arm of chromosome		
pat	Paternal origin		
q	Long arm of chromosome		
r	Ring chromosome	46,X,r(X)	Female with ring X chromosome
rob	Robertsonian translocation	rob(14;21) (q10;q10)	Breakage and reunion have occurred at band 14q10 and band 21q10 in the centromeric regions of chromosomes 14 and 21
t	Translocation	46, XX, t (2; 8) (q22;p21)	Female with balanced translocation between chromosomes 2 and 8, with breaks in bands 2q22 and 8p21
+	Gain of	47,XX, +21	Female with trisomy 21
−	Loss of	45,XY, −22	Male with monosomy 22
/	Mosaicism	46, XX/47, XX, +21	Female with two populations of cells, one with a normal karyotype and one with trisomy 21

(From SHAFFER LG, MCGOWAN-JORDAN J, SCHMID M. ISCN 2013: An international system for human cytogenetic nomenclature[M]. Basel: Karger, 2013.)

4.2.1 Gene Dosage, Balance and Imbalance

For chromosome and genomic disorders, it is the quantitative aspects of gene expression that underlie disease, in contrast to single-gene disorders, in which pathogenesis often reflects qualitative aspects of a gene's function. The clinical consequences of any particular chromosome abnormality will depend on the resulting imbalance of parts of the genome, the specific genes contained in or affected by the abnormality, and the likelihood of its transmission to the next generation.

The central concept for thinking about chromosome and genomic disorders is that of **gene dosage** and its balance or imbalance. This same concept applies generally to considering some single-gene disorders and their underlying mutational basis. However, it takes on uniform importance for chromosome abnormalities, where we are generally more concerned with the dosage of genes within the relevant chromosomal region than with the actual normal or abnormal sequence of those genes. Here, the sequence of the genes is typically quite unremarkable and would not lead to any clinical condition except for the fact that their dosage is incorrect.

Most genes in the human genome are present in two doses and are expressed from both copies. Some genes, however, are expressed from only a single copy (e.g., imprinted genes and X-linked genes subject to X inactivation). Extensive analysis of clinical cases has demonstrated that the relative dosage of these genes is critical for normal development. One or three doses instead of two is generally not conducive to normal function for a gene or set of genes that are typically expressed from two copies. Similarly, abnormalities of genomic imprinting or X inactivation that cause the anomalous expression of two copies of a gene or set of genes instead of one invariably lead to clinical disorders.

4.2.2 Abnormalities of Chromosome Number

A chromosome complement with any chromosome number other than 46 is said to be **heteroploid**. An exact multiple of the haploid chromosome number (n) is called **euploid**, and any other chromosome number is **aneuploid**.

(1) Triploidy and Tetraploidy

In addition to the diploid (2n) number characteristic of normal somatic cells, two other euploid chromosome complements, **triploid** (3n) and **tetraploid** (4n), are occasionally observed in clinical material. Both triploidy and tetraploidy have been seen in fetuses. Triploidy is observed in 1% to 3% of recognized conceptions. Triploid infants can be liveborn, although they do not survive long. Among the few that survive at least to the end of the first trimester of pregnancy, most result from fertilization of an egg by two sperm (dispermy). Other cases result from failure of one of the meiotic divisions in either sex, resulting in a diploid egg or sperm. The phenotypic manifestation of a triploid karyotype depends on the source of the extra chromosome set. Triploids with an extra set of maternal chromosomes are typically aborted spontaneously early in pregnancy, whereas those with an extra set of paternal chromosomes typically have an abnormal degenerative placenta (resulting in a so-called **partial hydatidiform mole**), with a small fetus. Tetraploids are always 92,XXXX or 92,XXYY and likely result from failure of completion of an early cleavage division of the zygote.

(2) Aneuploidy

Aneuploidy is the most common and clinically significant type of human chromosome disorder, occurring in at least 5% of all clinically recognized pregnancies. Most aneuploid patients have either **trisomy** (three instead of the normal pair of a particular chromosome) or, less often, **monosomy** (only one representative of a particular chromosome). Either trisomy or monosomy can have severe phenotypic consequences.

Trisomy can exist for any part of the genome, but trisomy for a whole chromosome is only occasionally compatible with life. By far the most common type of trisomy in liveborn infants is **trisomy** 21, the chromosome constitution seen in 95% of patients with **Down syndrome** (karyotype 47, XX, +21 or 47, XY, +21) (see Fig. 4-9). Other trisomies observed in liveborns include trisomy 18 and trisomy 13. It is notable that these autosomes (13, 18, and 21) are the three with the lowest number of genes located on them. Presumably, trisomy for autosomes with a greater number of genes is lethal in most instances. Monosomy for an entire chromosome is almost always lethal. An important exception is monosomy for the X chromosome, as seen in **Turner syndrome**. These conditions are considered in greater detail in Chapter 5.

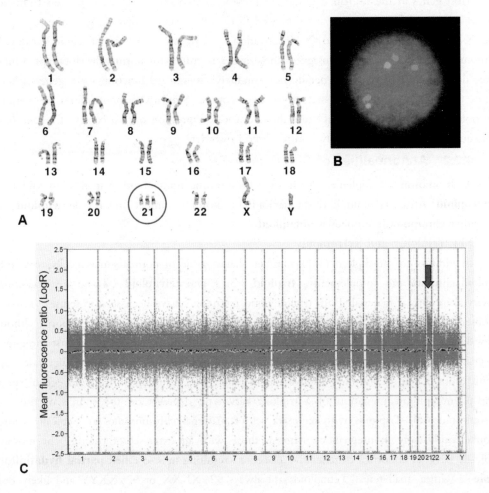

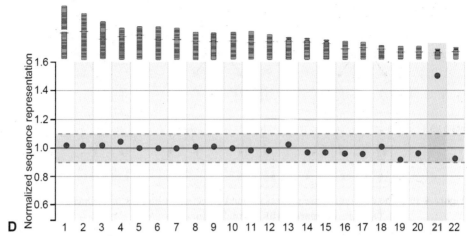

D

Figure 4-9   Chromosomal and genomic approaches to the diagnosis of trisomy 21

(A) Karyotype from a male patient with Down syndrome, showing three copies of chromosome 21. (B) Interphase fluorescence in situ hybridization analysis using locus-specific probes from chromosome 21 (*red*, three spots) and from a control autosome (*green*, two spots). (C) Detection of trisomy 21 in a female patient by whole-genome chromosomal microarray. Increase in the fluorescence ratio for sequences from chromosome 21 are indicated by the *red arrow*. (D) Detection of trisomy 21 by whole-genome sequencing and overrepresentation of sequences from chromosome 21. Normalized sequence representation for individual chromosomes (± SD) in chromosomally normal samples is indicated by the *gray shaded* region. A normalized ratio of approximately 1.5 indicates three copies of chromosome 21 sequences instead of two, consistent with trisomy 21.

Although the causes of aneuploidy are not fully understood, the most common chromosomal mechanism is **meiotic nondisjunction**. This refers to the failure of a pair of chromosomes to disjoin properly during one of the two meiotic divisions, usually during meiosis I. The genomic consequences of nondisjunction during meiosis I and meiosis II are different (see Fig. 4-10). If the error occurs during meiosis I, the gamete with 24 chromosomes contains both the paternal and the maternal members of the pair. If it occurs during meiosis II, the gamete with the extra chromosome contains both copies of either the paternal or the maternal chromosome. (Strictly speaking, these statements refer only to the paternal or maternal centromere, because recombination between homologous chromosomes has usually taken place in the preceding meiosis I, resulting in some genetic differences between the chromatids and thus between the corresponding daughter chromosomes.)

Proper disjunction of a pair of homologous chromosomes in meiosis I appears relatively straightforward (see Fig. 4-10). In reality, however, it involves a feat of complex engineering that requires precise temporal and spatial control over alignment of the two homologues, their tight connections to each other (synapsis), their interactions with the meiotic spindle, and, finally, their release and subsequent movement to opposite poles and to different daughter cells. The propensity of a chromosome pair to nondisjoin has been strongly associated with aberrations in the frequency or placement, or both, of recombination events in meiosis I, which are critical for maintaining proper synapsis. A chromosome pair with too few (or even no) recombinations, or with recombination too close to the centromere or telomere, may be more susceptible to nondisjunction than a chromosome pair with a more typical number and distribution of recombination events.

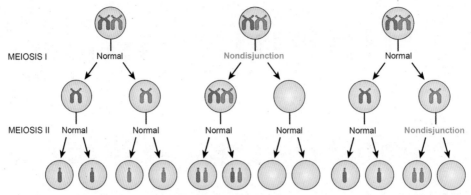

Figure 4-10   The different consequences of nondisjunction at meiosis Ⅰ (*center*) and meiosis Ⅱ (*right*), compared with normal disjunction (*left*)

If the error occurs at meiosis Ⅰ, the gametes either contain a representative of both members of the chromosome 21 pair or lack a chromosome 21 altogether. If nondisjunction occurs at meiosis Ⅱ, the abnormal gametes contain two copies of one parental chromosome 21 (and no copy of the other) or lack a chromosome 21.

In some cases, aneuploidy can also result from premature separation of sister chromatids in meiosis Ⅰ instead of meiosis Ⅱ. If this happens, the separated chromatids may by chance segregate to the oocyte or to the polar body, leading to an unbalanced gamete.

Nondisjunction can also occur in a mitotic division after formation of the zygote. If this happens at an early cleavage division, clinically significant **mosaicism** may result. In some malignant cell lines and some cell cultures, mitotic nondisjunction can lead to highly abnormal karyotypes.

4.2.3   Abnormalities of Chromosome Structure

Structural rearrangements result from chromosome breakage, recombination, or exchange, followed by reconstitution in an abnormal combination. Whereas rearrangements can take place in many ways, they are together less common than aneuploidy. Overall, structural abnormalities are present in approximately 1 in 375 newborns (see Fig. 4-8). Like numerical abnormalities, structural rearrangements may be present in all cells of a person or in mosaic form.

Structural rearrangements are classified as **balanced**, if the genome has the normal complement of chromosomal material, or **unbalanced**, if there is additional or missing material. Clearly these designations depend on the resolution of the method(s) used to analyze a particular rearrangement (see Fig. 4-1). Some that appear balanced at the level of high-resolution banding, for example, may be unbalanced when studied with chromosomal microarrays or by DNA sequence analysis. Some rearrangements are stable, capable of passing through mitotic and meiotic cell divisions unaltered, whereas others are unstable. Some of the more common types of structural rearrangements observed in human chromosomes are illustrated schematically in Figure 4-11.

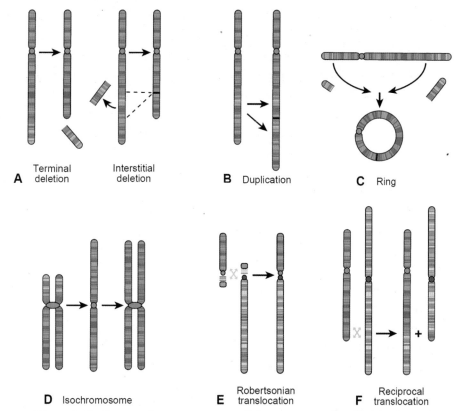

Figure 4-11   Structural rearrangements of chromosomes, described in the text

(A) Terminal and interstitial deletions, each generating an acentric fragment that is typically lost. (B) Duplication of a chromosomal segment, leading to partial trisomy. (C) Ring chromosome with two acentric fragments. (D) Generation of an isochromosome for the long arm of a chromosome. (E) Robertsonian translocation between two acrocentric chromosomes, frequently leading to a pseudodicentric chromosome. Robertsonian translocations are nonreciprocal, and the short arms of the acrocentrics are lost. (F) Translocation between two chromosomes, with reciprocal exchange of the translocated segments.

(1) Unbalanced Rearrangements

Unbalanced rearrangements are detected in approximately 1 in 1,600 live births (see Fig. 4-8). The phenotype is likely to be abnormal because of deletion or duplication of multiple genes, or (in some cases) both. Duplication of part of a chromosome leads to **partial trisomy** for the genes within that segment; deletion leads to **partial monosomy**. As a general concept, any change that disturbs normal gene dosage balance can result in abnormal development. A broad range of phenotypes can result, depending on the nature of the specific genes whose dosage is altered in a particular case.

Large structural rearrangements involving imbalance of at least a few megabases can be detected at the level of routine chromosome banding, including high-resolution karyotyping. Detection of smaller changes, however, generally requires higher resolution analysis, involving FISH or chromosomal microarray analysis.

① Deletions and Duplications

Deletions involve loss of a chromosome segment, resulting in chromosome imbalance (see

Fig. 4-11). A carrier of a chromosomal deletion (with one normal homologue and one deleted homologue) is monosomic for the genetic information on the corresponding segment of the normal homologue. The clinical consequences generally reflect **haploinsufficiency** (literally, the inability of a single copy of the genetic material to carry out the functions normally performed by two copies), and, where examined, their severity reflects the size of the deleted segment and the number and function of the specific genes that are deleted. Cytogenetically visible autosomal deletions have an incidence of approximately 1 in 7,000 live births. Smaller, submicroscopic deletions detected by microarray analysis are much more common, but as mentioned earlier, the clinical significance of many such variants has yet to be fully determined.

A deletion may occur at the end of a chromosome (**terminal**) or along a chromosome arm (**interstitial**). Deletions may originate simply by chromosome breakage and loss of the acentric segment. Numerous deletions have been identified in the course of prenatal diagnosis or in the investigation of dysmorphic patients or patients with intellectual disability.

In general, duplication appears to be less harmful than deletion. However, because duplication in a gamete results in chromosomal imbalance (i.e., partial trisomy), and because the chromosome breaks that generate it may disrupt genes, duplication often leads to some phenotypic abnormality.

② Marker and Ring Chromosomes

Very small, unidentified chromosomes, called **marker chromosomes**, are occasionally seen in chromosome preparations, frequently in a mosaic state. They are usually in addition to the normal chromosome complement and are thus also referred to as **supernumerary chromosomes** or **extra structurally abnormal chromosomes**. The prenatal frequency of de novo supernumerary marker chromosomes has been estimated to be approximately 1 in 2,500. Because of their small and indistinctive size, higher resolution genome analysis is usually required for precise identification.

Larger marker chromosomes contain genomic material from one or both chromosome arms, creating an imbalance for whatever genes are present. Depending on the origin of the marker chromosome, the risk for a fetal abnormality can range from very low to 100%. For reasons not fully understood, a relatively high proportion of such markers derive from chromosome 15 and from the sex chromosomes.

Many marker chromosomes lack telomeres and are **ring chromosomes** that are formed when a chromosome undergoes two breaks and the broken ends of the chromosome reunite in a ring structure (see Fig. 4-11). Some rings experience difficulties at mitosis, when the two sister chromatids of the ring chromosome become tangled in their attempt to disjoin at anaphase. There may be breakage of the ring followed by fusion, and larger and smaller rings may thus be generated. Because of this mitotic instability, it is not uncommon for ring chromosomes to be found in only a proportion of cells.

③ Isochromosomes

An isochromosome is a chromosome in which one arm is missing and the other duplicated in a mirror-image fashion (see Fig. 4-11). A person with 46 chromosomes carrying an isochromosome therefore has a single copy of the genetic material of one arm (partial monosomy) and three copies of the genetic material of the other arm (partial trisomy).

Although isochromosomes for a number of autosomes have been described, the most common isochromosome involves the long arm of the X chromosome—designated i (X) (q10)—in a proportion of individuals with Turner syndrome. Isochromosomes are also frequently seen in karyotypes of both solid tumors and hematological malignant neoplasms.

④ **Dicentric Chromosomes**

A dicentric chromosome is a rare type of abnormal chromosome in which two chromosome segments, each with a centromere, fuse end to end. Dicentric chromosomes, despite their two centromeres, can be mitotically stable if one of the two centromeres is inactivated epigenetically or if the two centromeres always coordinate their movement to one or the other pole during anaphase. Such chromosomes are formally called **pseudodicentric**. The most common pseudodicentrics involve the sex chromosomes or the acrocentric chromosomes (so-called Robertsonian translocations).

(2) **Balanced Rearrangements**

Balanced chromosomal rearrangements are found in as many as 1 in 500 individuals (see Fig. 4-8) and do not usually lead to a phenotypic effect because all the genomic material is present, even though it is arranged differently (see Fig. 4-11). As noted earlier, it is important to distinguish here between truly balanced rearrangements and those that appear balanced cytogenetically but are really unbalanced at the molecular level. Because of the high frequency of copy number polymorphisms around the genome, collectively adding up to differences of many megabases between genomes of unrelated individuals, the concept of what is balanced or unbalanced is subject to ongoing investigation and continual refinement.

Even when structural rearrangements are truly balanced, they can pose a threat to the subsequent generation because carriers are likely to produce a significant frequency of unbalanced gametes and therefore have an increased risk for having abnormal offspring with unbalanced karyotypes. Depending on the specific rearrangement, that risk can range from 1% to as high as 20%. There is also a possibility that one of the chromosome breaks will disrupt a gene, leading to mutation. Especially with the use of whole-genome sequencing to examine the nature of apparently balanced rearrangements in patients who present with significant phenotypes, this is an increasingly well-documented cause of disorders in carriers of balanced translocations. Such translocations can be a useful clue to the identification of the gene responsible for a particular genetic disorder.

① **Translocations**

Translocation involves the exchange of chromosome segments between two chromosomes. There are two main types: reciprocal and nonreciprocal.

Reciprocal Translocations

This type of rearrangement results from breakage or recombination involving nonhomologous chromosomes, with reciprocal exchange of the broken-off or recombined segments (see Fig. 4-11). Usually only two chromosomes are involved, and because the exchange is reciprocal, the total chromosome number is unchanged. Such translocations are usually without phenotypic effect. However, like other balanced structural rearrangements, they are associated with a high risk for unbalanced gametes and abnormal progeny. They come to attention either during prenatal diagnosis or when the parents of a clinically abnormal child with an unbalanced translocation are karyotyped. Balanced translocations are more commonly found in couples who have had two or more spontaneous abortions and in infertile males than in the general population.

The existence of translocations presents challenges for the process of chromosome pairing and homologous recombination during meiosis. When the chromosomes of a carrier of a balanced reciprocal translocation pair at meiosis, as shown in Figure 4-12, they must form a **quadrivalent** to ensure proper alignment of homologous sequences (rather than the typical bivalents seen with normal chromosomes). In typical segregation, two of the four chromosomes in the quadrivalent go to each pole at anaphase. However, the chromosomes can segregate from this configuration in several ways, depending on which chromosomes go to which pole. **Alternate segregation**, the usual type of meiotic segregation, produces balanced gametes that have either a normal chromosome complement or contain the two reciprocal chromosomes. Other segregation patterns, however, always yield unbalanced gametes (see Fig. 4-12).

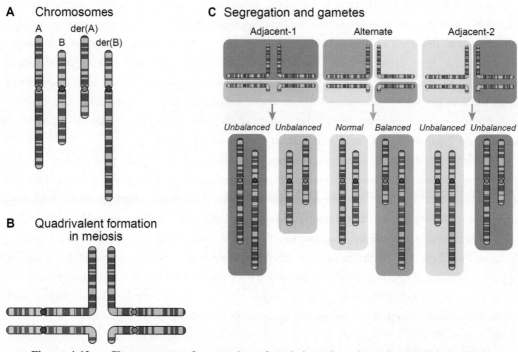

Figure 4-12   Chromosomes of a carrier of a balanced reciprocal translocation pair throughout meiosis

(A) Diagram illustrating a balanced translocation between two chromosomes, involving a reciprocal exchange between the distal long arms of chromosomes A and B. (B) Formation of a quadrivalent in meiosis is necessary to align the homologous segments of the two derivative chromosomes and their normal homologues. (C) Patterns of segregation in a carrier of the translocation, leading to either balanced or unbalanced gametes, shown at the bottom. Adjacent-1 segregation (in *red*, top chromosomes to one gamete, bottom chromosomes to the other) leads only to unbalanced gametes. Adjacent-2 segregation (in *green*, left chromosomes to one gamete, right chromosomes to the other) also leads only to unbalanced gametes. Only alternate segregation (in *gray*, upper left/lower right chromosomes to one gamete, lower left/upper right to the other) can lead to balanced gametes.

Robertsonian Translocations

Robertsonian translocations are the most common type of chromosome rearrangement observed in our species and involve two acrocentric chromosomes that fuse near the centromere region with loss of the short arms (see Fig. 4-11). Such translocations are nonreciprocal, and the resulting karyotype has only 45 chromosomes, including the translocation chromosome, which in effect is made up of the long arms of two acrocentric chromosomes. Because, as noted earlier, the short arms of all five pairs of acrocentric chromosomes consist largely of various classes of satellite DNA, as well as hundreds of copies of ribosomal RNA genes, loss of the short arms of two acrocentric chromosomes is not deleterious. Thus, the karyotype is considered to be balanced, despite having only 45 chromosomes. Robertsonian translocations are typically, although not always, pseudodicentric (see Fig. 4-11), reflecting the location of the breakpoint on each acrocentric chromosome.

Although Robertsonian translocations can involve all combinations of the acrocentric chromosomes, two—designated rob(13;14)(q10;q10) and rob(14;21)(q10;q10)—are relatively common. The translocation involving 13q and 14q is found in approximately 1 person in 1,300 and is thus by far the single most common chromosome rearrangement in our species. Rare individuals with two copies of the same type of Robertsonian translocation have been described. These phenotypically normal individuals have only 44 chromosomes and lack any normal copies of the involved acrocentrics, replaced by two copies of the translocation.

Although a carrier of a Robertsonian translocation is phenotypically normal, there is a risk for unbalanced gametes and therefore for unbalanced offspring. The risk for unbalanced offspring varies according to the particular Robertsonian translocation and the sex of the carrier parent. Carrier females in general have a higher risk for transmitting the translocation to an affected child. The chief clinical importance of this type of translocation is that carriers of a Robertsonian translocation involving chromosome 21 are at risk for producing a child with translocation Down syndrome, as will be explored further in Chapter 5.

② **Insertions**

An insertion is another type of nonreciprocal translocation that occurs when a segment removed from one chromosome is inserted into a different chromosome, either in its usual orientation with respect to the centromere or inverted. Because they require three chromosome breaks, insertions are relatively rare. Abnormal segregation in an insertion carrier can produce offspring with duplication or deletion of the inserted segment, as well as normal offspring and balanced carriers. The average risk for producing an abnormal child can be up to 50%, and prenatal diagnosis is therefore indicated.

③ **Inversions**

An inversion occurs when a single chromosome undergoes two breaks and is reconstituted with the segment between the breaks inverted. Inversions are of two types (see Fig. 4-13): **paracentric**, in which both breaks occur in one arm (Greek *para*, beside the centromere); and **pericentric**, in which there is a break in each arm (Greek *peri*, around the centromere). Pericentric inversions can be easier to identify cytogenetically when they change the proportion of the chromosome arms as well as the banding pattern.

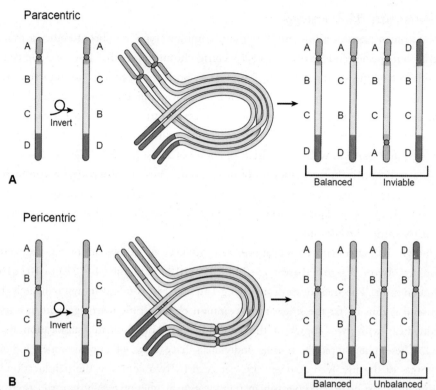

Figure 4-13   Crossing over within inversion loops formed at meiosis Ⅰ in carriers of a chromosome with segment B-C inverted (order A-C-B-D, instead of the normal order A-B-C-D)

(A) Paracentric inversion. Gametes formed after the second meiosis usually contain either a normal (A-B-C-D) or a balanced (A-C-B-D) copy of the chromosome because the acentric and dicentric products of the crossover are inviable. (B) Pericentric inversion. Gametes formed after the second meiosis may be balanced (normal or inverted) or unbalanced. Unbalanced gametes contain a copy of the chromosome with a duplication or a deficiency of the material flanking the inverted segment (A-B-C-A or D-B-C-D).

An inversion does not usually cause an abnormal phenotype in carriers because it is a balanced rearrangement. Its medical significance is for the progeny. A carrier of either type of inversion is at risk for producing abnormal gametes that may lead to unbalanced offspring because, when an inversion is present, a loop needs to form to allow alignment and pairing of homologous segments of the normal and inverted chromosomes in meiosis Ⅰ (see Fig. 4-13). When recombination occurs within the loop, it can lead to the production of unbalanced gametes: gametes with balanced chromosome complements (either normal or possessing the inversion) and gametes with unbalanced complements are formed, depending on the location of recombination events. When the inversion is paracentric, the unbalanced recombinant chromosomes are acentric or dicentric and typically do not lead to viable offspring (see Fig. 4-13). Thus, the risk that a carrier of a paracentric inversion will have a liveborn child with an abnormal karyotype is very low indeed.

A pericentric inversion, on the other hand, can lead to the production of unbalanced gametes with both **duplication** and **deficiency** of chromosome segments (see Fig. 4-13). The duplicated and deficient segments are the segments that are distal to the inversion. Overall, the risk for a carrier of a pericentric inversion leading to a child with an unbalanced karyotype is estimated to be 5% to 10%. Each pericentric inversion, however, is associated with a particular risk, typically reflecting the size and content of the duplicated and deficient segments.

4.2.4 Incidence of Chromosome Anomalies

The incidence of different types of chromosomal aberration has been measured in a number of large population surveys and was summarized earlier in Figure 4-8. The major numerical disorders of chromosomes observed in liveborns are three autosomal trisomies (trisomy 21, trisomy 18, and trisomy 13) and four types of sex chromosomal aneuploidy: Turner syndrome (usually 45,X), Klinefelter syndrome (47,XXY), 47,XYY, and 47,XXX (see Chapter 5). Triploidy and tetraploidy account for only a small percentage of cases, typically in spontaneous abortions. The classification and incidence of chromosomal defects measured in these surveys can be used to consider the fate of 10,000 conceptuses, as presented in Table 4-2.

Table 4-2　Outcome of 10,000 Pregnancies

Outcome	Pregnancies	Spontaneous Abortions (%)	Live Births
Total	10,000	1,500 (15)	8,500
Normal chromosome	9,200	750 (8)	8,450
Abnormal chromosome	800	750 (94)	50
Specific Abnormalities			
Triploid or tetraploid	170	170 (100)	0
45,X	140	139 (99)	1
Trisomy 16	112	112 (100)	0
Trisomy 18	20	19 (95)	1
Trisomy 21	45	35 (78)	10
Trisomy, other	209	208 (99.5)	1
47,XXY 47,XXX 47,XYY	19	4 (21)	15
Unbalanced rearrangements	27	23 (85)	4
Balanced rearrangements	19	3 (16)	16
Other	39	37 (95)	2

Note: These estimates are based on observed frequencies of chromosome abnormalities in spontaneous abortuses and in liveborn infants. It is likely that the frequency of chromosome abnormalities in all conceptuses is much higher than this, because many spontaneously abort before they are recognized clinically.

(1) Live Births

As mentioned earlier, the overall incidence of chromosome abnormalities in newborns has been found to be approximately 1 in 154 births (0.65%) (see Fig. 4-8). Most of the autosomal abnormalities can be diagnosed at birth, but most sex chromosome abnormalities, with the exception of Turner syndrome, are not recognized clinically until puberty. Unbalanced rearrangements are likely to come to clinical attention because of abnormal appearance and delayed physical and mental development in the chromosomally abnormal individual. In contrast, balanced rearrangements are rarely identified clinically unless a carrier of a rearrangement gives birth to a child with an unbalanced chromosome complement and family studies are initiated.

(2) Spontaneous Abortions

The overall frequency of chromosome abnormalities in spontaneous abortions is at least 40% to 50%, and the kinds of abnormalities differ in a number of ways from those seen in liveborns. Somewhat surprisingly, the single most common abnormality in abortuses is 45, X (the same abnormality found in Turner syndrome), which accounts for nearly 20% of chromosomally abnormal spontaneous abortuses but less than 1% of chromosomally abnormal live births (see Table 4-2). Another difference is the distribution of kinds of trisomy. For example, trisomy 16 is not seen at all in live births but accounts for approximately one third of trisomies in abortuses.

4.3 Chromosome and Genome Analysis in Cancer

We have focused in this chapter on constitutional chromosome abnormalities that are seen in most or all of the cells in the body and derive from chromosome or regional mutations that have been transmitted from a parent (either inherited or occurring de novo in the germline of a parent) or that have occurred in the zygote in early mitotic divisions.

However, such mutations also occur in somatic cells throughout life and are a hallmark of cancer, both in hematological neoplasias (e.g., leukemias and lymphomas) and in the context of solid tumor progression. An important area in cancer research is the delineation of chromosomal and genomic changes in specific forms of cancer and the relation of the breakpoints of the various structural rearrangements to the process of oncogenesis. The chromosome and genomic changes seen in cancer cells are numerous and diverse. The association of cytogenetic and genome analysis with tumor type and with the effectiveness of therapy is already an important part of the management of patients with cancer.

Review Points:

1. Abnormalities of Chromosome Number: euploidy (Polyploidy) is the category of chromosome changes which involve the addition or loss of complete sets of chromosomes. Aneuploidy is the category of chromosome changes which do not involve whole sets. It is usually the consequence of a failure of a single chromosome (or bivalent) to complete division.

2. Structural aberrations: structural rearrangements are defined as balanced, if the chromosome set has the normal complement of chromosomal material, or unbalanced, if there is additional or missing material. Some rearrangements are stable, capable of passing through mitotic and meiotic cell divisions unaltered, whereas others are unstable. To be stable, a rearranged chromosome must have normal structural elements, including a functional centromere and two telomeres.

3. Translocation: translocation involves the exchange or chromosome segments between two, usually nonhomolo-gous, chromosomes. There are two main types: reciprocal and Robertsonian.

4. When the chromosomes of a carrier of a balanced reciprocal translocation pair at meiosis, a quadrivalent (cross-shaped) figure is formed. At anaphase, the chromosomes usually segregate from this configuration in one of three ways, described as alternate, adjacent-1, and adjacent-2 segregation. Alternate segregation, the usual type of meiotic segregation, produces gametes that have either a normal chromosome complement or the two reciprocal chromo-somes; both types of gamete are balanced. In adjacent-1 segregation, homologous centromeres go to separate daugh-ter cells, whereas in adjacent-2 segregation (which is rare), homologous centromeres pass to the same daughter cell. Both adjacent-1 and adjacent-2 segregation yield unbalanced gametes.

Study Questions:

1. A spontaneously aborted fetus is found to have trisomy 18.
   a. What proportion of fetuses with trisomy 18 are lost by spontaneous abortion?
   b. What is the risk that the parents will have a liveborn child with trisomy 18 in a future pregnancy?
2. A newborn child with Down syndrome, when karyotyped, is found to have two cell lines: 70% of her cells have the typical 47,XX,+21 karyotype, and 30% are normal 46,XX. When did the nondisjunctional event probably occur? What is the prognosis for this child?
3. Which of the following persons is or is expected to be phenotypically normal?
   a. A female with 47 chromosomes, including a small supernumerary chromosome derived from the centromeric region of chromosome 15.
   b. A female with the karyotype 47,XX,+13.
   c. A male with deletion of a band on chromosome 4.
   d. A person with a balanced reciprocal translocation.
   e. A person with a pericentric inversion of chromosome 6.
   What kinds of gametes can each of these individuals produce? What kinds of offspring might result, assuming that the other parent is chromosomally normal?
4. For each of the following, state whether chromosome or genome analysis is indicated or not. For which family members, if any? For what kind of chromosome abnormality might the family in each case be at risk?
   a. A pregnant 29-year-old woman and her 41-year-old husband, with no history a pregnant 41-year-old woman and her 29-year-old husband, with no history of genetic defects.

b. A couple whose only child has Down syndrome.

c. A couple whose only child has cystic fibrosis.

d. A couple who has two boys with severe intellectual disability.

5. Explain the nature of the chromosome abnormality and the method of detection indicated by the following no-menclature.

    a. inv(X)(q21q26)

    b. 46,XX,del(1)(1qter → p36.2:)

    c. 46,XX,rob(13;21)(q10;q10),+21

    d. 45,XY,rob(13;21)(q10;q10)

CHAPTER 5
Chromosome Disease

Purpose and Requirement:

In this chapter, students should be able to assay "karyotype" and describe the medical aspects of chromosome abnormalities, especially some specific syndromes, such as Down Syndrome, Fragile X Syndrome, Klinefelter Syndrome and Cri du Chat Syndrome.

In this chapter, we present several of the most common and best understood chromosomal and genomic disorders encountered in clinical practice, building on the general principles of clinical cytogenetics and genome analysis introduced in the previous chapter. Each of the disorders presented here illustrates the principles of **dosage balance and imbalance** at the level of chromosomes and subchromosomal regions of the genome. Because a wide range of phenotypes seen in clinical medicine involve chromosome and subchromosomal mutations, we include in this chapter the spectrum of disorders that are characterized by intellectual disability or by abnormal or ambiguous sexual development. Although many such disorders can be determined by single genes, the clinical approach to evaluation of such phenotypes frequently includes detailed chromosome and genome analysis.

5.1 Mechanisms of Abnormalities

In this section, we consider abnormalities that illustrate the major chromosomal and genomic mechanisms that underlie genetic imbalance of entire chromosomes or chromosomal regions. Overall, we distinguish five different categories of such abnormalities, each of which can lead to disorders of clinical significance:

- Disorders due to **abnormal chromosome segregation** (nondisjunction).
- Disorders due to **recurrent chromosomal syndromes**, involving deletions or duplications at genomic hot spots.
- Disorders due to **idiopathic chromosomal abnormalities**, typically de novo.
- Disorders due to **unbalanced familial chromosomal abnormalities**.
- Disorders due to chromosomal and genomic events that reveal regions of **genomic imprinting**.

The distinguishing features of the underlying mechanisms are summarized in Table 5-1. Although the categories of defects that result from these mechanisms can involve any chromosomes, we introduce them here in the context of autosomal abnormalities.

Table 5-1 Mechanisms of Chromosome Abnormalities and Genomic Imbalance

Category	Underlying Mechanism	Consequences/Examples
Abnormal chromosome segregation	Nondisjunction	Aneuploidy (Down syndrome, Klinefelter syndrome) Uniparental disomy
Recurrent chromosomal syndromes	Recombination at segmental duplications	Duplication/deletion syndromes Copy number variation
Idiopathic chromosome abnormalities	Sporadic, variable breakpoints	Deletion syndromes (cri du chat syndrome, 1p36 deletion syndrome)
	De novo balanced translocations	Gene disruption
Unbalanced familial abnormalities	Unbalanced segregation	Offspring of balanced translocations Offspring of pericentric inversions
Syndromes involving genomic imprinting	Any event that reveals imprinted gene(s)	Prader-Willi/Angelman syndromes

5.2 Aneuploidy

The most common mutation in our species involves errors in chromosome segregation, typically leading to production of an abnormal gamete that has two copies or no copies of the chromosome involved in the nondisjunction event. Not withstanding the high frequency of such errors in meiosis and, to a lesser extent, in mitosis, there are only three well-defined nonmosaic chromosome disorders compatible with postnatal survival in which there is an abnormal dose of an entire autosome: **trisomy 21** (Down syndrome), **trisomy 18**, and **trisomy 13**. It is surely no coincidence that these chromosomes are the ones with the smallest number of genes among all autosomes. Imbalance for more gene-rich chromosomes is presumably incompatible with long-term survival, and aneuploidy for some of these is frequently associated with pregnancy loss.

Each of these autosomal trisomies is associated with growth retardation, intellectual disability, and multiple congenital anomalies (see Table 5-2). Nevertheless, each has a fairly distinctive phenotype that is immediately recognizable to an astute clinician in the newborn nursery. Trisomy 18 and trisomy 13 are both less common than trisomy 21. Survival beyond the first year is rare, in contrast to Down syndrome, in which average life expectancy is over 50 years of age.

The developmental abnormalities characteristic of any one trisomic state must be determined by the extra dosage of the particular genes on the additional chromosome. Knowledge of the specific relationship between the extra chromosome and the consequent developmental abnormality has been limited to date. Current research, however, is beginning to localize specific genes on the extra chromosome that are responsible for specific aspects of the abnormal phenotype, through direct or indirect modulation of patterning events during early development. The principles of gene dosage and the likely role of imbalance for individual genes that underlie specific developmental aspects of the phenotype apply to all aneuploid conditions. These are illustrated here in the context of Down syndrome, whereas the other conditions are summarized in Table 5-2.

Table 5-2   Features of Autosomal Trisomies Compatible With Postnatal Survival

Feature	Trisomy 21	Trisomy 18	Trisomy 13
Incidence (live births)	1 in 850	1 in 6,000~8,000	1 in 12,000~20,000
Clinical presentation	Hypotonia, short stature, loose skin on nape, palmar crease, clinodactyly	Hypertonia, prenatal growth deficiency, characteristic fist clench, rocker-bottom feet	Microcephaly, sloping forehead, characteristic fist clench, rocker-bottom feet, polydactyly
Dysmorphic facial features	Flat occiput, epicanthal folds, Brushfield spots	Receding jaw, low-set ears	Ocular abnormalities, cleft lip and palate
Intellectual disability	Moderate to mild	Severe	Severe
Other common features	Congenital heart disease Duodenal atresia Risk for leukemia Risk for premature dementia	Severe heart malformations; Feeding difficulties	Severe CNS malformations; Congenital heart defects
Life expectancy	55 yr	Typically less than a few months; almost all <1 yr	50% die within first month, >90% within first year

Note: CNS, Central nervous system.

➢ Down Syndrome

Down syndrome is by far the most common and best known of the chromosome disorders and is the single most common genetic cause of moderate intellectual disability. Approximately 1 child in 850 is born with Down syndrome, and among liveborn children or fetuses of mothers 35 years of age or older, the incidence of trisomy 21 is far higher (see Fig. 5-1).

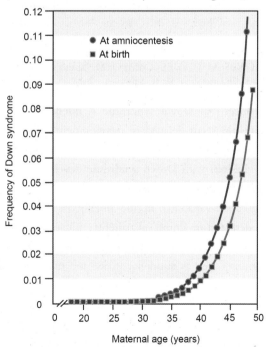

Figure 5-1   Maternal age dependence on incidence of trisomy 21 at birth and at time of amniocentesis

(From HOOK E B, CROSS P K, SCHREINEMACHERS D M. Chromosomal abnormality rates at amniocentesis and in live-born infants[J]. The journal of the american medical association, 1983, 249(15):2034-2038.)

Down syndrome can usually be diagnosed at birth or shortly thereafter by its dysmorphic features, which vary among patients but nevertheless produce a distinctive phenotype (see Fig. 5-2). Hypotonia may be the first abnormality noticed in the newborn. In addition to characteristic dysmorphic facial features (see Fig. 5-2), the patients are short in stature and have brachycephaly with a flat occiput. The neck is short, with loose skin on the nape. The hands are short and broad, often with a single transverse palmar crease ("simian crease") and incurved fifth digits (termed clinodactyly).

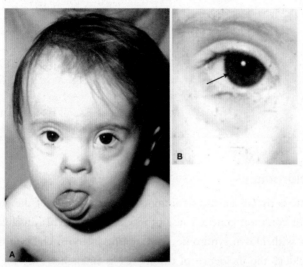

Figure 5-2 Phenotype of Down syndrome

(A) Young infant. The nasal bridge is flat; ears are low-set and have a characteristic folded appearance; the eyes show characteristic epicanthal folds and upslanting palpebral fissures; the mouth is open, showing a protruding tongue. (B) Brushfield spots around the margin of the iris (*arrow*).
(From JONES K L, JONES M C, DEL CAMPO M. Smith's recognizable patterns of human malformation[M]. 7th ed. Philadelphia: W.B. Saunders, 2013.)

A major cause for concern in Down syndrome is intellectual disability. Even though in early infancy the child may not seem delayed in development, the delay is usually obvious by the end of the first year. Although the extent of intellectual disability varies among patients from moderate to mild, many children with Down syndrome develop into interactive and even self-reliant persons, and many attend local schools.

There is a high degree of variability in the phenotype of Down syndrome individuals. Specific abnormalities are detected in almost all patients, but others are seen only in a subset of cases. Congenital heart disease is present in at least one third of all liveborn Down syndrome infants. Certain malformations, such as duodenal atresia and tracheoesophageal fistula, are much more common in Down syndrome than in other disorders.

Only approximately 20% to 25% of trisomy 21 conceptuses survive to birth. Among Down syndrome conceptuses, those least likely to survive are those with congenital heart disease. Approximately one fourth of the liveborn infants with heart defects die before their first birthday. There is a fifteen fold increase in the risk for leukemia among Down syndrome patients who survive the neonatal period. Premature dementia, associated with the neuropathological findings characteristic of Alzheimer disease (cortical atrophy, ventricular dilatation, and neurofibrillar tangles), affects nearly all Down syndrome patients, several decades earlier than the typical age at onset of Alzheimer disease in the general population.

As a general principle, it is important to think of this constellation of clinical findings, their variation, and likely outcomes in terms of gene imbalance—the relative overabundance of specific gene products. Their impact on various critical pathways in particular tissues and cell types, both early in development and throughout life. And the particular alleles present in a particular patient's genome, both for genes on the trisomic chromosome and for the many other genes inherited from his or her parents.

(1) The Chromosomes in Down Syndrome

The clinical diagnosis of Down syndrome usually presents no particular difficulty. Nevertheless, karyotyping is necessary for confirmation and to provide a basis for genetic counseling. Although the specific abnormal karyotype responsible for Down syndrome usually has little effect on the phenotype of the patient, it is essential for determining the recurrence risk.

① Trisomy 21

In at least 95% of all patients, the Down syndrome karyotype has 47 chromosomes, with an extra copy of chromosome 21. This trisomy results from meiotic nondisjunction of the chromosome 21 pair. As noted earlier, the risk for having a child with trisomy 21 increases with maternal age, especially after the age of 30 years (see Fig. 5-1). The meiotic error responsible for the trisomy usually occurs during maternal meiosis (approximately 90% of cases), predominantly in meiosis I, but approximately 10% of cases occur in paternal meiosis, often in meiosis II. Typical trisomy 21 is a sporadic event, and thus recurrences are infrequent.

Approximately 2% of Down syndrome patients are mosaic for two cell populations—one with a normal karyotype and one with a trisomy 21 karyotype. The phenotype may be milder than that of typical trisomy 21, but there is wide variability in phenotypes among mosaic patients, presumably reflecting the variable proportion of trisomy 21 cells in the embryo during early development.

② Robertsonian Translocation

Approximately 4% of Down syndrome patients have 46 chromosomes, one of which is a Robertsonian translocation between chromosome 21q and the long arm of one of the other acrocentric chromosomes (usually chromosome 14 or 22). The translocation chromosome replaces one of the normal acrocentric chromosomes, and the karyotype of a Down syndrome patient with a Robertsonian translocation between chromosomes 14 and 21 is therefore 46,XX or XY, rob (14;21) (q10;q10), +21. Despite having 46 chromosomes, patients with a Robertsonian translocation involving chromosome 21 are trisomic for genes on the entirety of 21q.

A carrier of a Robertsonian translocation, involving, for example, chromosomes 14 and 21, has only 45 chromosomes. One chromosome 14 and one chromosome 21 are missing and are replaced by the translocation chromosome. The gametes that can be formed by such a carrier are shown in Figure 5-3, and such carriers are at risk for having a child with translocation Down syndrome.

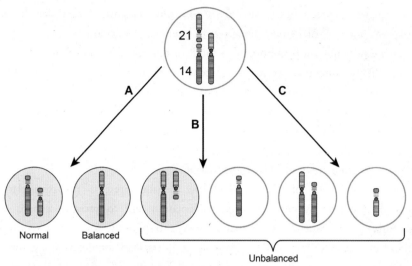

Figure 5-3   Chromosomes of gametes that theoretically can be produced by a carrier of a Robertsonian translocation, rob (14;21)

(A) Normal and balanced complements. (B) Unbalanced, one product with both the translocation chromosome and the normal chromosome 21, and the reciprocal product with chromosome 14 only. (C) Unbalanced, one product with both the translocation chromosome and chromosome 14, and the reciprocal product with chromosome 21 only. Theoretically, there are six possible types of gamete, but three of these appear unable to lead to viable offspring. Only the three shaded gametes at the left can lead to viable offspring. Theoretically, the three types of gametes will be produced in equal numbers, and thus the theoretical risk for a Down syndrome child should be 1 in 3. However, extensive population studies have shown that unbalanced chromosome complements appear in only approximately 10% to 15% of the progeny of carrier mothers and in only a few percent of the progeny of carrier fathers who have translocations involving chromosome 21.

Unlike standard trisomy 21, translocation Down syndrome shows no relation to maternal age but has a relatively high recurrence risk in families when a parent, especially the mother, is a carrier of the translocation. For this reason, karyotyping of the parents and possibly other relatives is essential before accurate genetic counseling can be provided.

21q21q Translocation

A 21q21q translocation chromosome is seen in a few percent of Down syndrome patients and is thought to originate as an isochromosome. It is particularly important to evaluate if a parent is a carrier because all gametes of a carrier of such a chromosome must either contain the 21q21q chromosome, with its double dose of chromosome 21 genetic material, or lack it and have no chromosome 21 representative at all. The potential progeny, therefore, inevitably have either Down syndrome or monosomy 21, which is rarely viable. Mosaic carriers are at an increased risk for recurrence, and thus prenatal diagnosis should be considered in any subsequent pregnancy.

③ Partial Trisomy 21

Very rarely is down syndrome diagnosed in a patient in whom only a part of the long arm of chromosome 21 is present in triplicate. These patients are of particular significance because they can show what region of chromosome 21 is likely to be responsible for specific components of the Down syndrome phenotype and what regions can be triplicated without causing that aspect of the phenotype. The most notable success has been identification of a less than 2-Mb region that is critical for the heart defects seen in approximately 40% of Down syndrome patients. Sorting out the specific genes crucial to the expression of the Down syndrome phenotype from those that merely happen to be syntenic with them on chromosome 21 is critical for determining the pathogenesis of the various clinical findings.

(2) Risk for Down Syndrome

A frequent problem in genetic counseling is to assess the risk for the birth of a Down syndrome child. The risk depends chiefly on the mother's age but also on both parents' karyotypes, as discussed previously. Down syndrome can be detected prenatally by karyotyping, by chromosomal microarray analysis, or by genome-wide sequencing of chorionic villus or amniotic fluid cells. Screening for Down syndrome is also possible now by **noninvasive prenatal screening** (**NIPS**) of cell-free fetal DNA in maternal plasma. Although all pregnancies should be offered prenatal diagnosis, a decision to undergo invasive methods of prenatal testing balances the risk that a fetus has Down syndrome and the risk that the procedure of amniocentesis or chorionic villus sampling used to obtain fetal tissue for chromosome analysis will lead to fetal loss. However, with NIPS emerging as a screening test for Down syndrome and other relatively common aneuploid conditions, this paradigm and counseling considerations are likely to change in the years ahead.

The population incidence of Down syndrome in live births is currently estimated to be approximately 1 in 850, reflecting the maternal age distribution for all births and the proportion of older mothers who make use of prenatal diagnosis and selective termination. At approximately the age of 30 years, the risk begins to rise sharply, approaching 1 in 10 births in the oldest maternal age-group (see Fig. 5-1). Even though younger mothers have a much lower risk, their birth rate is much higher, and therefore more than half of the mothers of all Down syndrome babies are younger than 35 years. The risk for Down syndrome due to translocation or partial trisomy is unrelated to maternal age. The paternal age appears to have no influence on the risk.

(3) Recurrence Risk

The recurrence risk for trisomy 21 or any other autosomal trisomy, after one such child has been born in a family, is approximately 1% overall. The risk is approximately 1.4% for mothers younger than 30 years, and it is the same as the age-related risk for older mothers. That is, there is a slight but significant increase in risk for the younger mothers but not for the older mothers, whose risk is already elevated. The reason for the increased risk for the younger mothers is not known. A history of trisomy 21 elsewhere in the family, although often a cause of maternal anxiety, does not appear to significantly increase the risk for having a Down syndrome child. The recurrence risk for Down syndrome due to a translocation is much higher, as described previously.

5.3 Idiopathic Chromosome Abnormalities

Whereas the abnormalities just described are mediated by the landscape of specific genomic features in particular chromosomal regions, many other chromosome abnormalities are due to deletions or rearrangements that have no definitive mechanistic basis (see Table 5-1). There are many reports of cytogenetically detectable abnormalities in dysmorphic patients involving events such as deletions, duplications, or translocations of one or more chromosomes in the karyotype. Overall, cytogenetically visible autosomal deletions occur with an estimated incidence of 1 in 7,000 live births. Most of these have been seen in only a few patients and are not associated with recognized clinical syndromes. Others, however, are sufficiently common to allow delineation of clearly recognizable syndromes in which a series of patients have similar abnormalities.

The defining mechanistic feature of this class of abnormalities is that the underlying chromosomal event is idiopathic (see Table 5-1). Most of them occur de novo and have highly variable breakpoints in the particular chromosomal region, thus distinguishing them as a class from those discussed in the previous section.

5.3.1 Autosomal Deletion Syndromes

One long-recognized syndrome is the **cri du chat syndrome**, in which there is either a terminal or interstitial deletion of part of the short arm of chromosome 5. This deletion syndrome was given its common name because crying infants with this disorder sound like a mewing cat. The facial appearance, shown in Figure 5-4, is distinctive and includes microcephaly, hypertelorism, epicanthal folds, low-set ears, sometimes with preauricular tags, and micrognathia. The overall incidence of the deletion is estimated to be as high as 1 in 15,000 live births.

Most cases of cri du chat syndrome are sporadic; only 10% to 15% of the patients are the offspring of translocation carriers. The breakpoints and extent of the deleted segment of chromosome 5p is highly variable among different patients, but the critical region missing in all patients with the phenotype has been identified as band 5p15. Many of the clinical findings have been attributed to haploinsufficiency for a gene or genes within specific regions. The degree of intellectual impairment usually correlates with the size of the deletion, although genomic studies suggest that haploinsufficiency for particular regions within 5p14-p15 may contribute disproportionately to severe intellectual disability (see Fig. 5-4).

Although many large deletions can be appreciated by routine karyotyping, detection of other idiopathic deletions requires more detailed analysis by microarrays; this is particularly true for abnormalities involving subtelomeric bands of many chromosomes, which can be difficult to visualize well by routine chromosome banding. For example, one of the most common idiopathic abnormalities, the **chromosome 1p36 deletion syndrome**, has a population incidence of 1 in 5,000 and involves a wide range of different breakpoints, all within the terminal 10 Mb of chromosome 1p. Approximately 95% of cases are de novo, and many (e.g., the case illustrated in Fig. 5-4) are not detectable by routine chromosome analysis.

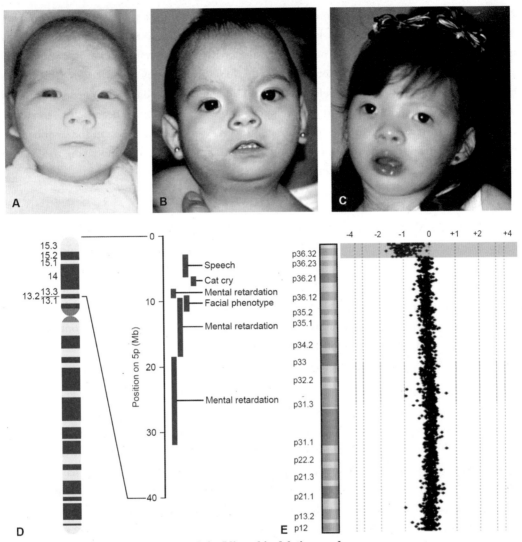

Figure 5-4 Idiopathic deletion syndromes

(A-C) Three different children with cri du chat syndrome, which results from deletion of part of chromosome 5p. Note, even among unrelated individuals, the characteristic facies with hypertelorism, epicanthus, and retrognathia. (D) Phenotype-karyotype map of chromosome 5p, based on chromosomal microarray analysis of a series of del(5p) patients. (E) Chromosomal microarray analysis of approximately 5-Mb deletion in band 1p36.3 (*red*), which is undetectable by conventional karyotyping.

(B and C from JONES K L, JONES M C, DEL CAMPO M. Smith's recognizable patterns of human malformation[M]. 7th ed. Philadelphia: W.B. Saunders, 2013. D from ZHANG X X, SNIJDERS A, SEGRAVES R, et al. High-resolution mapping of genotype-phenotype relationships in cri du chat syndrome using array comparative genomic hybridization[J]. American journal of human genetics, 2005,76(2):312-326.)

5.3.2 Balanced Translocations With Developmental Phenotypes

Reciprocal translocations are relatively common. Most are balanced and involve the precise exchange of chromosomal material between nonhomologous chromosomes. As such, they usually do not have an obvious phenotypic effect. However, among the approximately 1 in

2,000 newborns who has a de novo balanced translocation, the risk for a congenital abnormality is empirically elevated several-fold, leading to the suggestion that some balanced translocations involve direct disruption of a gene or genes by one or both of the translocation breakpoints.

Detailed analysis of a number of such cases by FISH, microarrays, and targeted or whole-genome sequencing has identified defects in protein-coding or noncoding RNA genes in patients with various phenotypes, ranging from developmental delay to congenital heart defects to autism spectrum disorders. Although the clinical abnormalities in these cases can be ascribed to mutations in individual genes located at the site of the translocations, the underlying mechanism in each case is the chromosomal rearrangement itself (see Table 5-1).

5.4　The Sex Chromosomes and Their Abnormalities

The X and Y chromosomes have long attracted interest because they differ between the sexes, because they have their own specific patterns of inheritance, and because they are involved in primary sex determination. They are structurally distinct and subject to different forms of genetic regulation, yet they pair in male meiosis. For all these reasons, they require special attention. In this section, we review the common sex chromosome abnormalities and their clinical consequences, the current state of knowledge concerning the control of sex determination, and abnormalities of sex development.

5.4.1　The Chromosomal Basis of Sex Determination

The different sex chromosome constitution of normal human male and female cells has been appreciated for more than 50 years. Soon after cytogenetic analysis became feasible, the fundamental basis of the XX/XY system of sex determination became apparent. Males with Klinefelter syndrome have 47 chromosomes with two X chromosomes as well as a Y chromosome (karyotype 47,XXY), whereas most Turner syndrome females have only 45 chromosomes with a single X chromosome (karyotype 45,X). These findings unambiguously establish the crucial role of the Y chromosome in normal male development. Furthermore, compared with the dramatic consequences of autosomal aneuploidy, these karyotypes underscore the relatively modest effect of varying the number of X chromosomes in either males or females. The basis for both observations can be explained in terms of the unique biology of the Y and X chromosomes.

The process of sex determination can be thought of as occurring in distinct but interrelated steps (see Fig. 5-5):

- Establishment of **chromosomal sex** (i.e., XY or XX) at the time of fertilization.
- Initiation of alternate pathways to differentiation of one or the other **gonadal sex**, as determined normally by the presence or absence of the testis-determining gene on the Y chromosome.
- Continuation of **sex-specific differentiation** of internal and external sexual organs.
- Especially after puberty, development of distinctive secondary sexual characteristics to create the corresponding **phenotypic sex**, as a male or female.

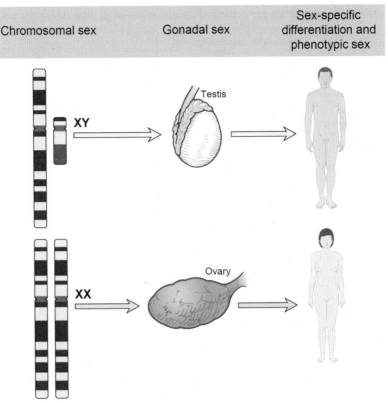

Figure 5-5　The process of sex determination and development

The establishment of chromosomal sex at fertilization; commitment to the male or female pathway of gonadal differentiation; sex-specific differentiation of internal and external genitalia and development of secondary sexual characteristics (phenotypic sex). Whereas the sex chromosomes play a determining role in specifying chromosomal sex, many genes located on both the sex chromosomes and the autosomes are involved in sex determination and subsequent sexual differentiation.

Whereas the sex chromosomes play a determining role in specifying chromosomal and gonadal sex, a number of genes located on both the sex chromosomes and the autosomes are involved in sex determination and subsequent sexual differentiation. In most instances, the role of these genes has come to light as a result of patients with various conditions known as **disorders of sex development**, and many of these are discussed later in this chapter.

5.4.2　The Y Chromosome

The structure of the Y chromosome and its role in sex development has been determined at both the molecular and genomic levels (see Fig. 5-6). In male meiosis, the X and Y chromosomes normally pair by segments at the ends of their short arms and undergo recombination in that region. The pairing segment includes the **pseudoautosomal region** of the X and Y chromosomes, so called because the X- and Y-linked copies of this region are essentially identical to one another and undergo homologous recombination in meiosis I, like pairs of autosomes. (The second, smaller pseudoautosomal segment is located at the distal ends of Xq and Yq.) By comparison with autosomes and the X chromosome, the Y chromosome is relatively gene poor and contains fewer than 100 genes (some of which belong to multigene families), specifying only approximately two dozen distinct proteins. Notably, the functions of a high proportion of these genes are restricted to gonadal and genital development.

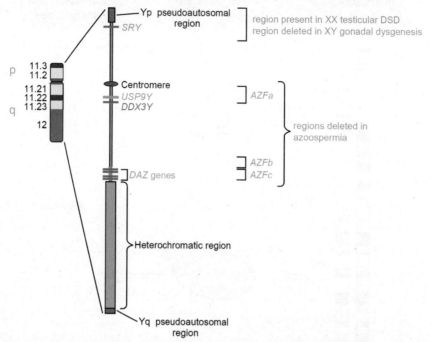

Figure 5-6 The Y chromosome in sex determination and in disorders of sex development (DSDs)
Individual genes and regions implicated in sex determination, DSDs, and defects of spermatogenesis are indicated, as discussed in the text.

(1) Embryology of the Reproductive System

The effect of the Y chromosome on the embryological development of the male and female reproductive systems is summarized in Figure 5-7. By the sixth week of development in both sexes, the primordial germ cells have migrated from their earlier extraembryonic location to the paired genital ridges, where they are surrounded by the sex cords to form a pair of primitive gonads. Up to this time, the developing gonad is ambipotent, regardless of whether it is chromosomally XX or XY.

Development into an ovary or a testis is determined by the coordinated action of a sequence of genes in finely balanced pathways that lead to ovarian development when no Y chromosome is present but tip to the side of testicular development when a Y is present. Under normal circumstances, the ovarian pathway is followed unless a particular Y-linked gene, originally designated testis-determining factor (TDF), diverts development into the male pathway.

If no Y chromosome is present, the gonad begins to differentiate to form an ovary, beginning as early as the eighth week of gestation and continuing for several weeks. The cortex develops, the medulla regresses, and oogonia begin to develop within follicles (see Fig. 5-7). Beginning at approximately the third month, the oogonia enter meiosis I, but this process is arrested at dictyotene until ovulation occurs many years later.

In the presence of a normal Y chromosome (with the *TDF* gene), however, the medullary tissue forms typical testes with seminiferous tubules and Leydig cells that, under the stimulation of chorionic gonadotropin from the placenta, become capable of androgen secretion (see Fig. 5-7). Spermatogonia, derived from the primordial germ cells by successive mitoses, line the walls of the seminiferous tubules, where they reside together with supporting Sertoli cells, awaiting the onset of puberty to begin spermatogenesis.

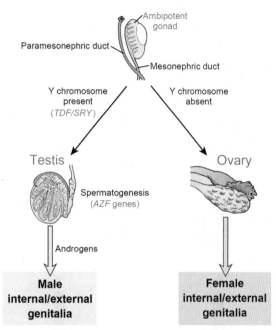

Figure 5-7   Scheme of developmental events in sex determination and differentiation of the male and female gonads from the ambipotent gonad

While the primordial germ cells are migrating to the genital ridges, thickenings in the ridges indicate the developing genital ducts, the **mesonephric** (also called **wolffian**) and **paramesonephric** (also called **müllerian**) ducts, under the influence of hormones produced by specific cell types in the developing gonad. Duct formation is usually completed by the third month of gestation.

In the early embryo, the external genitalia consist of a genital tubercle, paired labioscrotal swellings, and paired urethral folds. From this undifferentiated state, male external genitalia develop under the influence of androgens, beginning at around 12 weeks of gestation. In the absence of a testis (or, more specifically, in the absence of androgens), female external genitalia are formed regardless of whether an ovary is present.

(2) **SRY is the Major Testis-Determining Gene**

The earliest cytogenetic studies established the male-determining function of the Y chromosome. In the ensuing three decades, chromosomal and genomic analysis of individuals with different submicroscopic abnormalities of the Y chromosome and well-studied disorders of sex development allowed identification of the primary testis-determining region on Yp.

Whereas the X and Y chromosomes normally exchange in meiosis I within the Xp/Yp pseudoautosomal region, in rare instances, genetic recombination occurs outside of the pseudoautosomal region (see Fig. 5-8). This leads to two rare but highly informative abnormalities—males with a 46, XX karyotype and females with a 46, XY karyotype—that involve an inconsistency between chromosomal sex and gonadal sex, as we will explore in greater detail later in this chapter.

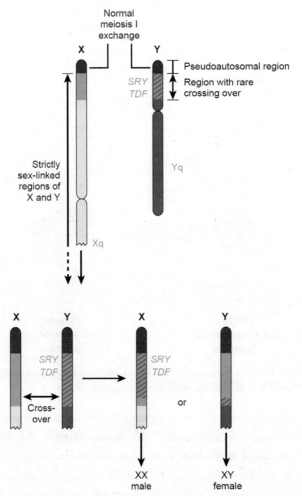

Figure 5-8   Etiological factors of phenotypic males with a 46, XX karyotype or phenotypic females with a 46, XY karyotype by aberrant exchange between X- and Y-linked sequences

X and Y chromosomes normally re-combine within the Xp/Yp pseudoautosomal segment in male meiosis. If recombination occurs below the pseudoau-tosomal boundary, between the X-specific and Y-specific portions of the chromosomes, sequences responsible for male gonadal sex determination (including the SRY gene) may be translocated from the Y to the X. Fertilization by a sperm containing such an X chromosome leads to a phenotypic male with XX testicular DSD. In contrast, fertilization by a sperm containing a Y chromosome that has lost SRY will lead to a phenotypic female with XY complete gonadal dysgenesis.

The *SRY* gene (sex-determining region on the Y) lies near the pseudoautosomal boundary on the Y chromosome. It is present in many males with an otherwise normal 46, XX karyotype and is deleted or mutated in a proportion of females with an otherwise normal 46, XY karyotype, thus strongly implicating *SRY* in normal male sex determination (see Fig. 5-8).

SRY is expressed only briefly early in development in cells of the germinal ridge just before differentiation of the testis. *SRY* encodes a DNA-binding protein that is likely to be a transcription factor, which up-regulates a key autosomal gene, *SOX9*, in the ambipotent gonad, leading ultimately to testes differentiation. Thus, by all available genetic and developmental criteria, *SRY* is equivalent to the *TDF* gene on the Y chromosome. If *SRY* is absent or not functioning properly, then the female sex differentiation pathway ensues (see Fig. 5-7).

Although there is clear evidence demonstrating the critical role of *SRY* in normal male sexual development, the presence or absence of *SRY/TDF* does not explain all cases of abnormal sex determination. Other genes are involved in the sex determination pathway and are discussed later in this chapter.

(3) Y-Linked Genes in Spermatogenesis

The prevalence of Y chromosome deletions and microdeletions in the general male population is reported to be approximately 1 in 2,000 to 3,000 males. However, microdeletions in the male-specific portion of Yq are found in a significant proportion of men with low sperm count, ranging from cases of nonobstructive azoospermia (no sperm detectable in semen) to severe oligospermia (<5 million/mL; normal range, 20 to 40 million/mL). These findings suggest that one or more genes, termed azoospermia factors (AZF), are located on the Y chromosome, and three such regions on Yq (AZFa, AZFb, and AZFc) have been defined (see Fig. 5-6).

Genomic analysis of these microdeletions led to identification of a series of genes that appear to be important in spermatogenesis. For example, the 3. 5-Mb-long AZFc deletion region contains seven different families of genes that are expressed only in the testis, including four copies of the *DAZ* genes (deleted in azoospermia) that encode nearly identical RNA-binding proteins expressed only in the premeiotic germ cells of the testis. De novo deletions of AZFc arise in approximately 1 in 4,000 males and account for approximately 12% of azoospermic males and approximately 6% of males with severe oligospermia. Deletion of only two of the four *DAZ* genes has been associated with milder oligospermia. Similar to the other genomic disorders described earlier in this chapter, they are mediated by recombination between segmentally duplicated sequences. AZFa and AZFb deletions, although less common, also involve recombination. The Yq microdeletions are not syndromic, however; they are responsible only for a defect in spermatogenesis in otherwise normal males. The explanation is that all of the genes involved in the AZF deletions are expressed only in the testis and have no functions in other tissues or cell types.

Overall, approximately 2% of otherwise healthy males are infertile because of severe defects in sperm production, and it appears likely that de novo deletions or mutations of genes on Yq account for a significant proportion of these. Thus men with idiopathic infertility should be karyotyped, and Y chromosome molecular testing and genetic counseling may be appropriate before the initiation of assisted reproduction by intracytoplasmic sperm injection for such couples, mostly because of the risk for passing a Yq microdeletion responsible for infertility to the infertile couple's sons.

5.4.3　The X Chromosome

Aneuploidy for the X chromosome is among the most common of cytogenetic abnormalities. The relative tolerance of human development for X chromosome abnormalities can be explained in terms of **X chromosome inactivation**, the process by which most genes on one of the two X chromosomes in females are silenced epigenetically. Here we discuss the chromosomal and genomic mechanisms of X inactivation and their implications for human and medical genetics.

X Chromosome Inactivation

The principle of X inactivation is that in somatic cells in normal females (but not in normal males), one X chromosome is inactivated early in development, thus equalizing the expression of X-linked genes in the two sexes. In normal female development, because the choice of which X chromosome is to be inactivated is a random one that is then maintained clonally, females are mosaic with respect to X-linked gene expression.

There are many epigenetic features that distinguish the active and inactive X chromosomes in somatic cells (see Table 5-3). These features can be useful diagnostically for identifying the inactive X chromosome(s) in clinical material. In patients with extra X chromosomes (whether male or female), any X chromosome in excess of one is inactivated (see Fig. 5-9). Thus all diploid somatic cells in both males and females have a single active X chromosome, regardless of the total number of X or Y chromosomes present.

The X chromosome contains approximately 1,000 genes, but not all of these are subject to inactivation. Notably, the genes that continue to be expressed, at least to some degree, from the inactive X are not distributed randomly along the X chromosome. Many more genes "escape" inactivation on distal Xp (as many as 50%) than on Xq (just a few percent). This finding has important implications for genetic counseling in cases of partial X chromosome aneuploidy, because imbalance for genes on Xp may have greater clinical significance than imbalance for genes on Xq, where the effect is largely mitigated by X inactivation.

Table 5-3　Epigenetic and Chromosomal Features of X Chromosome Inactivation in Somatic Cells

Feature	Active X	Inactive X
Gene expression	Yes; similar to male X	Most genes silenced; $\approx 15\%$ expressed to some degree
Chromatin state	Euchromatin	Facultative heterochromatin; Barr body
Noncoding RNA	*XIST* gene silenced	*XIST* RNA expressed from Xi only; associates with Barr body
DNA replication timing	Synchronous with autosomes	Late-replicating in S phase
Histone variants	Similar to autosomes and male X	Enriched for macroH2A
Histone modifications	Similar to autosomes and male X	Enriched for heterochromatin marks; deficient in euchromatin marks

Sexual phenotype	Karyotype	No. of active X's	No. of inactive X's
Male	46,XY; 47,XYY	1	0
	47,XXY; 48,XXYY	1	1
	48,XXXY; 49,XXXYY	1	2
	49,XXXXY	1	3
Female	45,X	1	0
	46,XX	1	1
	47,XXX	1	2
	48,XXXX	1	3
	49,XXXXX	1	4

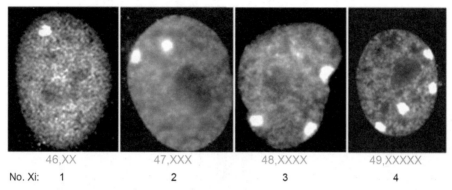

46,XX	47,XXX	48,XXXX	49,XXXXX
No. Xi: 1	2	3	4

Figure 5-9 Sex chromosome constitution and X chromosome inactivation

Top, In individuals with extra X chromosomes, any X in excess of one is inactivated, regardless of sex and regardless of the number of Y chromosomes present. Thus the number of inactive X chromosomes in diploid cells is always one less than the total number of X chromosomes. *Bottom*, Detection of inactive X chromosomes (Xi) in interphase nuclei from females with 46,XX, 47,XXX, 48,XXXX, and 49,XXXXX karyotypes. Regions of bright fluorescence indicate the presence of the histone variant macroH2A associated with inactive X chromosomes (see Table 5-3).

① Patterns of X Inactivation

X inactivation is normally random in female somatic cells and leads to mosaicism for two cell populations expressing alleles from one or the other X (see Fig. 5-10). Where examined, most females have approximately equal proportions of cells expressing alleles from the maternal or paternal X (i.e., approximately 50 : 50), and approximately 90% of phenotypically normal females fall within a distribution that extends from approximately 25 : 25 to approximately 75 : 25 (see Fig. 5-10). Such a distribution presumably reflects the expected range of outcomes for a random event (i.e., the choice of which X will be the inactive X) involving a relatively small number of cells during early embryogenesis. For individuals who are carriers for X-linked single-gene disorders, this X inactivation ratio can influence the clinical phenotype, depending on what proportion of cells in relevant tissues or cell types express the deleterious allele on the active X.

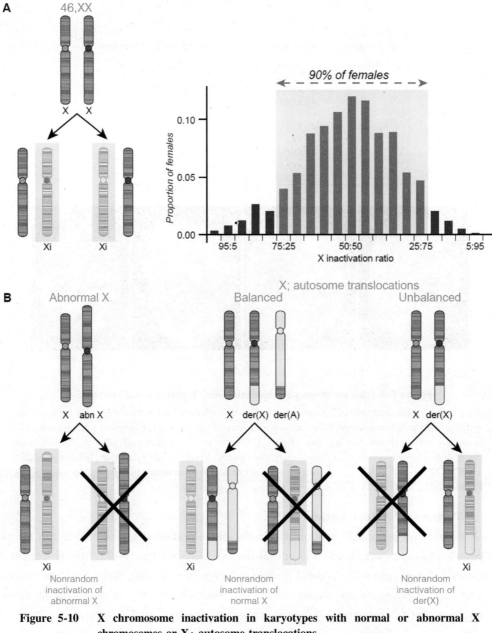

Figure 5-10　X chromosome inactivation in karyotypes with normal or abnormal X chromosomes or X; autosome translocations

(A) Normal female cells (46,XX) undergo random X inactivation, resulting in a mosaic of two cell populations (*left*) in which either the paternal or maternal X is the inactive X (Xi, indicated by *shaded box*). In phenotypically normal females, the ratio of the two cell populations has a mode at 50 : 50, but with variation observed in the population (*right*), some with an excess of cells expressing alleles from the paternal X and others with an excess of cells expressing alleles from the maternal X.
(B) Individuals carrying a structurally abnormal X (abn X) or X; autosome translocation in a balanced or unbalanced state show nonrandom X inactivation in which virtually all cells have the same X inactive. The other cell population is inviable or at a growth disadvantage because of genetic imbalance and is thus underrepresented or absent. der(X) and der(A) represent the two derivatives of the X; autosome translocation.
(B from AMOS-LANDGRAF J M, COTTLE A, PLENGE R M, et al. X chromosome-inactivation patterns of 1,005 phenotypically unaffected females [J]. The american journal of human genetics, 2006,79(3):493−499.)

However, there are exceptions to the distribution expected for random X inactivation when the karyotype involves a **structurally abnormal X chromosome**. For example, in nearly all patients with unbalanced structural abnormalities of an X chromosome (including deletions, duplications, and isochromosomes), the structurally abnormal chromosome is always the inactive X. Because the initial inactivation event early in embryonic development is likely random, the patterns observed after birth probably reflect secondary selection against genetically unbalanced cells that are inviable (see Fig. 5-10). Because of this preferential inactivation of the abnormal X, such X chromosome anomalies have less of an impact on phenotype than unbalanced abnormalities of similar size or gene content involving autosomes.

Nonrandom inactivation is also observed in most cases of **X; autosome translocations** (see Fig. 5-10). If such a translocation is balanced, the normal X chromosome is preferentially inactivated, and the two parts of the translocated chromosome remain active, again likely reflecting selection against cells in which critical autosomal genes have been inactivated. In the unbalanced offspring of a balanced carrier, however, only the translocation product carrying the **X inactivation center** is present, and this chromosome is invariably inactivated; the normal X is always active. These nonrandom patterns of inactivation have the general effect of minimizing, but not always eliminating, the clinical consequences of the particular chromosomal defect. Because patterns of X inactivation are strongly correlated with clinical outcome, determination of an individual's X inactivation pattern by cytological or molecular analysis (see Table 5-3) is indicated in all cases involving X; autosome translocations.

② The X Inactivation Center

Inactivation of an X chromosome depends on the presence of the X inactivation center region (*XIC*) on that chromosome, whether it is a normal X chromosome or a structurally abnormal X. Detailed analysis of structurally abnormal, inactivated X chromosomes led to the identification of the *XIC* within an approximately 800-kb candidate region in proximal Xq, in band Xq13.2 (see Fig. 5-11), which coordinates many, if not all, of the critical steps necessary to initiate and promulgate the silenced chromatin state along the near-entirety of the X chosen to become the inactive X. This complex series of events requires a noncoding RNA gene, *XIST*, that appears to be a key master regulatory locus for the onset of X inactivation. It is one of a suite of noncoding RNA genes in the interval, others of which may operate in the regulation of *XIST* expression and in other early events in the X inactivation process.

5.4.4 Cytogenetic Abnormalities of the Sex Chromosomes

Sex chromosome abnormalities are among the most common of all human genetic disorders, with an overall incidence of approximately 1 in 400 live births. Like abnormalities of the autosomes, they can be either numerical or structural and can be present in all cells or in mosaic form. As a group, disorders of the sex chromosomes tend to occur as isolated events without apparent predisposing factors, except for an effect of late maternal age in the cases that originate from errors of maternal meiosis I. There are a number of clinical indications that raise the possibility of a sex chromosome abnormality and thus the need for chromosomal or genomic studies. These indications include delay in onset of puberty, primary or secondary amenorrhea, infertility, and ambiguous genitalia.

The most common sex chromosome abnormalities involve aneuploidy for the X and/or Y chromosomes. The phenotypes associated with these chromosomal defects are, in general, less severe than those associated with comparable autosomal disorders because, as discussed earlier, X chromosome inactivation, as well as the low gene content of the Y, minimize the clinical consequences of sex chromosome imbalance. By far the most common sex chromosome defects in liveborn infants and in fetuses are the trisomic types (XXY, XXX, and XYY), but all three are rare in spontaneous abortions. In contrast, monosomy for the X (Turner syndrome) is less frequent in liveborn infants but is the most common chromosome anomaly reported in spontaneous abortions.

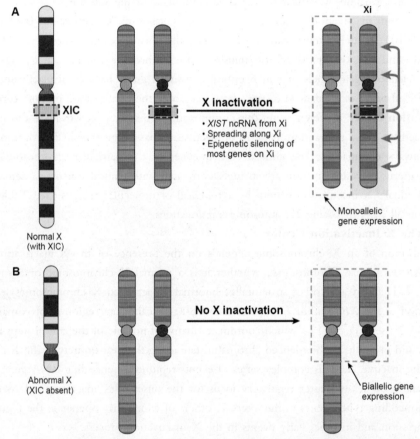

Figure 5-11 X chromosome inactivation and dependence on X inactivation center (XIC)
(A) On normal X chromosomes, XIC lies within an approximately 800-kb candidate region in Xq13.2 that contains a number of noncoding RNA (ncRNA) genes, including *XIST*, the master X inactivation control gene. In early development in XX embryos, the *XIST* RNA spreads along the length of one X, which will become the inactive X (Xi), with epigenetic silencing of most genes on that X chromosome, resulting in monoallelic expression of most, but not all X-linked genes. (B) On structurally abnormal X chromosomes that lack the XIC, X inactivation cannot occur and genes present on the abnormal X are expressed biallelically. Although a fairly large abnormal X is shown here for illustrative purposes, in fact only very small such fragments are observed in female patients, who invariably display significant congenital anomalies, suggesting that biallelic expression of larger numbers of X-linked genes is inconsistent with normal development and is likely inviable.

Sex Chromosome Aneuploidy

The incidence and major features of the four conditions associated with sex chromosome aneuploidy are compared in Tables 5-4 and 5-5. These well-defined syndromes are important causes of infertility, abnormal development, or both, and thus warrant a more detailed description. The effects of these chromosome abnormalities on development have been studied in long-term multicenter studies of hundreds of affected individuals, some of whom have been monitored for more than 40 years. As a group, those with sex chromosome aneuploidy show reduced levels of psychosocial adaptation, educational achievement, occupational performance, and economic independence, and on average they score slightly lower on intelligence (IQ) tests than their peers. However, each group shows high variability, making it impossible to generalize to specific cases. In fact, the overall impression is a high degree of normalcy, particularly in adulthood, which is remarkable among those with major chromosomal anomalies. Because almost all patients with sex chromosome abnormalities have only mild developmental abnormalities, a parental decision regarding potential termination of a pregnancy in which the fetus is found to have this type of defect can be a very difficult and even controversial one.

Table 5-4 Incidence of Sex Chromosome Abnormalities

Sex	Disorder	Karyotype	Approximate Incidence
Male	Klinefelter syndrome	47,XXY	1/600 males
		48,XXXY	1/25,000 males
		Others (48,XXYY; 49,XXXYY; mosaics)	1/10,000 males
	47,XYY syndrome	47,XYY	1/1,000 males
	Other X or Y chromosome abnormalities		1/1,500 males
	XX testicular DSD	46,XX	1/20,000 males
		Overall incidence: 1/300 males	
Female	Turner syndrome	45,X	1/4,000 females
		46,X,i(Xq)	1/50,000 females
		Others (deletions, mosaics)	1/15,000 females
	Trisomy X	47,XXX	1/1,000 females
	Other X chromosome abnormalities		1/3,000 females
	XY gonadal dysgenesis	46,XY	1/20,000 females
	Androgen insensitivity syndrome	46,XY	1/20,000 females
		Overall incidence: 1/650 females	

Note: DSD, Disorder of sex development.

(From MILUNSKY A. Genetic disorders of the fetus[M]. 4th ed. Baltimore: Johns Hopkins University Press, 1998.)

Here, we use **Klinefelter syndrome** to illustrate the major principles of sex chromosome aneuploidy.

Klinefelter Syndrome (47,XXY)

Klinefelter patients are almost always infertile because of the failure of germ cell development, and patients are often identified clinically for the first time because of infertility. As such, Klinefelter syndrome is classified among **disorders of sex development**, as we shall see in the next section. Klinefelter syndrome is relatively common among infertile males (approximately 4%) or males with oligospermia or azoospermia (approximately 10%). In adulthood, persistent androgen deficiency may result in decreased muscle tone, a loss of libido, and decreased bone mineral density.

The incidence of Klinefelter syndrome is estimated to be as high as 1 in 600 male births.

Approximately half the cases result from nondisjunction in paternal meiosis I because of a failure of normal Xp/Yp recombination in the pseudoautosomal region. Among cases of maternal origin, most result from errors in maternal meiosis I. Maternal age is increased in such cases. Approximately 15% of Klinefelter patients have mosaic karyotypes, most commonly 46,XY/47,XXY. As a group, such mosaic patients have variable phenotypes, and some may have normal testicular development.

Although there is wide phenotypic variation among patients with this and other sex chromosome aneuploidies, some consistent phenotypic differences have been identified between patients with Klinefelter syndrome and chromosomally normal males (see Table 5-5). Verbal comprehension and ability are below those of 46,XY males. Patients with Klinefelter syndrome have a several-fold increased risk for learning difficulties, especially in reading, that may require educational intervention. Language difficulties may lead to shyness, unassertiveness, apparent immaturity, and an increased risk for depression. Although most Klinefelter males form normal adult relationships, many of the affected boys have relatively poor psychosocial adjustment. Because of the relatively mild yet variable phenotype, many cases are presumed to go undetected.

Table 5-5   Features of Sex Chromosome Aneuploidy Conditions

Feature	47,XXY Klinefelter Syndrome	47,XYY	47,XXX Trisomy X	45,X Turner Syndrome
Prevalence	1 in 600 male births	1 in 1,000 male births	1 in 1,000 female births	1 in 2,500 to 4,000 female births
Clinical phenotype	Tall male	Tall, but otherwise typical male appearance	Hypotonia, delayed milestones; language and learning difficulties; tend to be taller than average	Short stature, webbed neck, lymphedema; risk for cardiac abnormalities
Cognition/intelligence	Verbal IQ reduced to low-normal range; educational difficulties	Verbal IQ reduced to low-normal range; language delay; reading difficulties	Normal to low-normal range (both verbal and performance IQ decreased)	Typically normal, but performance IQ lower than verbal IQ
Behavioral phenotype	No major disorders; tendency to poor social adjustments, but normal adult relationships	Subset with specific behavioral problems likely associated with lower IQ	Typically, no behavioral problems; some anxiety and low self-esteem; reduced social skills	Typically normal, but impaired social adjustment
Sex development/fertility	Hypogonadism, azoospermia, infertility	Normal	Reduced fertility in some Premature ovarian failure	Gonadal dysgenesis, delayed maturation, infertility
Variant karyotypes	See Table 5-4		48,XXXX; 49,XXXXX Increased severity with additional X's	46,Xi(Xq); 45,X/ 46,XX mosaics; other mosaics

Review Points:

1. Down syndrome (also named trisomy 21). Karyotype: 46, XX(XY), +21.

Clinical Feature: mental retardation, a flat face, sparse, an abnormal pattern of palm creases, straight hair, and short stature.

2. Cri du Chat syndrome. also named 5P-syndrome.

Clinical Feature: Low birth weight, abnormal larynx development, adults have small heads, round face, small chin. Widely set eyes, poor muscle tone: difficulty walking and talking correctly, hyperactivity. Aggression, tantrums and severe mental retardation.

3. Klinefelter Syndrome. Karyotype: 47, XXY.

Clinical Feature: reduced sexual maturity and secondary sexual characteristics, breast swelling, no sperm, slow to learn.

4. Fragile X Syndrome.

Clinical Feature: large ears, long face, and prominent jaw large testes and the learning difficulties.

Study Questions:

1. In a woman with a 47,XXX karyotype, what types of gametes would theoretically be formed and in what proportions? What are the theoretical karyotypes and phenotypes of her progeny? What are the actual karyotypes and phenotypes of her progeny?

2. Individuals carrying a copy of the inv(9) described in the text are clinically normal. Provide two possible explanations.

3. The birth incidence rates of 47,XXY and 47,XYY males are approximately equal. Is this what you would expect on the basis of the possible origins of the two abnormal karyotypes? Please explain.

4. How can a person with an XX karyotype differentiate as a phenotypically normal male?

5. What are the expected clinical consequences of the following deletions? If the same amount of DNA is deleted in each case, why might the severity of each be different?

    a. 46,XX,del(13)(pter→p11.1:)

    b. 46,XY,del(Y)(pter→q12:)

    c. 46,XX,del(5)(p15)

    d. 46,XX,del(X)(q23q26)

6. Provide possible explanations for the fact that persons with X chromosome aneuploidy are clinically not completely normal.

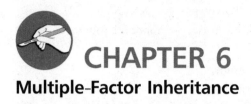

CHAPTER 6
Multiple-Factor Inheritance

Purpose and Requirement:

The chapter goals are to comprehend the multiple-factor hypothesis, give priority to the concepts about minor gene, additive effect, quantitative traits, quality traits, threshold, heritability, and complex diseases, and grasp the method of estimating heritability and recurrence risk of polygenetic diseases.

Common diseases such as congenital birth defects, myocardial infarction, cancer, neuropsychiatric disorders, diabetes, and Alzheimer disease cause morbidity and premature mortality in nearly two of every three individuals during their lifetimes (see Table 6-1). Many of these diseases "run in families"—cases seem to cluster among the relatives of affected individuals more frequently than in the general population. However, their inheritance generally does not follow one of the mendelian patterns seen in the single-gene disorders described in Chapter 3. This is because such diseases rarely result simply from inheriting one or two alleles of major effect at a single locus, as is the case for dominant and recessive mendelian disorders. Instead, they are thought to result from complex interactions among a number of genetic variants that alter susceptibility to disease, combined with certain environmental exposures and perhaps chance events as well, all of which acting together may trigger, accelerate, or protect against the disease process. For this reason, these disorders are considered to be **multifactorial** in origin, and the familial clustering generates a pattern of inheritance that is referred to as **complex**.

Table 6-1 Frequency of Different Types of Genetic Disease

Type	Incidence at Birth (per 1,000)	Prevalence at Age 25 (per 1,000)	Population Prevalence (per 1,000)
Disorders due to genome and chromosome mutations	6	1.8	3.8
Disorders due to single-gene mutations	10	3.6	20
Disorders with multifactorial inheritance	≈50	≈50	≈600

The familial clustering and complex inheritance seen with multifactorial disorders can be explained by recognizing that family members share a greater proportion of their genetic information and environmental exposures than individuals chosen at random in the population. Thus the relatives of an affected individual are more likely to experience the same **gene-gene** and **gene-environment interactions** that led to disease in the proband than are individuals who are unrelated to the proband.

In this chapter, we first address the question of how we infer that gene variants in the population predispose to such common diseases. We then describe how studies of familial aggregation and twin studies are used by geneticists to quantify the relative contributions of genetic variation and environment and show how these tools have been applied to multifactorial diseases. Finally, we devote the remainder of the chapter to describing a few examples of complex disorders where information is beginning to emerge about the specific nature of the genetic and environmental contributions to disease.

As we shall see in this chapter, the individual genes, the particular variants in those genes, and the environmental factors that interact with these variants have not yet been fully identified for the vast majority of common multifactorial diseases. A more detailed understanding of the approaches that geneticists use to identify the genetic factors underlying complex disease first requires a full appreciation of the distribution of genetic variation in different populations.

Ultimately, finding the genes and their variants that interact with the environment to contribute to susceptibility will give us a better understanding of the underlying processes leading to common multifactorial diseases and, perhaps, better tools for prevention or treatment.

6.1 Qualitative and Quantitative Traits

Multifactorial diseases with complex inheritance can be classified either as discrete **qualitative** traits or as continuous **quantitative** traits. A qualitative trait is the simpler of the two. A disease, such as lung cancer or rheumatoid arthritis, is either present or absent in an individual. Distinguishing between individuals who either have a disease or not is usually straightforward, but it may sometimes require detailed examination or specialized testing if the manifestations are subtle.

In contrast, a quantitative trait is a measurable physiological or biochemical quantity, such as height, blood pressure, serum cholesterol concentration, or body mass index, that varies among different individuals within a population. Although a quantitative trait varies continuously across a range of values, there are certain disease diagnoses, such as short stature, hypertension, hypercholesterolemia, or obesity, that are defined based on whether the value of the trait falls outside the so-called **normal range**, defined as an arbitrary interval around the population average. Frequently the normal range is derived by using the **normal distribution**, which is described in the next section, as an approximation for the distribution of the values of a quantitative trait in the population. Note that the term *normal* is used here in two different ways. Asserting that a physiological quantity has a "normal" distribution in the population and stating that an individual's value is in the "normal" range are different uses of the same word, one statistical and the other a measure of conformity to what is typically observed.

➤ The Normal Distribution

As is often the case with physiological quantities, such as systolic blood pressure, a graph of the number (or the fraction) of individuals in the population (Y-axis) having a particular quantitative value (X-axis) approximates the familiar, bell-shaped curve known as the **normal** (or **gaussian**) **distribution** (see Fig. 6-1A). The position of the peak and the width of the curve of the normal distribution are governed by two quantities, the **mean** (μ) and the **variance** (σ^2), respectively. The mean is the arithmetic average of the values, and because more people have values for the trait near the average, the curve ordinarily has its peak at the mean value. The variance (or its square root, σ, the **standard deviation**, abbreviated SD) is a measure of how much spread there is in the values to either side of the mean and therefore determines the breadth of the curve.

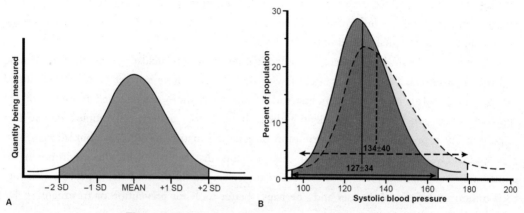

Figure 6-1   Distribution of quantitative trait variation

(A) The normal gaussian distribution, with mean (average) and standard deviations (SDs) indicated. For many traits, the "normal" range is considered the mean ± 2 SD, as indicated by the *shaded* region. (B) Distribution of systolic blood pressure in approximately 3,300 men aged 40 to 45 (*solid line*) and approximately 2,200 men aged 50 to 55 (*dotted line*). The mean and ± 2 SD are shown above *double-headed arrows*.

Any physiological quantity that can be measured across a sample of a population is a **quantitative phenotype**, and the mean and variance for that sample can be calculated and used to approximate the underlying mean and variance of the population from which the sample was drawn. For example, the systolic blood pressure of thousands of men in two different age-groups is shown in Figure 6-1B. The systolic blood pressure of the younger cohort is nearly symmetrical. In the older age-group, however, the curve becomes more "skewed" (asymmetrical), with more individuals with systolic blood pressures above the mean than below, indicating a tendency toward hypertension in that age-group.

The normal distribution provides guidelines for setting the limits of the normal range. A normal range is often defined as the values of a quantitative trait that are seen in approximately 95% of the population. Basic statistical theory states that when the values of a quantitative trait in a population follow the bell-shaped curve (i.e., are normally distributed), approximately 5% of the population will have measurements more than 2 SD above or below the population mean. For a given individual, however, it may still be perfectly "normal" (i.e., the individual is in good health), despite being a value outside the "normal" range.

6.2   Familial Aggregation and Correlation

6.2.1   Allele Sharing Among Relatives

The more closely related two individuals are in a family, the more alleles they have in common, inherited from their common ancestors. The most extreme examples of two individuals having alleles in common are identical (**monozygotic** [MZ]) twins, who have the same alleles at every locus. The next most closely related individuals in a family are **first-degree relatives**, such as a parent and child or a pair of sibs, including fraternal (**dizygotic** [DZ]) twins. In a parent-child pair, the child has exactly one allele out of two (50% of alleles) in common with each parent at every locus, that is, the allele the child inherited from that parent. Siblings (including DZ twins) also have 50% of their alleles in common with their other siblings, but this is only on average. This is because a pair of sibs inherits the same two alleles at a locus one fourth of the time, no alleles in common one fourth of the time, and one allele in common one half of the time (see Fig. 6-2). At any one locus therefore, the average number of alleles an individual is expected to share with a sibling is given by:

$$1/4(2 \text{ alleles}) + 1/4(0 \text{ allele}) + 1/2(1 \text{ allele}) = 0.5 + 0 + 0.5 = 1 \text{ allele}$$

The more distantly related two members of a family are, the fewer alleles they will have in common, inherited from a common ancestor.

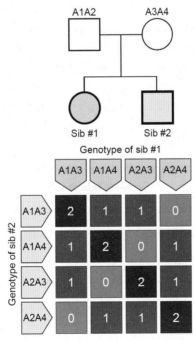

Figure 6-2   Allele sharing at an arbitrary locus between sibs concordant for a disease

The parents' genotypes are shown as A1A2 for the father and A3A4 for the mother. All four possible genotypes for sib #1 are given across the top of the table, and all four possible genotypes for sib #2 are given along the left side of the table. The numbers inside the boxes represent the number of alleles both sibs have in common for all 16 different combinations of genotypes for both sibs. For example, the upper left-hand corner has the number 2 because sib #1 and sib #2 both have the genotype A1A3 and so have both A1 and A3 alleles in common. The bottom left-hand corner contains the number 0 because sib #1 has genotype A1A3, whereas sib #2 has genotype A2A4, so there are no alleles in common.

6.2.2　Familial Aggregation in Qualitative Traits

If certain alleles increase the chance of developing a disease, one would expect an affected individual to have a greater-than-expected number of affected relatives compared to what would be predicted from the frequency of the disease in the general population (**familial aggregation of disease**). This is because the more closely related the family members are to the affected relative, the more they will share the relevant alleles and the greater their chance of also being affected. Here, we will present two approaches to measuring familial aggregation: relative risk ratios and family history case-control studies.

Relative Risk Ratio

One way to measure familial aggregation of a disease is by comparing the frequency of the disease in the relatives of an affected proband with its frequency (prevalence) in the general population. The **relative risk ratio** λ_r (where the subscript "r" refers to relatives) is defined as:

$$\lambda_r = \frac{\text{Prevalence of the disease in the relatives of an affected person}}{\text{Prevalence of the disease in the general population}}$$

The value of λ_r as a measure of familial aggregation depends both on how frequently a disease is found to have recurred in a relative of an affected individual (the numerator) and on the population prevalence (the denominator). The larger λ_r is, the greater is the familial aggregation. The population prevalence enters into the calculation because the more common a disease is, the greater is the likelihood that aggregation may be just a coincidence based on drawing alleles from the overall gene pool rather than a result of sharing the alleles that predispose to disease because of familial inheritance. A value of $\lambda_r = 1$ indicates that a relative is no more likely to develop the disease than is any individual in the population, whereas a value greater than 1 indicates that a relative is more likely to develop the disease. In practice, one measures λ for a particular class of relatives (e.g., r=s for sibs or r=p for parents). Examples of relative risk ratios determined for various diseases in samples of siblings (thus, λ_s) are shown in Table 6-2.

Table 6-2　Risk Ratios λ_s for Siblings of Probands With Diseases With Familial Aggregation and Complex Inheritance

Disease	Relationship	λ_s
Schizophrenia	Siblings	12
Autism	Siblings	150
Manic-depressive (bipolar) disorder	Siblings	7
Type 1 diabetes mellitus	Siblings	35
Crohn disease	Siblings	25
Multiple sclerosis	Siblings	24

6.2.3　Family History Case-Control Studies

Another approach to assessing familial aggregation is the **case-control study**, in which patients with a disease (the cases) are compared with suitably chosen individuals without the disease (the controls), with respect to family history of disease (as well as other factors, such as environmental exposures, occupation, geographical location, parity, and previous illnesses). To assess a possible genetic contribution to familial aggregation of a disease, the frequency with which the disease is found in the extended families of the cases (**positive family history**) is compared with the frequency of positive family history among suitable controls, matched for age and ethnicity, but who do not have the disease. Spouses are often used as controls in this situation because they usually match the cases in age and ethnicity and share the same household environment. Other frequently used controls are patients with unrelated diseases matched for age, occupation, and ethnicity. Thus, for example, in a study of **multiple sclerosis** (**MS**), approximately 3.5% of first-degree relatives of patients with MS also had MS, a prevalence that was much higher than among first-degree relatives of matched controls without MS (0.2%). Thus the odds of having a first-degree relative with MS were 18 times higher among MS patients than among controls. One can conclude therefore that substantial familial aggregation is occurring in MS, thereby providing evidence of a genetic predisposition to this disease.

6.2.4 Measuring the Genetic Contribution to Quantitative Traits

Just as a hereditary contribution to a disease increases familial aggregation for that disease, sharing of alleles that govern a particular quantitative trait affects the distribution of values of that trait in family members. The more sharing of alleles that govern a quantitative trait there is among relatives, the more similar the value of the trait will be among family members compared to what would be expected from the variance of the trait measured in the general population. The effect of genetic variation on quantitative traits is often measured and reported in two related ways: **correlation** between relatives and **heritability**.

(1) **Familial Correlation**

The tendency for the values of a physiological measurement to be more similar among relatives than it is in the general population is measured by determining the degree of **correlation** of particular physiological quantities among relatives. The **coefficient of correlation** (symbolized by the letter r) is a statistical measure of correlation applied to a pair of measurements, such as, for example, a child's serum cholesterol level and that of a parent. Accordingly, a **positive correlation** would exist between the cholesterol measurements in a group of patients and the cholesterol levels in their relatives if it is found that the higher a patient's level, the proportionately higher is the level in the patient's relatives. When a correlation exists, a graph of values in the proband and his or her relatives, in which each point represents a proband-relative pair of values, will tend to cluster around a straight line. In such examples, the value of r can range from 0 when there is no correlation to +1 for perfect positive correlation. In the example of serum cholesterol, Figure 6-3 shows a modest positive correlation ($r=0.294$) between serum cholesterol level of mothers aged 30 to 39 and those of their male children aged 4 to 9. In contrast, a **negative correlation** exists when the greater the increase in the patient's measurement, the lower the measurement is in the patient's relatives. The measurements are still correlated, but in the opposite direction. In such a case, the value of r can range from 0 to −1 for a perfect negative correlation.

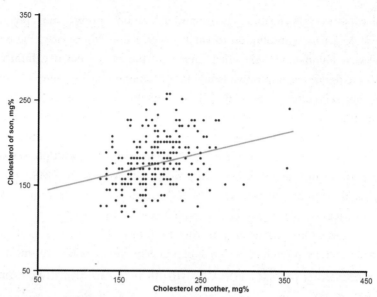

Figure 6-3 **Plot of serum cholesterol levels in a group of mothers aged 30 to 39 and in their male children aged 4 to 9**

Each dot represents a mother-son pair of measurements. The straight line is a "best fit" through the data points.

(2) Heritability

The concept of **heritability** of a quantitative trait (symbolized as H^2) was developed in an attempt to determine how much the genetic differences between individuals in a population contribute to variability of that trait in the population. H^2 is defined as the fraction of the total phenotypic variance of a quantitative trait that is due to allelic variation in the broadest sense, regardless of the mechanism by which the various alleles affect the phenotype. The higher the heritability, the greater is the contribution of genetic differences among people to the variability of the trait in the population. The value of H^2 varies from 0, if genotype contributes nothing to the total phenotypic variance in a population, to 1, if genotype is totally responsible for the phenotypic variance in that population.

Heritability of a human trait is a theoretical quantity that is usually estimated from the correlation between measurements of that trait among relatives of known degrees of relatedness, such as parents and children, siblings, or, as we shall see later in this chapter, twins.

6.3 Determining the Relative Contributions of Genes and Environment to Complex Disease

6.3.1 Distinguishing Between Genetic and Environmental Influences Using Family Studies

For both qualitative and quantitative traits, similarities among family members are most likely the result of overlapping genotype and common exposure to nongenetic (i. e., environmental) factors such as socioeconomic status, local environment, dietary habits, or cultural behaviors, all of which are frequently shared among family members but are generally considered to be of nongenetic origin. Given evidence of familial aggregation of a disease or correlation of a quantitative trait, geneticists attempt to separate the relative contributions of genotype and environment to the phenotype using a variety of approaches. One approach is to compare λ_r measurements or quantitative trait correlations between relatives who are of varying degrees of relatedness to the proband. For example, if genes predispose to a disease, one would expect λ_r to be greatest for MZ twins, to be somewhat smaller for first-degree relatives such as sibs or parent-child pairs, and to continue to decrease as allele-sharing decreases among the more distant relatives in a family.

To illustrate this approach, consider **cleft lip with or without cleft palate**, or CL(P), one of the most common congenital malformations, affecting 1.4 per 1,000 newborns worldwide. CL(P) originates as a failure of fusion of embryonic tissues that will go to make up the upper lip and the hard palate at approximately the 35th day of gestation. It is a multifactorial disorder with complex inheritance; for reasons that are not well understood, approximately 60% to 80% of those affected with CL(P) are males. Despite the similarity in names, CL(P) is usually etiologically distinct from isolated cleft palate (i.e., without cleft lip).

CL(P) is heterogeneous and includes forms in which the clefting is only one feature of a syndrome that includes other anomalies, known as **syndromic CL(P)**, as well as forms that are not associated with other birth defects, which are known as **nonsyndromic CL(P)**. Syndromic CL(P) can be inherited as a mendelian single-gene disorder or can be caused by chromosome disorders (especially trisomy 13 and 4p⁻ deletion syndrome) or teratogenic exposure (rubella embryopathy, thalidomide, or anticonvulsants). Nonsyndromic CL(P) can also be inherited as a single-gene disorder but more commonly is a sporadic occurrence and demonstrates some degree of familial aggregation without an obvious mendelian inheritance pattern.

The risk for CL(P) in a child increases as a function of the number of relatives the child has who are affected with CL(P) and the more closely related they are to the child (see Table 6-3). The simplest explanation for this is that the more closely related one is to the proband and, the more probands there are in the family, the more likely one is to share disease susceptibility alleles with the probands. Therefore one's risk for the disorder increases.

Table 6-3   Risk for Cleft Lip With or Without Cleft Palate in a Child Depending on the Number of Affected Parents and Other Relatives

Affected Relatives	Risk for CL(P) (%)		
	No. of Affected Parents		
	0	1	2
None	0.1	3	34
One sibling	3	11	40
Two siblings	8	19	45
One sibling and one second-degree relative	6	16	43
One sibling and one third-degree relative	4	14	44

Note: CL(P), Cleft lip with or without cleft palate.

Another approach is to compare the disease relative risk ratio in biological relatives of the proband with that in biologically unrelated family members (e.g., adoptees or spouses), all living in the same household environment. Returning to MS, for example, λ_r is 190 for MZ twins and 20 to 40 for first-degree biological relatives (parents, children, and sibs). In contrast, λ_r is 1 for the adopted siblings of an affected individual, suggesting that most of the familial aggregation in MS is genetic rather than the result of a shared environment. A similar analysis can be carried out for quantitative traits such as blood pressure: no correlation exists between a child's blood pressure and that of his adopted siblings, in contrast to the positive correlation with blood pressure of biological siblings, all living in the same household.

6.3.2 Distinguishing Between Genetic and Environmental Influences Using Twin Studies

Of all methods used to separate genetic and environmental influences, geneticists have relied most heavily on twin studies.

(1) Twinning

MZ and DZ twins are "experiments of nature" that provide an excellent opportunity to separate environmental and genetic influences on phenotypes in humans. MZ twins arise from the cleavage of a single fertilized zygote into two separate zygotes early in embryogenesis. They occur in approximately 0.3% of all births, without significant differences among different ethnic groups. At the time the zygote cleaves in two, MZ twins start out with identical genotypes at every locus and are therefore often thought of as having identical genotypes and gene expression patterns.

In contrast, DZ twins arise from the simultaneous fertilization of two eggs by two sperm. Genetically, DZ twins are siblings who share a womb and, like all siblings, share, on average, 50% of the alleles at all loci. DZ twins are of the same sex half the time and of opposite sex the other half. In contrast to MZ twins, DZ twins occur with a frequency that varies as much as fivefold in different populations, from a low of 0.2% among Asians to more than 1% of births in parts of Africa and among African Americans.

The striking difference between MZ and DZ twins in their genetic makeup is most easily seen by comparing the pattern for a type of so-called DNA fingerprint in twins (see Fig. 6-4). This method of **DNA fingerprinting** is generated by simultaneously examining many DNA fragments of varying lengths that share a particular DNA sequence (minisatellite) and are located throughout the genome. MZ twins show an indistinguishable pattern, whereas many differences are seen between DZ twins, whether of same sex or not.

Disease Concordance in Monozygotic and Dizygotic Twins

When twins have the same disease, they are said to be **concordant** for that disorder. Conversely, when only one member of the pair of twins is affected and the other is not, the relatives are **discordant** for the disease. An examination of how frequently MZ twins are concordant for a disease is a powerful method for determining whether genotype alone is sufficient to produce a particular disease. The differences between a disease that is mendelian from one that shows complex inheritance are immediately evident. Using **sickle cell disease** as an example of a mendelian disorder, if one MZ twin has sickle cell disease, the other twin will always have the disease as well. In contrast, as an example of a multifactorial disorder, when one MZ twin has **type 1 diabetes mellitus** (previously known as insulin-dependent or juvenile diabetes), the other twin will also have type 1 diabetes in only approximately 40% of such twin pairs. Disease concordance less than 100% in MZ twins is strong evidence that nongenetic factors play a role in the disease. Such factors could include environmental influences, such as exposure to infection or diet, as well as other effects, such as somatic mutation, effects of aging, or epigenetic changes in gene expression in one twin compared with the other.

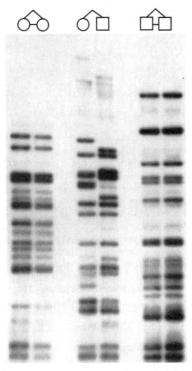

Figure 6-4   DNA fingerprinting of twins by detecting a variable number tandem repeat polymorphism

A class of polymorphism that has many alleles in loci around the genome due to variation in the number of copies repeated in tandem. Each pair of lanes contains DNA from a set of twins. The twins of the first and third sets have identical DNA fingerprints, indicating that they are identical (MZ) twins. The twins of the set in the middle have clearly distinguishable DNA fingerprints, confirming that they are fraternal (DZ) twins.

MZ and same-sex DZ twins share a common intrauterine environment and sex and are usually reared together in the same household by the same parents. Thus a comparison of concordance for a disease between MZ and same-sex DZ twins shows how frequently disease occurs when relatives who experience the same prenatal and often the same postnatal environment have the same alleles at every locus (MZ twins), compared with only 50% of their alleles in common (DZ twins). Greater concordance in MZ versus DZ twins is strong evidence of a genetic component to the disease, as shown in Table 6-4 for a number of disorders.

Table 6-4　Concordance Rates in MZ and DZ Twins for Various Multifactorial Disorders

Disorder	Concordance (%)[*]	
	MZ	DZ
Nontraumatic epilepsy	70	6
Multiple sclerosis	18	2
Type 1 diabetes	40	5
Schizophrenia	46	15
Bipolar disease	62	8
Osteoarthritis	32	16
Rheumatoid arthritis	12	3
Psoriasis	72	15
Cleft lip with or without cleft palate	30	2
Systemic lupus erythematosus	22	0

Note: * Rounded to the nearest percent. DZ, Dizygotic; MZ, monozygotic.

(2) Estimating Heritability from Twin Studies

Just as twin data may be used to assess the separate roles of genes and environment in qualitative disease traits, twins are also used to estimate the heritability of a quantitative trait using the correlation in the values of a physiological measurement in MZ and DZ twins. If one assumes that the alleles affecting the trait exert their effect additively (which is certainly overly simplistic and probably incorrect in many, if not all cases), MZ twins, who share 100% of their alleles, have twice the amount of allele sharing compared to that of DZ twins, who share 50% of their alleles on average. H^2, introduced earlier in this chapter, can therefore be approximated by taking twice the difference in the correlation coefficient r for a quantitative trait between MZ twins (r_{MZ}) and r between same-sex DZ twins (r_{DZ}) (as given by Falconer's formula):

$$H^2 = 2 \times (r_{MZ} - r_{DZ})$$

If the variability of the trait is determined chiefly by environment, the correlation within pairs of DZ twins will be similar to that seen between pairs of MZ twins. There will be little difference in the value of r for MZ and DZ twins. Thus, $r_{MZ} - r_{DZ} \approx 0$, and H^2 will approach 0. At the other extreme, however, if the variability is determined exclusively by genetic makeup, the correlation coefficient r between MZ pairs will approach 1, whereas r between DZ twins will be half of that. Now, $r_{MZ} - r_{DZ} \approx 1/2$, and therefore H^2 will be approximately $2 \times (1/2) = 1$.

Twins Reared Apart

Although a rare occurrence, twins are sometimes separated at birth for social reasons and placed in different homes, thus providing an opportunity to observe individuals of identical or half-identical genotypes reared in different environments. Such studies have been used primarily in research in psychiatric disorders, substance abuse, and eating disorders, in which strong environmental influences within the family are believed to play a role in the development of disease. For example, in one study of obesity, the **body mass index** (BMI; weight/height^2, expressed in kg/m^2) was measured in MZ and DZ twins reared in the same household versus those reared apart (see Table 6-5). Although the average BMI among MZ or DZ twins was similar, regardless of whether they were reared together or apart, the pairwise correlation for BMI between a pair of twins was much higher for the MZ than the DZ twins. Also interesting is that the higher correlation between MZ versus DZ twins was independent of whether the twins were reared together or apart, which suggests that genotype has a highly significant impact on adult weight and consequently on the risk for obesity and its complications.

Table 6-5 Pairwise Correlation of BMI Between MZ and DZ Twins Reared Together and Apart

Twin Type	Rearing	Men			Women		
		No. of Pairs	BMI*	Pairwise Correlation	No. of Pairs	BMI*	Pairwise Correlation
Monozygotic	Apart	49	24.8±2.4	0.70	44	24.2±3.4	0.66
	Together	66	24.2±2.9	0.74	88	23.7±3.5	0.66
Dizygotic	Apart	75	25.1±3.0	0.15	143	24.9±4.1	0.25
	Together	89	24.6±2.7	0.33	119	23.9±3.5	0.27

Note: * Mean ± 1 SD. BMI, Body mass index; DZ, dizygotic; MZ, monozygotic.

6.3.3 Limitations of Familial Aggregation and Heritability Estimates From Family and Twin Studies

(1) Potential Sources of Bias

There are a number of difficulties in measuring and interpreting λ_s. One is that studies of familial aggregation of disease are subject to various forms of **bias**. There is **ascertainment bias**, which arises when families with more than one affected sibling are more likely to come to a researcher's attention, thereby inflating the sibling recurrence risk λ_s. Ascertainment bias is also a problem for twin studies. Many studies rely on asking one twin with a particular disease to recruit the other twin to participate in a study (**volunteer-based ascertainment**), rather than ascertaining them first as twins through a twin registry and only then examining their health status (**population-based ascertainment**). Volunteer-based ascertainment can give biased results because twins, particularly MZ twins who may be emotionally close, are more likely to volunteer if they are concordant than if they are not, which inflates the concordance rate.

Similarly, because case-control studies of family history often rely, for practical reasons, on taking a history from the proband rather than examining all the relatives directly, there may be **recall bias**, in which a proband may be more likely to know of family members with the same or similar disease, than would the controls. Such biases will inflate the level of familial aggregation.

Other difficulties arise in measuring and interpreting heritability. The same trait may yield different measurements of heritability in different populations because of different allele frequencies or diverse environmental conditions. For example, heritability measurements of height would be lower when measured in a population with widespread famine that stunts growth in childhood as compared to the same population after food becomes plentiful.

Heritability of a trait should therefore not be thought of as an intrinsic, universally applicable measure of "how genetic" the trait is, because it depends on the population and environment in which the estimate is being made. Although heritability estimates are still made in genetic research, most geneticists consider them to be only crude estimates of the role of genetic variation in causing phenotypic variation.

(2) Potential Genetic or Epigenetic Differences

Despite the evident power of twin studies, one must caution against thinking of such studies as perfectly controlled experiments that compare individuals who share either half or all of their genetic variation and are exposed either to the same or to different environments. Studies of MZ twins assume the twins are genetically identical. Although this is mostly true, genotype and gene expression patterns may come to differ between MZ twins because of genetic or epigenetic changes that occur after the cleavage event that produced the MZ twin embryos. There are a number of ways that MZ twins may differ in their genotypes or patterns of gene expression. Genotype may differ due to somatic rearrangements and/or rare somatic mutations that occur after the cleavage event. Epigenetic changes may occur in response to environmental or stochastic factors, thus leading to differences in gene expression between MZ twins. (Female MZ twins have an additional source of variability, because of the stochastic nature of X inactivation patterns in various tissues.)

(3) Other Limitations

Another problem may arise when assuming that the environmental exposure of MZ and DZ twins has been held constant when they are reared together but not when twins are reared apart. Environmental exposures, including even intrauterine environment, may vary for twins reared in the same family. For example, MZ twins frequently share a placenta, and there may be a disparity between the twins in blood supply, intrauterine development, and birth weight. For late-onset diseases, such as neurodegenerative disease of late adulthood, the assumption that MZ and DZ twins are exposed to similar environments throughout their adult lives becomes less and less valid, and thus a difference in concordance provides less strong evidence for genetic factors in disease causation. Conversely, one assumes that by determining disease concordance in MZ twins reared apart, one is measuring the effect of different environments on the same genotype. However, the environment of twins reared apart may actually not be as different as one might suppose. Thus no twin study is a perfectly controlled assessment of genetic versus environmental influence.

Finally, caution is necessary when generalizing from twin studies. The most extreme situation would be when the phenotype being studied is only sometimes genetic in origin. That is, nongenetic phenocopies may exist. If genotype alone causes the disease in half the pairs of twins (MZ twin concordance of 100%) in your sample and a nongenetic phenocopy affects only one twin of the other half of twin pairs in your sample (MZ twin concordance of 0%), twin studies will show an intermediate level of 50% concordance that really applies to neither form of the disease.

6.4 Examples of Common Multifactorial Diseases With a Genetic Contribution

In this section and the next, we turn to considering examples of several common conditions that illustrate general concepts of multifactorial disorders and their complex inheritance, as summarized here.

Characteristics of Inheritance of Complex Diseases:

- Genetic variation contributes to diseases with complex inheritance, but these diseases are not single-gene disorders and do not demonstrate a simple mendelian pattern of inheritance.

- Diseases with complex inheritance often demonstrate familial aggregation because relatives of an affected individual are more likely to have disease-predisposing alleles in common with the affected person than with unrelated individuals.

- Diseases with complex inheritance are more common among the close relatives of a proband and become less common in relatives who are less closely related and therefore share fewer predisposing alleles. Greater concordance for disease is expected among monozygotic versus dizygotic twins.

- However, pairs of relatives who share disease-predisposing genotypes at relevant loci may still be discordant for phenotype (show lack of penetrance) because of the crucial role of nongenetic factors in disease causation. The most extreme examples of lack of penetrance despite identical genotypes are discordant monozygotic twins.

6.4.1 Multifactorial Congenital Malformations

Many common congenital malformations, occurring as isolated defects and not as part of a syndrome, are multifactorial and demonstrate complex inheritance (see Table 6-6). Among these, **congenital heart malformations** are some of the most common and serve to illustrate the current state of understanding of other categories of congenital malformation.

Table 6-6 Some Common Congenital Malformations With Multifactorial Inheritance

Malformation	Approximate Population Incidence (per 1,000)
Cleft lip with or without cleft palate	0.4~1.7
Cleft palate	0.4
Congenital dislocation of hip	2.0[*]
Congenital heart defects	4.0~8.0
Ventricular septal defect	1.7
Patent ductus arteriosus	0.5
Atrial septal defect	1.0
Aortic stenosis	0.5
Neural tube defects	2.0~10.0
Spina bifida and anencephaly	Variable
Pyloric stenosis	1.0, [†]5.0[*]

Note: [*] Per 1,000 males. [†] Per 1,000 females.

Congenital heart defects (CHDs) occur at a frequency of approximately 4 to 8 per 1,000 births. They are a heterogeneous group, caused in some cases by single-gene or chromosomal mechanisms and in others by exposure to teratogens, such as rubella infection or maternal diabetes. The cause is usually unknown, however, and the majority of cases are believed to be multifactorial in origin.

There are many types of CHDs, with different population incidences and empirical risks. It is known that when heart defects recur in a family, however, the affected children do not necessarily have exactly the same anatomical defect but instead show recurrence of lesions that are similar with regard to developmental mechanisms. By using developmental mechanisms as a classification scheme, five main groups of CHDs can be distinguished:

- Flow lesions.
- Defects in cell migration.
- Defects in cell death.
- Abnormalities in extracellular matrix.
- Defects in targeted growth.

The subtype of congenital heart malformations known as flow lesions illustrates the familial aggregation and elevated risk for recurrence in relatives of an affected individual, all characteristic of a complex trait (see Table 6-7). Flow lesions, which constitute approximately 50% of all CHDs, include hypoplastic left heart syndrome, coarctation of the aorta, atrial septal defect of the secundum type, pulmonary valve stenosis, a common type of ventricular septal defect, and other forms (see Fig. 6-5). Up to 25% of patients with flow lesions, particularly tetralogy of Fallot, may have the deletion of chromosome region 22q11 seen in the **velocardiofacial syndrome**.

Certain CHDs are inherited as multifactorial traits. Until more is known, the figures shown in Table 6-7 can be used as estimates of the recurrence risk for flow lesions in first-degree relatives. There is, however, a rapid falloff in risk (to levels not much higher than the population risk) in second- and third-degree relatives of index patients with flow lesions. Similarly, relatives of index patients with types of CHDs other than flow lesions can be offered reassurance that their risk is no greater than that of the general population. For further reassurance, many CHDs can now be assessed prenatally by ultrasonography.

Table 6-7   Population Incidence and Recurrence Risks for Various Flow Lesions

Defect	Population Incidence (%)	Frequency in Sibs (%)	λ_s
Ventricular septal defect	0.170	4.3	25
Patent ductus arteriosus	0.083	3.2	38
Atrial septal defect	0.066	3.2	48
Aortic stenosis	0.044	2.6	59

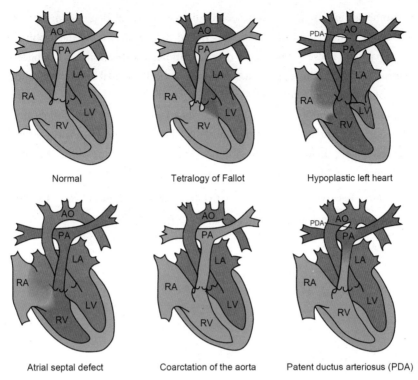

Figure 6-5   Diagram of various flow lesions seen in congenital heart disease

Blood on the left side of the circulation is shown in *red*, on the right side in *blue*. Abnormal admixture of oxygenated and deoxygenated blood is *purple*. AO, Aorta; LA, left atrium; LV, left ventricle; PA, pulmonary artery; RA, right atrium; RV, right ventricle.

6.4.2   Neuropsychiatric Disorders

Mental illnesses are some of the most common and perplexing of human diseases, affecting 4% of the human population worldwide. The annual cost in medical care and social services exceeds $150 billion in the United States alone. Among the most severe of the mental illnesses are schizophrenia and bipolar disease (manic-depressive illness).

Schizophrenia affects 1% of the world's population. It is a devastating psychiatric illness, with onset commonly in late adolescence or young adulthood, and is characterized by abnormalities in thought, emotion, and social relationships, often associated with delusional thinking and disordered mood. A genetic contribution to schizophrenia is supported by both twin and family aggregation studies. MZ concordance in schizophrenia is estimated to be 40% to 60%; DZ concordance is 10% to 16%. The recurrence risk ratio is elevated in first- and second-degree relatives of schizophrenic patients (see Table 6-8).

Although there is considerable evidence of a genetic contribution to schizophrenia, only a subset of the genes and alleles that predispose to the disease has been identified to date. A major exception is the small percentage (<2%) of all schizophrenia that is found in individuals with interstitial deletions of particular chromosomes, such as the 22q11 deletion responsible for the velocardiofacial syndrome. It is estimated that 25% of patients with 22q11 deletions develop schizophrenia, even in the absence of many or most of the other physical signs of the syndrome. The mechanism by which a deletion of 3 Mb of DNA on 22q11 causes mental illness in patients with this syndrome is unknown. Chromosomal microarrays have been used to scan the entire genome for other deletions and duplications, many too small to be detectable by standard cytogenetic approaches. These studies have revealed numerous deletions and duplications (copy number variants [CNVs]) throughout the genome in both normal individuals and individuals with a variety of psychiatric and neurodevelopmental disorders. In particular, small (1- to 1.5-Mb) interstitial deletions at 1q21.1, 15q11.2, and 15q13.3 have been implicated repeatedly in a small fraction of patients with schizophrenia. For the vast majority of patients with schizophrenia, however, genetic lesions are not known, and counseling therefore relies on empirical risk figures (see Table 6-8).

Table 6-8   Recurrence Risks and Relative Risk Ratios in Schizophrenia Families

Relation to Individual Affected by Schizophrenia	Recurrence Risk (%)	λ_r
Child of two schizophrenic parents	46	23
Child	9~16	11.5
Sibling	8~14	11
Nephew or niece	1~4	2.5
Uncle or aunt	2	2
First cousin	2~6	4
Grandchild	2~8	5

Bipolar disease is predominantly a mood disorder in which episodes of mood elevation, grandiosity, high-risk dangerous behavior, and inflated self-esteem (mania) alternate with periods of depression, decreased interest in what are normally pleasurable activities, feelings of worthlessness, and suicidal thinking. The prevalence of bipolar disease is 0.8% , approximately equal to that of schizophrenia, with a similar age at onset. The seriousness of this condition is underscored by the high (10% to 15%) rate of suicide in affected patients.

A genetic contribution to bipolar disease is strongly supported by twin and family aggregation studies. MZ twin concordance is 40% to 60%. DZ twin concordance is 4% to 8%. Disease risk is also elevated in relatives of affected individuals (see Table 6-9). One striking aspect of bipolar disease in families is that the condition has variable expressivity. Some members of the same family demonstrate classic bipolar illness, others have depression alone (unipolar disorder) , and others carry a diagnosis of a psychiatric syndrome that involves both thought and mood (**schizoaffective disorder**). Even less is known about genes and alleles that predispose to bipolar disease than is known for schizophrenia. In particular, although an increase in de novo deletions or duplications has been identified in bipolar psychosis, recurrent CNVs involving particular regions of the genome have not been identified. Counseling therefore typically relies on empirical risk figures (see Table 6-9).

Table 6-9   Recurrence Risks and Relative Risk Ratios in Bipolar Disorder Families

Relation to Individual Affected with Bipolar Disease	Recurrence Risk (%) *	λ_r
Child of two parents with bipolar disease	50~70	75
Child	27	34
Sibling	20~30	31
Second-degree relative	5	6

Note: * Recurrence of bipolar, unipolar, or schizoaffective disorder.

6.4.3   Coronary Artery Disease

Coronary artery disease (CAD) kills approximately 500,000 individuals in the United States yearly and is one of the most frequent causes of morbidity and mortality in the developed world. CAD due to atherosclerosis is the major cause of the nearly 1,500,000 cases of myocardial infarction (MI) and the more than 200,000 deaths from acute MI occurring annually. In the aggregate, CAD costs more than \$143 billion in health care expenses alone each year in the United States, not including lost productivity. For unknown reasons, males are at higher risk for CAD both in the general population and within affected families.

Family studies have repeatedly supported a role for heredity in CAD, particularly when it occurs in relatively young individuals. The pattern of increased risk suggests that when the proband is female or young, there is likely to be a greater genetic contribution to MI in the family, thereby increasing the risk for disease in the proband's relatives. For example, the recurrence risk (see Table 6-10) in male first-degree relatives of a female proband is sevenfold greater than that in the general population, compared with the 2.5-fold increased risk in female relatives of a male proband. When the proband is young (<55 years) and female, the risk for CAD is more than 11 times greater than that of the general population. Having multiple relatives affected at a young age increases risk substantially as well. Twin studies also support a role for genetic variants in CAD (see Table 6-11).

Table 6-10   Risk for Coronary Artery Disease in Relatives of a Proband

Proband	Increased Risk for CAD in a Family Member *
Male	3-fold in male first-degree relatives 2.5-fold in female first-degree relatives
Female	7-fold in male first-degree relatives
Female <55 years of age	11.4-fold in male first-degree relatives
Two male relatives <55 years of age	13-fold in first-degree relatives

Note: * Relative to the risk in the general population. CAD, Coronary artery disease.

(Data from SILBERBERG J S, WLODARCZYK J, FRYER J, et al. Risk associated with various definitions of family history of coronary heart disease: The Newcastle family history study II [J]. American journal of epidemiology, 1998,147(12):1133−1139.)

Table 6-11 Twin Concordance Rates and Relative Risks for Fatal Myocardial Infarction When Proband Had Early Fatal Myocardial Infarction*

Sex of the Twins	Concordance MZ Twins	Increased Risk[†] in a MZ Twin	Concordance DZ Twins	Increased Risk[†] in a DZ Twin
Male	0.39	6- to 8-fold	0.26	3-fold
Female	0.44	15-fold	0.14	2.6-fold

Note: * Early myocardial infarction defined as age <55 years in males, age <65 years in females. † Relative to the risk in the general population. DZ, Dizygotic; MZ, monozygotic.

(Data from MARENBERG M E, RISCH N, BERKMAN L F, et al. Genetic susceptibility to death from coronary heart disease in a study of twins[J]. The new england journal of medicine, 1994,330(15):1041−1046.)

A few mendelian disorders leading to CAD are known. **Familial hypercholesterolemia**, an autosomal dominant defect of the low-density lipoprotein (LDL) receptor, is one of the most common of these but accounts for only approximately 5% of survivors of MI. Most cases of CAD show multifactorial inheritance, with both nongenetic and genetic predisposing factors. There are many stages in the evolution of atherosclerotic lesions in the coronary artery. What begins as a fatty streak in the intima of the artery evolves into a fibrous plaque containing smooth muscle, lipid, and fibrous tissue. These intimal plaques become vascular and may bleed, ulcerate, and calcify, thereby causing severe vessel narrowing as well as providing fertile ground for thrombosis, resulting in sudden, complete occlusion and MI. Given the many stages in the evolution of atherosclerotic lesions in the coronary artery, it is not surprising that many genetic differences affecting the various pathological processes involved could predispose to or protect from CAD (see Fig. 6-6). Additional risk factors for CAD include other disorders that are themselves multifactorial with genetic components, such as hypertension, obesity, and diabetes mellitus. The metabolic and physiological derangements represented by these disorders also contribute to enhancing the risk for CAD. Finally, diet, physical activity, systemic inflammation, and smoking are environmental factors that also play a major role in influencing the risk for CAD. Given all the different processes, metabolic derangements, and environmental factors that contribute to the development of CAD, it is easy to imagine that genetic susceptibility to CAD could be a complex multifactorial condition.

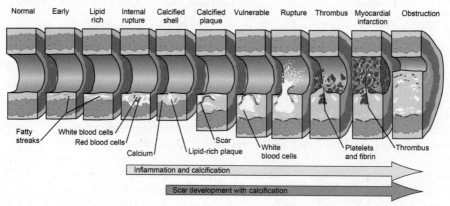

Figure 6-6 Sections of coronary artery demonstrating the steps leading to coronary artery disease
Genetic and environmental factors operating at any or all of the steps in this pathway can contribute to the development of this complex, common disease.

CAD is often an incidental finding in family histories of patients with other genetic diseases. In view of the high recurrence risk, physicians and genetic counselors may need to consider whether first-degree relatives of patients with CAD should be evaluated further and offered counseling and therapy, even when CAD is not the primary genetic problem for which the patient or relative has been referred. Such an evaluation is clearly indicated when the proband is young, particularly if the proband is female.

6.5   Examples of Multifactorial Traits for Which Specific Genetic and Environmental Factors are Known

Up to this point, we have described some of the epidemiological approaches involving family and twin studies that are used to assess the extent to which there may be a genetic contribution to a complex trait. It is important to realize, however, that studies of familial aggregation, disease concordance, or heritability do not specify how many loci there are, which loci and alleles are involved, or how a particular genotype and set of environmental influences interact to cause a disease or to determine the value of a particular physiological measurement. In most cases, all we can show is that there is some genetic contribution and estimate its magnitude. There are, however, a few multifactorial diseases with complex inheritance for which we have begun to identify the genetic and, in some cases, environmental factors responsible for increasing disease susceptibility. We give a few examples in the next part of this chapter, illustrating increasing levels of complexity.

6.5.1   Modifier Genes in Mendelian Disorders

Allelic variation at a single locus can explain variation in the phenotype in many single-gene disorders. However, even for well-characterized mendelian disorders known to be due to defects in a single gene, variation at other gene loci may impact some aspect of the phenotype, illustrating features therefore of complex inheritance.

In **cystic fibrosis (CF)**, for example, whether or not a patient has pancreatic insufficiency requiring enzyme replacement can be explained largely by which mutant alleles are present in the *CFTR* gene. The correlation is imperfect, however, for other phenotypes. For example, the variation in the degree of pulmonary disease seen in CF patients remains unexplained by allelic heterogeneity. It has been proposed that the genotype at other genetic loci could act as **genetic modifiers**, that is, genes whose alleles have an effect on the severity of pulmonary disease seen in CF patients. For example, reduction in forced expiratory volume after one second (FEV_1), calculated as a percentage of the value expected for CF patients (a CF-specific FEV_1 percent), is a quantitative trait commonly used to measure deterioration in pulmonary function in CF patients. A comparison of CF-specific FEV_1 percent in affected MZ versus affected DZ twins provides an estimate of the heritability of the severity of lung disease in CF patients of approximately 50%. This value is independent of the specific *CFTR* allele(s) (because both kinds of twins will have the same CF mutations).

Two loci harboring alleles responsible for modifying the severity of pulmonary disease in CF are known: *MBL2*, a gene that encodes a serum protein called mannose-binding lectin; and the *TGFB1* locus encoding the cytokine transforming growth factor β (TGFβ). Mannose-binding lectin is a plasma protein in the innate immune system that binds to many pathogenic organisms and aids in their destruction by phagocytosis and complement activation. A number of common alleles that result in reduced blood levels of the lectin exist at the *MBL2* locus in European populations. Lower levels of mannose-binding lectin appear associated with worse outcomes for CF lung disease, perhaps because low levels of lectin result in difficulties with containing respiratory pathogens, particularly Pseudomonas. Alleles at the *TGFB1* locus that result in higher TGFβ production are also associated with worse outcome, perhaps because TGFβ promotes lung scarring and fibrosis after inflammation. Thus both *MBL2* and *TGFB1* are **modifier genes**, variants at which—while they do not cause CF—can modify the clinical phenotype associated with disease-causing alleles at the *CFTR* locus.

6.5.2 Digenic Inheritance

The next level of complexity is a disorder determined by the additive effect of the genotypes at two or more loci. One clear example of such a disease phenotype has been found in a few families of patients with a form of retinal degeneration called **retinitis pigmentosa** (**RP**) (see Fig. 6-7). Affected individuals in these families are heterozygous for mutant alleles at two different loci (**double heterozygotes**). One locus encodes the photoreceptor membrane protein peripherin and the other encodes a related photoreceptor membrane protein called Rom1. Heterozygotes for only one or the other of these mutations in these families are unaffected. Thus the RP in this family is caused by the simplest form of multigenic inheritance, inheritance due to the effect of mutant alleles at two loci, without any known environmental factors that influence disease occurrence or severity. The proteins encoded by these two genes are likely to have overlapping physiological function because they are both located in the stacks of membranous disks found in retinal photoreceptors. It is the additive effect of having an abnormality in two proteins with overlapping function that produces disease.

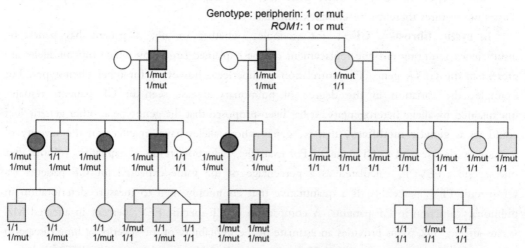

Figure 6-7 Pedigree of a family with retinitis pigmentosa due to digenic inheritance
Dark *blue* symbols are affected individuals. Each individual's genotypes at the peripherin locus (*first line*) and *ROM1* locus (*second line*) are written below each symbol. The normal allele is 1; the mutant allele is mut. *Light blue* symbols are unaffected, despite carrying a mutation in one or the other gene. (Redrawn from KAJIWARA K, BERSON E L, DRYJA T P. Digenic retinitis pigmentosa due to mutations at the unlinked peripherin/RDS and ROM1 loci[J]. Science, 1994,264(5165):1604-1608.)

A multigenic model has also been observed in a few families with **Bardet-Biedl syndrome**, a rare birth defect characterized by obesity, variable degrees of intellectual disability, retinal degeneration, polydactyly, and genitourinary malformations. Fourteen different genes have been found in which mutations cause the syndrome. Although inheritance is clearly autosomal recessive in most families, a few families appear to demonstrate digenic inheritance, in which the disease occurs only when an individual is homozygous for mutations at one of these 14 loci and is heterozygous for a mutation at another of the loci.

6.5.3 Gene-Environment Interactions in Venous Thrombosis

Another example of gene-gene interaction predisposing to disease is found in the group of conditions referred to as hypercoagulability states, in which venous or arterial clots form inappropriately and cause life-threatening complications of **thrombophilia**. With hypercoagulability, however, there is a third factor, an environmental influence that in the presence of the predisposing genetic factors, increases the risk for disease even more.

One such disorder is **idiopathic cerebral vein thrombosis**, a disease in which clots form in the venous system of the brain, causing catastrophic occlusion of cerebral veins in the absence of an inciting event such as infection or tumor. It affects young adults, and although quite rare (<1 per 100,000 in the population), it carries a high mortality rate (5% to 30%). Three relatively common factors—two genetic and one environmental—that lead to abnormal coagulability of the clotting system are each known to individually increase the risk for cerebral vein thrombosis (see Fig. 6-8):

- A missense variant in the gene for the clotting factor, factor V.
- A variant in the 3′ untranslated region (UTR) of the gene for the clotting factor prothrombin.
- The use of oral contraceptives.

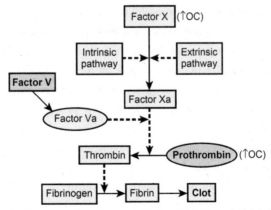

Figure 6-8 The clotting cascade relevant to factor V Leiden and prothrombin variants

Once factor X is activated, through either the intrinsic or extrinsic pathway, activated factor V promotes the production of the coagulant protein thrombin from prothrombin, which in turn cleaves fibrinogen to generate fibrin required for clot formation. Oral contraceptives (OC) increase blood levels of prothrombin and factor X as well as a number of other coagulation factors. The hypercoagulable state can be explained as a synergistic interaction of genetic and environmental factors that increase the levels of factor V, prothrombin, factor X and others to promote clotting. Activated forms of coagulation proteins are indicated by the letter a. *Solid arrows* are pathways; *dashed arrows* are stimulators.

A polymorphic allele of factor V, **factor V Leiden** (**FVL**), in which arginine is replaced by glutamine at position 506 (Arg506Gln), has a frequency of approximately 2.5% in white populations but is rarer in other population groups. This alteration affects a cleavage site used to degrade factor V, thereby making the protein more stable and able to exert its procoagulant effect for a longer duration. Heterozygous carriers of FVL, approximately 5% of the white population, have a risk for cerebral vein thrombosis that, although still quite low, is 7-fold higher than that in the general population. Homozygotes have a risk that is 8-fold higher.

The second genetic risk factor, a mutation in the **prothrombin** gene, changes a G to an A at position 20210 in the 3′ UTR of the gene (prothrombin g.20210G>A). Approximately 2.4% of white individuals are heterozygotes, but it is rare in other ethnic groups. This change appears to increase the level of prothrombin mRNA, resulting in increased translation and elevated levels of the protein. Being heterozygous for the prothrombin 20210G>A allele raises the risk for cerebral vein thrombosis 3- to 6-fold.

Finally, the use of **oral contraceptives** containing synthetic estrogen increases the risk for thrombosis 14- to 22-fold, independent of genotype at the factor V and prothrombin loci, probably by increasing the levels of many clotting factors in the blood. Although using oral contraceptives and being heterozygous for FVL cause only a modest increase in risk compared with either factor alone, oral contraceptive use in a heterozygote for prothrombin 20210G>A raises the relative risk for cerebral vein thrombosis 30- to 150-fold.

There is also interest in the role of FVL and prothrombin 20210G>A alleles in **deep venous thrombosis** (**DVT**) of the lower extremities, a condition that occurs in approximately 1 in 1,000 individuals per year, far more common than idiopathic cerebral venous thrombosis. Mortality due to DVT (primarily due to pulmonary embolus) can be up to 10%, depending on age and the presence of other medical conditions. Many environmental factors are known to increase the risk for DVT and include trauma, surgery (particularly orthopedic surgery), malignant disease, prolonged periods of immobility, oral contraceptive use, and advanced age.

The FVL allele increases the relative risk for a first episode of DVT 7-fold in heterozygotes. Heterozygotes who use oral contraceptives see their risk increased 30-fold compared with controls. Heterozygotes for prothrombin 20210G>A also have an increase in their relative risk for DVT of twofold to 3-fold. Notably, double heterozygotes for FVL and prothrombin 20210G>A have a relative increased risk of 20-fold—a risk approaching a few percent of the population.

Thus each of these three factors, two genetic and one environmental, on its own increases the risk for an abnormal hypercoagulable state. Having two or all three of these factors at the same time raises the risk even more, to the point that thrombophilia screening programs for selected populations of patients may be indicated in the future.

6.5.4 Type 1 Diabetes Mellitus

A common complex disease for which some of the underlying genetic architecture is being delineated is diabetes mellitus. Diabetes occurs in two major forms: type 1 (T1D) (sometimes referred to as insulin-dependent; IDDM) and type 2 (T2D) (sometimes referred to as non-insulin-dependent; NIDDM), representing approximately 10% and 88% of all cases, respectively. Familial aggregation is seen in both types of diabetes, but in any given family, usually only T1D or T2D is present. They differ in typical onset age, MZ twin concordance, and association with particular genetic variants at particular loci. Here, we focus on T1D to illustrate the major features of complex inheritance in diabetes.

T1D has an incidence in the white population of approximately 2 per 1,000 (0.2%), but this is lower in African and Asian populations. It usually manifests in childhood or adolescence. It results from autoimmune destruction of the β cells of the pancreas, which normally produce insulin. A large majority of children who will go on to have T1D develop multiple autoantibodies early in childhood against a variety of endogenous proteins, including insulin, well before they develop overt disease.

There is strong evidence for genetic factors in T1D: concordance among MZ twins is approximately 40%, which far exceeds the 5% concordance in DZ twins. The lifetime risk for T1D in siblings of an affected proband is approximately 7%, resulting in an estimated λs of ≈35. However, the earlier the age of onset of the T1D in the proband, the greater is λs.

(1) The Major Histocompatibility Complex

The major genetic factor in T1D is the major histocompatibility complex (MHC) locus, which spans some 3 Mb on chromosome 6 and is the most highly polymorphic locus in the human genome, with over 200 known genes (many involved in immune functions) and well over 2,000 alleles known in populations around the globe (see Fig. 6-9). On the basis of structural and functional differences, two major subclasses, the class Ⅰ and class Ⅱ genes, correspond to the **human leukocyte antigen (HLA)** genes, originally discovered by virtue of their importance in tissue transplantation between unrelated individuals. The HLA class Ⅰ (HLA-A, HLA-B, HLA-C) and class Ⅱ (HLA-DR, HLA-DQ, HLA-DP) genes encode cell surface proteins that play a critical role in the presentation of antigen to lymphocytes, which cannot recognize and respond to an antigen unless it is complexed with an HLA molecule on the surface of an antigen-presenting cell. Within the MHC, the HLA class Ⅰ and class Ⅱ genes are by far the most highly polymorphic loci (see Fig. 6-9).

The original studies showing an association between T1D and alleles designated as *HLA-DR*3 and *HLA-DR*4 relied on a serological method in use at that time for distinguishing between different HLA alleles, one that was based on immunological reactions in a test tube. This method has long been superseded by direct determination of the DNA sequence of different alleles, and sequencing of the MHC in a large number of individuals has revealed that the serologically determined "alleles" associated with T1D are not single alleles at all. Both *DR*3 and *DR*4 can be subdivided into a dozen or more alleles located at a locus now termed *HLA-DRB*1.

(2) Genes Other Than Class Ⅱ Major Histocompatibility Complex Loci in Type 1 Diabetes

The MHC haplotype alone accounts for only a portion of the genetic contribution to the risk for T1D in siblings of a proband. Family studies in T1D (see Table 6-12) suggest that even when siblings share the same MHC class Ⅱ haplotypes, the risk for disease is only approximately 17%, still well below the MZ twin concordance rate of approximately 40%. Thus there must be other genes, elsewhere in the genome, that contribute to the development of T1D, assuming that MZ twins and sibs have similar environmental exposures. Indeed, genetic association studies indicate that variation at nearly 50 different loci around the genome can increase susceptibility to T1D, although most have very small effects on increasing disease susceptibility.

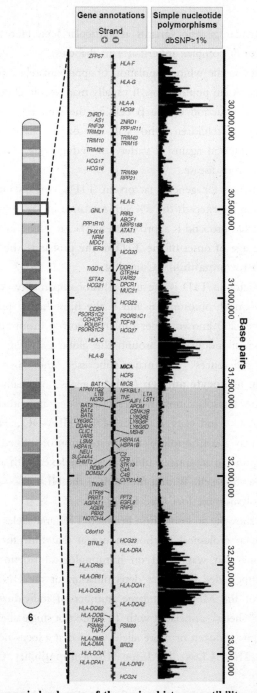

Figure 6-9　Genomic landscape of the major histocompatibility complex (MHC)

The classic MHC is shown on the short arm of chromosome 6, comprising the class I region (*yellow*) and class II region (*blue*), both enriched in human leukocyte antigen (HLA) genes. Sequence-level variation is shown for single nucleotide polymorphisms (SNPs) found with at least 1% frequency. Remarkably high levels of polymorphism are seen in regions containing the classic HLA genes where variation is enriched in coding exons involved in defining the antigen-binding cleft. Other genes (*pink*) in the MHC region show lower levels of polymorphism. dbSNP, minor allele frequency in the Single Nucleotide Polymorphism database.

(From TROWSDALE J, KNIGHT J C. Major histocompatibility complex genomics and human disease[J]. Annual review of genomics and human genetics, 2013, 14:301-323.)

Table 6-12 **Empirical Risks for Counseling in Type 1 Diabetes**

Relationship to Affected Individual	Risk for Development of Type 1 Diabetes (%)
None	0.2
MZ twin	40
Sibling	7
Sibling with no DR haplotypes in common	1
Sibling with 1 DR haplotype in common	5
Sibling with 2 DR haplotypes in common	17*
Child	4
Child of affected mother	3
Child of affected father	5

Note: * 20%~25% for particular shared haplotypes. MZ, Monozygotic.

It is important to stress, however, that genetic factors alone do not cause T1D because the MZ twin concordance rate is only approximately 40%, not 100%. Until a more complete picture develops of the genetic and nongenetic factors that cause T1D, risk counseling using HLA haplotyping must remain empirical (see Table 6-12).

6.5.5 Alzheimer Disease

Alzheimer disease (AD) is a fatal neurodegenerative disease that affects 1% to 2% of the United States population. It is the most common cause of dementia in older adults and is responsible for more than half of all cases of dementia. As with other dementias, patients experience a chronic, progressive loss of memory and other cognitive functions, associated with loss of certain types of cortical neurons. Age, sex, and family history are the most significant risk factors for AD. Once a person reaches 65 years of age, the risk for any dementia, and AD in particular, increases substantially with age and female sex (see Table 6-13).

Table 6-13 **Cumulative Age- and Sex-Specific Risks for Alzheimer Disease and Dementia**

Time Interval Past 65 Years of Age	Risk for Development of AD (%)	Risk for Development of Any Dementia (%)
65 to 80 years		
Male	6.3	10.9
Female	12	19
65 to 100 years		
Male	25	32.8
Female	28.1	45

Note: AD, Alzheimer disease.

AD can be diagnosed definitively only postmortem, on the basis of neuropathological findings of characteristic protein aggregates (β-amyloid plaques and neurofibrillary tangles). The most important constituent of the plaques is a small (39- to 42-amino acid) peptide, Aβ, derived from cleavage of a normal neuronal protein, the amyloid protein precursor. The secondary structure of Aβ gives the plaques the staining characteristics of amyloid proteins.

In addition to three rare autosomal dominant forms of the disease, in which disease onset is in the third to fifth decade, there is a common form of AD with onset after the age of 60 years (late onset). This form has no obvious mendelian inheritance pattern but does show familial aggregation and an elevated relative risk ratio ($\lambda_s \approx 4$) typical of disorders with complex inheritance. Twin studies have been inconsistent but suggest MZ concordance of approximately 50% and DZ concordance of approximately 18%.

The ε4 Allele of Apolipoprotein E

The major locus with alleles found to be significantly associated with common late-onset AD is *APOE*, which encodes apolipoprotein E. Apolipoprotein E is a protein component of the LDL particle and is involved in clearing LDL through an interaction with high-affinity receptors in the liver. Apolipoprotein E is also a constituent of amyloid plaques in AD and is known to bind the Aβ peptide. The *APOE* gene has three alleles, ε2, ε3, and ε4, due to substitutions of arginine for two different cysteine residues in the protein.

When the genotypes at the *APOE* locus were analyzed in AD patients and controls, a genotype with at least one ε4 allele was found two to three times more frequently among patients compared with controls in both the general U.S. and Japanese populations (see Table 6-14), with much less of an association in Hispanic and African American populations. Even more striking is that the risk for AD appears to increase further if both *APOE* alleles are ε4, through an effect on the age at onset of AD. Patients with two ε4 alleles have an earlier onset of disease than those with only one. In a study of patients with AD and unaffected controls, the age at which AD developed in the affected patients was earliest for ε4/ε4 homozygotes, next for ε4/ε3 heterozygotes, and significantly less for the other genotypes (see Fig. 6-10).

Table 6-14　Association of Apolipoprotein E ε4 Allele with Alzheimer Disease[*]

Genotype	Frequency			
	United States		Japan	
	AD	Control	AD	Control
ε4/ε4; ε4/ε3; or ε4/ε2	0.64	0.31	0.47	0.17
ε3/ε3; ε2/ε3; or ε2/ε2	0.36	0.69	0.53	0.83

Note: * Frequency of genotypes with and without the ε4 allele among Alzheimer disease (AD) patients and controls from the United States and Japan.

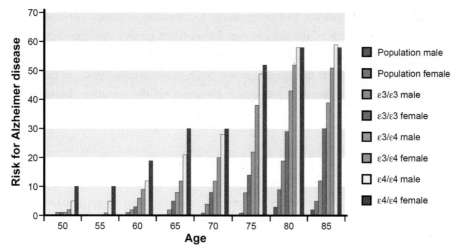

Figure 6-10   Chance of developing Alzheimer disease as a function of age for different APOE genotypes for each sex

At one extreme is the ε4/ε4 homozygote, who has ≈40% chance of remaining free of the disease by the age of 85 years, whereas an ε3/ε3 homozygote has ≈70% to ≈90% chance of remaining disease free at the age of 85 years, depending on the sex. General population risk is also shown for comparison.

(From ROBERTS J S, CUPPLES L A, RELKIN N R, et al. Genetic risk assessment for adult children of people with Alzheimer's disease: the Risk Evaluation and Education for Alzheimer's Disease (REVEAL) study[J]. Journal of geriatric psychiatry and neurology, 2005,18(4):250−255.)

In the population in general, the risk for developing AD by age 80 is approaching 10%. The ε4 allele is clearly a predisposing factor that increases the risk for development of AD by shifting the age at onset to an earlier age, such that ε3/ε4 heterozygotes have a 40% risk for developing the disease, and ε4/ε4 have a 60% risk by age 85. Despite this increased risk, other genetic and environmental factors must be important because a significant proportion of ε3/ε4 and ε4/ε4 individuals live to extreme old age with no evidence of AD. There are also reports of association between the presence of the ε4 allele and neurodegenerative disease after traumatic head injury (as seen in professional boxers, football players, and soldiers who have suffered blast injuries), indicating that at least one environmental factor, brain trauma, can interact with the ε4 allele in the pathogenesis of AD.

The ε4 variant of *APOE* represents a prime example of a predisposing allele: it predisposes to a complex trait in a powerful way but does not predestine any individual carrying the allele to the disease. Additional genes as well as environmental effects are also clearly involved; although several of these appear to have a significant effect, most remain to be identified. In general, testing of asymptomatic people for the *APOE* ε4 allele remains inadvisable because knowing that one is a heterozygote or homozygote for the ε4 allele does not mean one will develop AD, nor are there any interventions currently known that can affect the chance one will or will not develop AD.

6.6   The Challenge of Multifactorial Disease With Complex Inheritance

The greatest challenge facing medical genetics and genomic medicine going forward is unraveling the complex interactions between the variants at multiple loci and the relevant environmental factors that underlie the susceptibility to common multifactorial disease. This area of research is the central focus of the field of population-based genetic epidemiology. The field is developing rapidly, and it is clear that the genetic contribution to many more complex diseases in humans will be elucidated in the coming years. Such understanding will, in time, allow the development of novel preventive and therapeutic measures for the common disorders that cause such significant morbidity and mortality in the population.

Review Points:

1. Quantitative traits.

   The characteristics of quantitative traits, the genetic basis of quantitative traits, the significance of polygenic inheritance.

2. The statistical analyses on quantitative traits.

   Mean, variance, standard deviation, normal distribution.

3. Heritability.

   Estimating the heritability from Twin studies.

4. Characteristics of inheritance of complex diseases.

   Recurrence risk assessment of complex diseases.

Study Questions:

1. For a certain malformation, the recurrence risk in sibs and offspring of affected persons is 10%, the risk in nieces and nephews is 5%, and the risk in first cousins is 2.5%.

   a. Is this more likely to be an autosomal dominant trait with reduced penetrance or a multifactorial trait? Please explain.

   b. What other information might support your conclusion?

2. A large sex difference in affected persons is often a clue to X-linked inheritance. How would you establish that pyloric stenosis is multifactorial rather than X-linked?

3. A series of children with a particular congenital malformation includes both boys and girls. In all cases, the parents are normal. How would you determine whether the malformation is more likely to be multifactorial than autosomal recessive?

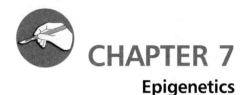

CHAPTER 7
Epigenetics

Purpose and Requirement:

The chapter goals are to comprehend epigenetic phenomena. The students are required to study epigenetic in hierarchies: In protein level, to comprehend histone modification and histone remodeler organization; In DNA level, to grasp DNA methylation; In RNA level, to study the main functions of non-coding RNAs in epigenetic field.

7.1 Epigenetic and Epigenomic Aspects of Gene Expression

Given the range of functions and fates that different cells in any organism must adopt over its lifetime, it is apparent that not all genes in the genome can be actively expressed in every cell at all times. As important as completion of the Human Genome Project has been for contributing to our understanding of human biology and disease, identifying the genomic sequences and features that direct developmental, spatial, and temporal aspects of gene expression remains a formidable challenge. Several decades of work in molecular biology have defined critical regulatory elements for many individual genes, as we saw in the previous section, and more recent attention has been directed toward performing such studies on a genome-wide scale.

In Chapter 2, we introduced general aspects of chromatin that package the genome and its genes in all cells. Here, we explore the specific characteristics of chromatin that are associated with active or repressed genes as a step toward identifying the regulatory code for expression of the human genome. Such studies focus on reversible changes in the chromatin landscape as determinants of gene function rather than on changes to the genome sequence itself and are thus called epigenetic or, when considered in the context of the entire genome, epigenomic (Greek *epi-*, over or upon).

The field of **epigenetics** is growing rapidly and is the study of heritable changes in cellular function or gene expression that can be transmitted from cell to cell (and even generation to generation) as a result of chromatinbased molecular signals (see Fig. 7-1). Complex epigenetic states can be established, maintained, and transmitted by a variety of mechanisms: modifications to the DNA, such as **DNA methylation**; numerous **histone modifications** that alter chromatin packaging or access; and substitution of specialized **histone variants** that mark chromatin associated with particular sequences or regions in the genome. These chromatin changes can be highly dynamic and transient, capable of responding rapidly and sensitively to changing needs in the cell, or they can be long lasting, capable of being transmitted through multiple cell divisions or even to subsequent generations. In either instance, the key concept is that epigenetic mechanisms do not alter the underlying DNA sequence, and this distinguishes them from genetic mechanisms, which are sequence based. Together, the epigenetic marks and the DNA sequence make up the set of signals that guide the genome to express its genes at the right time, in the right place, and in the right amounts.

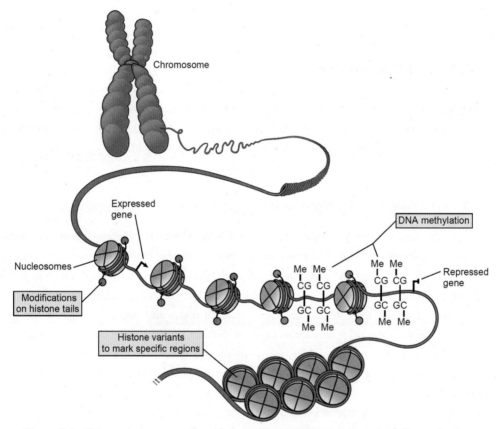

Figure 7-1 Schematic representation of chromatin and three major epigenetic mechanisms
DNA methylation at CpG dinucleotides, associated with gene repression; various modifications (indicated by different colors) on histone tails, associated with either gene expression or repression; and various histone variants that mark specific regions of the genome, associated with specific functions required for chromosome stability or genome integrity.

Increasing evidence points to a role for epigenetic changes in human disease in response to environmental or lifestyle influences. The dynamic and reversible nature of epigenetic changes permits a level of adaptability or plasticity that greatly exceeds the capacity of DNA sequence alone and thus is relevant both to the origins and potential treatment of disease. A number of large-scale epigenomics projects (akin to the original Human Genome Project) have been initiated to catalogue DNA methylation sites genome-wide (the so-called methylome), to evaluate CpG landscapes across the genome, to discover new histone variants and modification patterns in various tissues, and to document positioning of nucleosomes around the genome in different cell types, and in samples from both asymptomatic individuals and those with cancer or other diseases. These analyses are part of a broad effort (called the **ENCODE Project**, for Encyclopedia of DNA Elements) to explore epigenetic patterns in chromatin genomewide in order to better understand control of gene expression in different tissues or disease states.

7.1.1 DNA Methylation

DNA methylation involves the modification of cytosine bases by methylation of the carbon at the fifth position in the pyrimidine ring (see Fig. 7-2). Extensive DNA methylation is a mark of repressed genes and is a widespread mechanism associated with the establishment of specific programs of gene expression during cell differentiation and development. Typically, DNA methylation occurs on the C of CpG dinucleotides (see Fig. 7-1) and inhibits gene expression by recruitment of specific methyl-CpG-binding proteins that, in turn, recruit chromatin-modifying enzymes to silence transcription. The presence of 5-methylcytosine (5-mC) is considered to be a stable epigenetic mark that can be faithfully transmitted through cell division. However, altered methylation states are frequently observed in cancer, with hypomethylation of large genomic segments or with regional hypermethylation (particularly at CpG islands) in others.

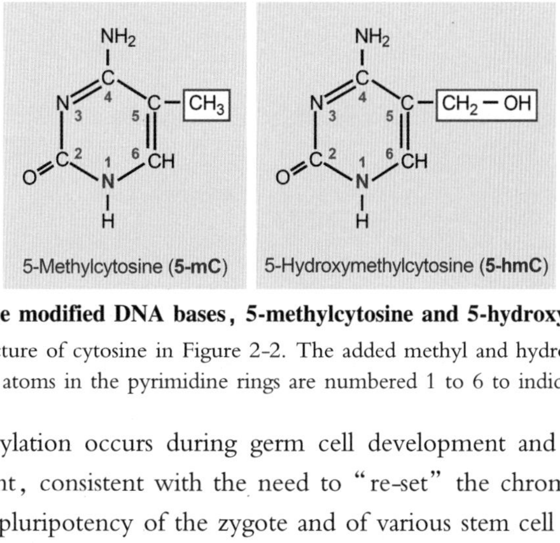

Figure 7-2   The modified DNA bases, 5-methylcytosine and 5-hydroxymethylcytosine
Compare to the structure of cytosine in Figure 2-2. The added methyl and hydroxymethyl groups are boxed in *purple*. The atoms in the pyrimidine rings are numbered 1 to 6 to indicate the 5-carbon.

Extensive demethylation occurs during germ cell development and in the early stages of embryonic development, consistent with the need to "re-set" the chromatin environment and restore totipotency or pluripotency of the zygote and of various stem cell populations. Although the details are still incompletely understood, these reprogramming steps appear to involve the enzymatic conversion of 5-mC to 5-hydroxymethylcytosine (5-hmC; see Fig. 7-2), as a likely intermediate in the demethylation of DNA. Overall, 5-mC levels are stable across adult tissues (approximately 5% of all cytosines), whereas 5-hmC levels are much lower and much more variable (0.1% to 1% of all cytosines). Interestingly, although 5-hmC is widespread in the genome, its highest levels are found in known regulatory regions, suggesting a possible role in the regulation of specific promoters and enhancers.

7.1.2 Histone Modifications

A second class of epigenetic signals consists of an extensive inventory of modifications to any of the core histone types, H2A, H2B, H3, and H4 (see Chapter 2). Such modifications include histone methylation, phosphorylation, acetylation, and others at specific amino acid residues, mostly located on the N-terminal "tails" of histones that extend out from the core nucleosome itself (see Fig. 7-1). These epigenetic modifications are believed to influence gene expression by affecting chromatin compaction or accessibility and by signaling protein complexes that—depending on the nature of the signal—activate or silence gene expression at that site. There are dozens of modified sites that can be experimentally queried genome-wide by using antibodies that recognize specifically modified sites—for example, histone H3 methylated at lysine position 9 (H3K9 methylation, using the one-letter abbreviation K for lysine) or histone H3 acetylated at lysine position 27 (H3K27 acetylation). The former is a repressive mark associated with silent regions of the genome, whereas the latter is a mark for activating regulatory regions.

Specific patterns of different histone modifications are associated with promoters, enhancers, or the body of genes in different tissues and cell types. The ENCODE Project, introduced earlier, examined 12 of the most common modifications in nearly 50 different cell types and integrated the individual chromatin profiles to assign putative functional attributes to well over half of the human genome. This finding implies that much more of the genome plays a role, directly or indirectly, in determining the varied patterns of gene expression that distinguish cell types than previously inferred from the fact that less than 2% of the genome is "coding" in a traditional sense.

7.1.3 Histone Variants

The histone modifications just discussed involve modification of the core histones themselves, which are all encoded by multigene clusters in a few locations in the genome. In contrast, the many dozens of histone variants are products of entirely different genes located elsewhere in the genome, and their amino acid sequences are distinct from, although related to, those of the canonical histones.

Different histone variants are associated with different functions, and they replace—all or in part—the related member of the core histones found in typical nucleosomes to generate specialized chromatin structures (see Fig. 7-1). Some variants mark specific regions or loci in the genome with highly specialized functions. For example, the CENP-A histone is a histone H3-related variant that is found exclusively at functional centromeres in the genome and contributes to essential features of centromeric chromatin that mark the location of kinetochores along the chromosome fiber. Other variants are more transient and mark regions of the genome with particular attributes. For example, H2A.X is a histone H2A variant involved in the response to DNA damage to mark regions of the genome that require DNA repair.

7.1.4 Chromatin Architecture

In contrast to the impression one gets from viewing the genome as a linear string of sequence, the genome adopts a highly ordered and dynamic arrangement within the space of the nucleus, correlated with and likely guided by the epigenetic and epigenomic signals just discussed. This three-dimensional landscape is highly predictive of the map of all expressed sequences in any given cell type (the **transcriptome**) and reflects dynamic changes in chromatin architecture at different levels (see Fig. 7-3). First, large chromosomal domains (up to millions of base pairs in size) can exhibit coordinated patterns of gene expression at the chromosome level, involving dynamic interactions between different intrachromosomal and interchromosomal points of contact within the nucleus. At a finer level, technical advances to map and sequence points of contact around the genome in the context of three-dimensional space have pointed to ordered loops of chromatin that position and orient genes precisely, exposing or blocking critical regulatory regions for access by RNA pol II, transcription factors, and other regulators. Lastly, specific and dynamic patterns of nucleosome positioning differ among cell types and tissues in the face of changing environmental and developmental cues (see Fig. 7-3). The biophysical, epigenomic, and/or genomic properties that facilitate or specify the orderly and dynamic packaging of each chromosome during each cell cycle, without reducing the genome to a disordered tangle within the nucleus, remain a marvel of landscape engineering.

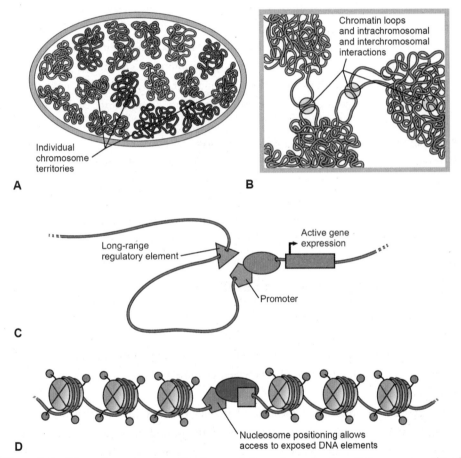

Figure 7-3 Three-dimensional architecture and dynamic packaging of the genome, viewed at increasing levels of resolution

(A) Within interphase nuclei, each chromosome occupies a particular territory, represented by the different colors. (B) Chromatin is organized into large subchromosomal domains within each territory, with loops that bring certain sequences and genes into proximity with each other, with detectable intrachromosomal and interchromosomal interactions. (C) Loops bring long-range regulatory elements (e.g., enhancers or locus-control regions) into association with promoters, leading to active transcription and gene expression. (D) Positioning of nucleosomes along the chromatin fiber provides access to specific DNA sequences for binding by transcription factors and other regulatory proteins.

7.2 Gene Expression as the Integration of Genomic and Epigenomic Signals

The gene expression program of a cell encompasses the specific subset of the approximately 20,000 proteincoding genes in the genome that are actively transcribed and translated into their respective functional products, the subset of the estimated 20,000 to 25,000 ncRNA genes that are transcribed, the amount of products produced, and the particular sequence (alleles) of those products. The gene expression profile of any particular cell or cell type in a given individual at a given time (whether in the context of the cell cycle, early development, or one's entire life span) and under a given set of circumstances (as influenced by environment, lifestyle, or disease) is thus the integrated sum of several different but interrelated effects, including the following:

- The primary sequence of genes, their allelic variants, and their encoded products.
- Regulatory sequences and their epigenetic positioning in chromatin.
- Interactions with the thousands of transcriptional factors, ncRNAs, and other proteins involved in the control of transcription, splicing, translation, and post-translational modification.
- Organization of the genome into subchromosomal domains.
- Programmed interactions between different parts of the genome.
- Dynamic three-dimensional chromatin packaging in the nucleus.

All of these orchestrate in an efficient, hierarchical, and highly programmed fashion. Disruption of any one—due to genetic variation, to epigenetic changes, and/or to disease-related processes—would be expected to alter the overall cellular program and its functional output.

7.3 Allelic Imbalance in Gene Expression

It was once assumed that genes present in two copies in the genome would be expressed from both homologues at comparable levels. However, it has become increasingly evident that there can be extensive imbalance between alleles, reflecting both the amount of sequence variation in the genome and the interplay between genome sequence and epigenetic patterns that were just discussed.

In Chapter 2, we introduced the general finding that any individual genome carries two different alleles at a minimum of 3 to 5 million positions around the genome, thus distinguishing by sequence the maternally and paternally inherited copies of that sequence position. Here, we explore ways in which those sequence differences reveal allelic imbalance in gene expression, both at autosomal loci and at X chromosome loci in females.

By determining the sequences of all the RNA products—the transcriptome—in a population of cells, one can quantify the relative level of transcription of all the genes (both protein-coding and noncoding) that are transcriptionally active in those cells. Consider, for example, the collection of protein-coding genes. Although an average cell might contain approximately 300,000 copies of mRNA in total, the abundance of specific mRNAs can differ over many orders of magnitude. Among genes that are active, most are expressed at low levels (estimated to be <10 copies of that gene's mRNA per cell), whereas others are expressed at much higher levels (several hundred to a few thousand copies of that mRNA per cell). Only in highly specialized cell types are particular genes expressed at very high levels (many tens of thousands of copies) that account for a significant proportion of all mRNA in those cells.

Now consider an expressed gene with a sequence variant that allows one to distinguish between the RNA products (whether mRNA or ncRNA) transcribed from each of two alleles, one allele with a T that is transcribed to yield RNA with an A and the other allele with a C that is transcribed to yield RNA with a G (see Fig. 7-4). By sequencing individual RNA molecules and comparing the number of sequences generated that contain an A or G at that position, one can infer the ratio of transcripts from the two alleles in that sample. Although most genes show essentially equivalent levels of biallelic expression, recent analyses of this type have demonstrated widespread unequal allelic expression for 5% to 20% of autosomal genes in the genome (see Table 7-1). For most of these genes, the extent of imbalance is twofold or less, although up to tenfold differences have been observed for some genes. This allelic imbalance may reflect interactions between genome sequence and gene regulation. For example, sequence changes can alter the relative binding of various transcription factors or other transcriptional regulators to the two alleles or the extent of DNA methylation observed at the two alleles (see Table 7-1).

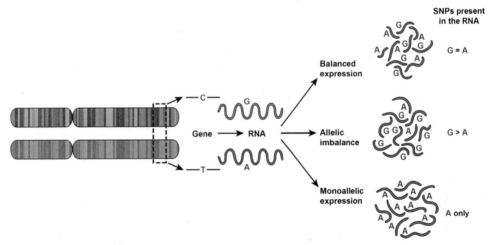

Figure 7-4   Allelic expression patterns for a gene sequence with a transcribed DNA variant (here, a C or a T) to distinguish the alleles

As described in the text, the relative abundance of RNA transcripts from the two alleles (here, carrying a G or an A) demonstrates whether the gene shows balanced expression (*top*), allelic imbalance (*center*), or exclusively monoallelic expression (*bottom*). Different underlying mechanisms for allelic imbalance are compared in Table 7-1. SNP, Single nucleotide polymorphism.

➤ Monoallelic Gene Expression

Some genes, however, show a much more complete form of allelic imbalance, resulting in monoallelic gene expression (see Fig. 7-4). Several different mechanisms have been shown to account for allelic imbalance of this type for particular subsets of genes in the genome: DNA rearrangement, random monoallelic expression, parent-of-origin imprinting, and, for genes on the X chromosome in females, X chromosome inactivation. Their distinguishing characteristics are summarized in Table 7-1.

(1) Somatic Rearrangement

A highly specialized form of monoallelic gene expression is observed in the genes encoding **immunoglobulins** and **T-cell receptors**, expressed in B cells and T cells, respectively, as part of the immune response. Antibodies are encoded in the germline by a relatively small number of genes that, during B-cell development, undergo a unique process of somatic rearrangement that involves the cutting and pasting of DNA sequences in lymphocyte precursor cells (but not in any other cell lineages) to rearrange genes in somatic cells to generate enormous antibody diversity. The highly orchestrated DNA rearrangements occur across many hundreds of kilobases but involve only one of the two alleles, which is chosen randomly in any given B cell (see Table 7-1). Thus expression of mature mRNAs for the immunoglobulin heavy or light chain subunits is exclusively monoallelic.

Table 7-1 Allelic Imbalance in Gene Expression

Type	Characteristics	Genes Affected	Basis	Developmental Origin
Unbalanced expression	Unequal RNA abundance from two alleles due to DNA variants and associated epigenetic changes; usually < twofold difference in expression	5% ~ 20% of autosomal genes	Sequence variants cause different levels of expression at the two alleles	Early embryogenesis
Monoallelic expression				
● Somatic rearrangement	Changes in DNA organization to produce functional gene at one allele, but not other	Immunoglobulin genes, T-cell receptor genes	Random choice of one allele	B- and T-cell lineages
● Random allelic silencing or activation	Expression from only one allele at a locus, due to differential epigenetic packaging at locus	Olfactory receptor genes in sensory neurons; other chemosensory or immune system genes; up to 10% of all genes in other cell types	Random choice of one allele	Specific cell types
● Genomic imprinting	Epigenetic silencing of allele(s) in imprinted region	> 100 genes with functions in development	Imprinted region marked epigenetically according to parent of origin	Parental germline
● X chromosome inactivation	Epigenetic silencing of alleles on one X chromosome in females	Most X-linked genes in females	Random choice of one X chromosome	Early embryogenesis

This mechanism of somatic rearrangement and random monoallelic gene expression is also observed at the T-cell receptor genes in the T-cell lineage. However, such behavior is unique to these gene families and cell lineages; the rest of the genome remains highly stable throughout development and differentiation.

(2) Random Monoallelic Expression

In contrast to this highly specialized form of DNA rearrangement, monoallelic expression typically results from differential epigenetic regulation of the two alleles. One well-studied example of random monoallelic expression involves the OR gene family. In this case, only a single allele of one OR gene is expressed in each olfactory sensory neuron; the many hundred other copies of the OR family remain repressed in that cell. Other genes with chemosensory or immune system functions also show random monoallelic expression, suggesting that this mechanism may be a general one for increasing the diversity of responses for cells that interact with the outside world. However, this mechanism is apparently not restricted to the immune and sensory systems, because a substantial subset of all human genes (5% to 10% in different cell types) has been shown to undergo random allelic silencing. These genes are broadly distributed on all autosomes, have a wide range of functions, and vary in terms of the cell types and tissues in which monoallelic expression is observed.

(3) Parent-of-Origin Imprinting

For the examples just described, the choice of which allele is expressed is not dependent on parental origin. Either the maternal or paternal copy can be expressed in different cells and their clonal descendants. This distinguishes random forms of monoallelic expression from **genomic imprinting**, in which the choice of the allele to be expressed is nonrandom and is determined solely by parental origin. Imprinting is a normal process involving the introduction of epigenetic marks (see Fig. 7-1) in the germline of one parent, but not the other, at specific locations in the genome. These lead to monoallelic expression of a gene or, in some cases, of multiple genes within the imprinted region.

Imprinting takes place during gametogenesis, before fertilization, and marks certain genes as having come from the mother or father (see Fig. 7-5). After conception, the parent-of-origin imprint is maintained in some or all of the somatic tissues of the embryo and silences gene expression on allele(s) within the imprinted region. Whereas some imprinted genes show monoallelic expression throughout the embryo, others show tissue-specific imprinting, especially in the placenta, with biallelic expression in other tissues. The imprinted state persists postnatally into adulthood through hundreds of cell divisions so that only the maternal or paternal copy of the gene is expressed. Yet, imprinting must be reversible: a paternally derived allele, when it is inherited by a female, must be converted in her germline so that she can then pass it on with a maternal imprint to her offspring. Likewise, an imprinted maternally derived allele, when it is inherited by a male, must be converted in his germline so that he can pass it on as a paternally imprinted allele to his offspring (see Fig. 7-5). Control over this conversion process appears to be governed by specific DNA elements called **imprinting control regions** or **imprinting centers** that are located within imprinted regions throughout the genome. Although their precise mechanism of action is not known, many appear to involve ncRNAs that initiate the epigenetic change in chromatin, which then spreads outward along the chromosome over the imprinted region. Notably, although the imprinted region can encompass more than a single gene, this form of monoallelic expression is confined to a delimited genomic segment, typically a few hundred kilobase pairs to a few megabases in overall size. This distinguishes genomic imprinting both from the more general form of random monoallelic expression (which appears to involve individual genes under locus-specific control) and from X chromosome inactivation (which involves genes along the entire chromosome).

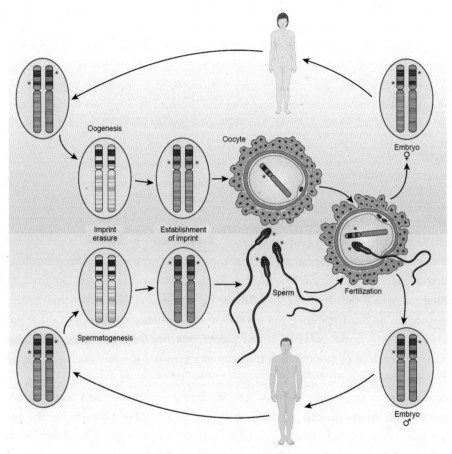

Figure 7-5 Genomic imprinting and conversion of maternal and paternal imprints during passage through male or female gametogenesis

Within a hypothetical imprinted region on a pair of homologous autosomes, paternally imprinted genes are indicated in *blue*, whereas a maternally imprinted gene is indicated in *red*. After fertilization, both male and female embryos have one copy of the chromosome carrying a paternal imprint and one copy carrying a maternal imprint. During oogenesis (*top*) and spermatogenesis (*bottom*), the imprints are erased by removal of epigenetic marks, and new imprints determined by the sex of the parent are established within the imprinted region. Gametes thus carry a monoallelic imprint appropriate to the parent of origin, whereas somatic cells in both sexes carry one chromosome of each imprinted type.

(4) X Chromosome Inactivation

The chromosomal basis for sex determination results in a dosage difference between typical males and females with respect to genes on the X chromosome. Here we discuss the chromosomal and molecular mechanisms of X chromosome inactivation, the most extensive example of random monoallelic expression in the genome and a mechanism of **dosage**

compensation that results in the epigenetic silencing of most genes on one of the two X chromosomes in females.

In normal female cells, the choice of which X chromosome is to be inactivated is a random one that is then maintained in each clonal lineage. Thus females are mosaic with respect to X-linked gene expression. Some cells express alleles on the paternally inherited X but not the maternally inherited X, whereas other cells do the opposite (see Fig. 7-6). This mosaic pattern of gene expression distinguishes most X-linked genes from imprinted genes, whose expression, as we just noted, is determined strictly by parental origin.

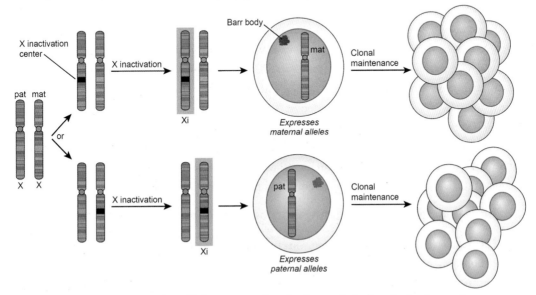

Figure 7-6   Random X chromosome inactivation early in female development
Shortly after conception of a female embryo, both the paternally and maternally inherited X chromosomes (pat and mat, respectively) are active. Within the first week of embryogenesis, one or the other X is chosen at random to become the future inactive X, through a series of events involving the X inactivation center (black box). That X then becomes the inactive X (Xi, indicated by the *shading*) in that cell and its progeny and forms the Barr body in interphase nuclei. The resulting female embryo is thus a clonal mosaic of two epigenetically determined cell types: one expresses alleles from the maternal X (*pink* cells), whereas the other expresses alleles from the paternal X (*blue* cells). The ratio of the two cell types is determined randomly but varies among normal females and among females who are carriers of X-linked disease alleles.

Although the inactive X chromosome was first identified cytologically by the presence of a heterochromatic mass (called the **Barr body**) in interphase cells, many epigenetic features distinguish the active and inactive X chromosomes, including DNA methylation, histone modifications, and a specific histone variant, macroH2A, that is particularly enriched in chromatin on the inactive X. As well as providing insights into the mechanisms of X inactivation, these features can be useful diagnostically for identifying inactive X chromosomes in clinical material.

Although X inactivation is clearly a chromosomal phenomenon, not all genes on the X chromosome show monoallelic expression in female cells. Extensive analysis of expression of nearly all X-linked genes has demonstrated that at least 15% of the genes show biallelic expression and are expressed from both active and inactive X chromosomes, at least to some extent. A proportion of these show significantly higher levels of mRNA production in female cells compared to male cells and are interesting candidates for a role in explaining sexually dimorphic traits.

A special subset of genes is located in the pseudoautosomal segments, which are essentially identical on the X and Y chromosomes and undergo recombination during spermatogenesis (see Chapter 2). These genes have two copies in both females (two X-linked copies) and males (one X-linked and one Y-linked copy) and thus do not undergo X inactivation. As expected, these genes show balanced biallelic expression, as one sees for most autosomal genes.

The X Inactivation Center and the XIST Gene

X inactivation occurs very early in female embryonic development, and determination of which X will be designated the inactive X in any given cell in the embryo is a random choice under the control of a complex locus called the **X inactivation center**. This region contains an unusual ncRNA gene, *XIST*, that appears to be a key master regulatory locus for X inactivation. *XIST* (an acronym for inactive X [Xi]-specific transcripts) has the novel feature that it is expressed only from the allele on the inactive X. It is transcriptionally silent on the active X in both male and female cells. Although the exact mode of action of *XIST* is unknown, X inactivation cannot occur in its absence. The product of *XIST* is a long ncRNA that stays in the nucleus in close association with the inactive X chromosome.

7.4 Variation in Gene Expression and Its Relevance to Medicine

The regulated expression of genes in the human genome involves a set of complex interrelationships among different levels of control, including proper gene dosage (controlled by mechanisms of chromosome replication and segregation), gene structure, chromatin packaging and epigenetic regulation, transcription, RNA splicing, and, for protein-coding loci, mRNA stability, translation, protein processing, and protein degradation. For some genes, fluctuations in the level of functional gene product, due either to inherited variation in the structure of a particular gene or to changes induced by nongenetic factors such as diet or the environment, are of relatively little importance. For other genes, even relatively minor changes in the level of expression can have dire clinical consequences, reflecting the importance of those gene products in particular biological pathways. The nature of inherited variation in the structure and function of chromosomes, genes, and the genome, combined with the influence of this variation on the expression of specific traits, is the very essence of medical and molecular genetics.

Review Points:

1. Epigenetic phenomena.

Homozygous twins share a common genotype and are genetically identical but show significant phenotypic discordances.

Epigenetic: All heritable changes in gene expression and chromatin organization that are independent of the DNA sequence itself.

Significance: A supplementary of Genetics and admit acquired factors in individual development.

2. Histone modifications.

Mechanisms exist to "open up" or "condense" chromatin. The types of Histone modification. Give priority to Histones acetylating.

3. Histone remodeler.

Four families: SWI/SNF, ISWI, CHD, INO80; Rebuild or remove histories from DNA. ATP needed.

4. DNA methylation.

The function of DNMT1 (Methylate original site during DNA replication), DNMT2 (Unclear) and DNMT3 (Methylate new site).

CG Island: CpG cluster exists in upstream 5' of structural gene and methylation of CpG regulates gene expression.

5. Non-coding RNAs.

RNA which is not used for making proteins (non-coding RNA) can be cleaved and used to inhibit protein-coding RNA, such as miRNA, siRNA.

Study Questions:

Consider different ways in which mutations or variation in the following might lead to human disease: epigenetic modifications, DNA methylation, miRNA genes, lncRNA genes.

CHAPTER 8
Genetics of Cancer

Purpose and Requirement:

The chapter goals are to comprehend the monoclonal origin hypothesis of tumor, multistep oncogenesis theory and two-hit theory. The function of oncogene and tumor suppressor gene should be grasped well, and also some basic concepts like proto-oncogene, cellular oncogene, and virus oncogene.

Cancer is one of the most common and serious diseases seen in clinical medicine. There are 14 million new cases of cancer diagnosed each year and over 8 millions deaths from the disease worldwide. Based on the most recent statistics available, cancer treatment costs $80 billion per year in direct health care expenditures in the United States alone. Cancer is invariably fatal if it is not treated. Identification of persons at increased risk for cancer before its development is an important objective of genetics research. And for both those with an inherited predisposition to cancer as well as those in the general population, early diagnosis of cancer and its early treatment are vital, and both are increasingly reliant on advances in genome sequencing and gene expression analysis.

8.1 Neoplasia

Cancer is the name used to describe the more virulent forms of **neoplasia**, a disease process characterized by uncontrolled cellular proliferation leading to a mass or tumor (**neoplasm**). The abnormal accumulation of cells in a neoplasm occurs because of an imbalance between the normal processes of cellular proliferation and cellular attrition. Cells proliferate as they pass through the cell cycle and undergo mitosis. Attrition, due to programmed cell death, removes cells from a tissue. For a neoplasm to be a cancer, however, it must also be **malignant**, which means that not only is its growth uncontrolled, it is also capable of invading neighboring tissues that surround the original site (the **primary** site) and can spread (**metastasize**) to more distant sites (see Fig. 8-1). Tumors that do not invade or metastasize are not cancerous but are referred to as **benign** tumors, although their abnormal function, size or location may make them anything but benign to the patient.

Cancer is not a single disease but rather comes in many forms and degrees of malignancy. There are three main classes of cancer:

- **Sarcomas**, in which the tumor has arisen in mesenchymal tissue, such as bone, muscle, or connective tissue, or in nervous system tissue.

- **Carcinomas**, which originate in epithelial tissue, such as the cells lining the intestine, bronchi, or mammary ducts.
- **Hematopoietic** and **lymphoid** malignant neoplasms, such as leukemia and lymphoma, which spread throughout the bone marrow, lymphatic system, and peripheral blood.

Within each of the major groups, tumors are classified by site, tissue type, histological appearance, degree of malignancy, chromosomal aneuploidy, and, increasingly, by which gene mutations and abnormalities in gene expression are found within the tumor.

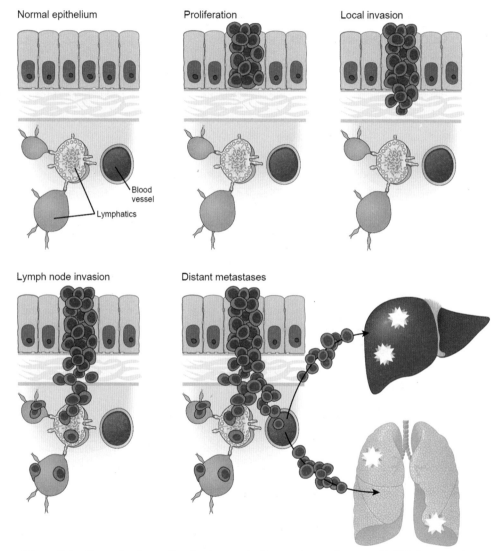

Figure 8-1 General scheme for development of a carcinoma in an epithelial tissue such as colonic epithelium

The diagram shows progression from normal epithelium to local proliferation, invasion across the lamina propria, spread to local lymph nodes, and final distant metastases to liver and lung.

In this chapter, we describe how genetic and genomic studies demonstrate that cancer is fundamentally a genetic disease. We describe the kinds of genes that have been implicated in initiating cancer and the mechanisms by which dysfunction of these genes can result in the disease. Second, we review a number of heritable cancer syndromes and demonstrate how insights gained into their pathogenesis have illuminated the basis of the much more common, sporadic forms of cancer. We also examine some of the special challenges that such heritable syndromes present for medical genetics and genetic counseling. Third, we illustrate ways in which genetics and genomics have changed both how we think about the causes of cancer and how we diagnose and treat the disease. Genomics—in particular the identification of mutations, altered epigenomic modifications, and abnormal gene expression in cancer cells—is vastly expanding our knowledge of why cancer develops and is truly changing cancer diagnosis and treatment.

8.2 Genetic Basis of Cancer

8.2.1 Driver and Passenger Gene Mutations

The application to the study of cancer of powerful new sequencing technologies for genome sequencing and RNA expression studies has brought remarkable new clarity to our understanding of the origins of cancer. By analyzing many thousands of samples obtained from more than 30 types of human cancer, researchers are building **The Cancer Genome Atlas**, a public catalog of mutations, epigenomic modifications, and abnormal gene expression profiles found in a wide variety of cancers. Although the project is still under way, the results to date from these studies are striking. The number of mutations present in a tumor can vary from just a few to many tens of thousands. Most mutations found through sequencing of tumor tissue appear to be random, are not recurrent in particular cancer types, and probably occur as the cancer develops, rather than directly causing the neoplasia to develop or progress. Such mutations are referred to as "**passenger**" **mutations**. However, a subset of a few hundred genes has been repeatedly found to be mutated at high frequency in many samples of the same type of cancer or even in multiple different types of cancers, mutated in fact far too frequently to simply be passenger mutations. These genes are thus presumed to be involved in the development or progression of the cancer itself and are therefore referred to as "**driver**" **genes**, that is, they harbor mutations (so-called **driver gene mutations**) that are likely to be causing a cancer to develop or progress. Although many driver genes are specific to particular tumor types, some, such as those in the *TP*53 gene encoding the p53 protein, are found in the vast majority of cancers of many different types. Although the most common driver genes are now known, it is likely that additional, less abundant driver genes will be identified as The Cancer Genome Atlas continues to grow.

8.2.2 Spectrum of Driver Gene Mutations

Many different genome alterations can act as driver gene mutations. In some cases, a single nucleotide change or small insertion or deletion can be a driver mutation. Large numbers of cell divisions are required to produce an adult organism of an estimated 10^{14} cells from a single-cell zygote. Given a frequency of 10^{-10} replication errors per base of DNA per cell division, and an estimated 10^{15} cell divisions during the lifetime of an adult, replication errors alone result in thousands of new single nucleotide or small insertion/deletion mutations in the genome in every cell of the organism. Some environmental agents, such as carcinogens in cigarette smoke or ultraviolet or X-irradiation, will increase the rate of mutations around the genome. If, by chance, mutations occur in critical driver genes in a particular cell, then the oncogenic process may be initiated.

Chromosome and subchromosomal mutations can also serve as driver mutations. Particular translocations are sometimes highly specific for certain types of cancer and involve specific genes (e.g., the *BCR-ABL* translocation in **chronic myelogenous leukemia**). In contrast, other cancers can show complex rearrangements in which chromosomes break into numerous pieces and rejoin, forming novel and complex combinations (a process known as "**chromosome shattering**"). Finally, large genomic alterations involving many kilobases of DNA can form the basis for loss of function or increased function of one or more driver genes. Large genomic alterations include deletions of a segment of a chromosome or multiplication of a chromosomal segment to produce regions with many copies of the same gene (**gene amplification**).

8.2.3 The Cellular Functions of Driver Genes

The nature of some driver gene mutations comes as no surprise: the mutations directly affect specific genes that regulate processes that are readily understood to be important in oncogenesis. These processes include cell-cycle regulation, cellular proliferation, differentiation and exit from the cell cycle, growth inhibition by cell-cell contacts, and programmed cell death (apoptosis). However, the effects of other driver gene mutations are not so readily understood and include genes that act more globally and indirectly affect the expression of many other genes. Included in this group are genes encoding products that maintain genome and DNA integrity or genes that affect gene expression, either at the level of transcription by epigenomic changes, at the post-transcriptional level through effects on messenger RNA (mRNA) translation or stability, or at the post-translational level through their effects on protein turnover (see Table 8-1). Other driver genes affect translation, for example, genes that encode **noncoding RNAs** from which regulatory **microRNAs** (**miRNAs**) are derived. Many miRNAs have been found to be either greatly overexpressed or down-regulated in various tumors, sometimes strikingly so. Because each

Table 8-1 Classes of Driver Genes Mutated in Cancer

Genes with Specific Effects on Cellular Proliferation or Apoptosis	Genes with Global Effects on Genome or DNA Integrity or on Gene Expression
Cell cycle regulation	Cienome integrity
Cell cycle checkpoint proteins	• Chromosome segregation
Cellular proliferation signaling	• Genome and gene mutation
• Transcription factors	• DNA repair
• Receptor and membrane-bound tyrosine kinases	• Telomere stability
• Growth factors	Gene expression: abnormal metabolites affecting activity of multiple genes/gene produers
• Intracellular serine-threonine kinases	Gene expression: epigenetic modifications of DNA/chromatin
• PI3 kinases	• DNA methylation and hydroxymethylation
• G proteins and G protein-coupled receptors	• Chromatin histone methylation, demethylation, and acetylation
• mTOR signaling	• Nucleosome remodeling
• WnoB-catenin signaling	• Chromatin accessibility and compaction (SWISNF complexes)
• Transcription factors	Gene expression: post-transcriptional alterations
Differentiation and lineage survival	• Aberrant mRNA splicing
• Transcription factors protecting specific cell lineages	• MicroRNAs affecting mRNA stability and translation
• Genes involved in exit from cell cycle into G_0	Gene expression: protein stability/turnover
Apoptosis	

Note: mRNA, Messenger RNA; mTOR, mammalian target of rapamycin; PI3, phosphatidylinositol-3.

miRNA may regulate as many as 200 different gene targets, overexpression or underexpression of miRNAs may have widespread oncogenic effects because many driver genes will be dysregulated. Noncoding miRNAs that impact gene expression and contribute to oncogenesis are referred to as **oncomirs**.

Figure 8-2 is a diagram outlining how mutations in specific regulators of growth and in global guardians of DNA and genome integrity perturb normal homeostasis (see Fig. 8-2A), leading to a vicious cycle causing loss of cell cycle control, uncontrolled proliferation, interrupted differentiation, and defects in apoptosis (see Fig. 8-2B).

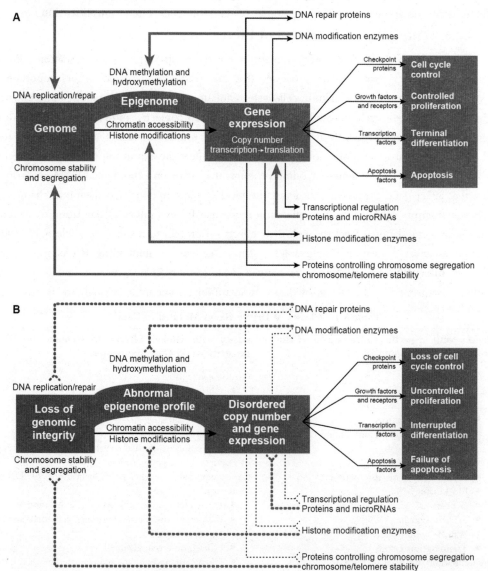

Figure 8-2 Overview of normal genetic pathways controlling normal tissue homeostasis
(A) The information encoded in the genome (*black arrows*) results in normal gene expression, as modulated by the epigenomic state. Many genes provide negative feedback (*purple arrows*) to ensure normal homeostasis. (B) Perturbations in neoplasia. Abnormalities in gene expression (*dotted black arrows*) lead to a vicious cycle of positive feedback (*dotted brown lines*) of progressively more disordered gene expression and genome integrity.

8.2.4 Activated Oncogenes and Tumor Suppressor Genes

Both classes of driver genes—those with specific effects on cellular proliferation or survival and those with global effects on genome or DNA integrity (see Table 8-1)—can be further subdivided into one of two functional categories depending on how, if mutated, they drive oncogenesis.

The first category includes **proto-oncogenes**. These are normal genes that, when mutated in very particular ways, become driver genes through alterations that lead to excessive levels of activity. Once mutated in this way, driver genes of this type are referred to as **activated oncogenes**. Only a single mutation at one allele can be sufficient for activation, and the mutations that activate a proto-oncogene can range from highly specific point mutations causing dysregulation or hyperactivity of a protein, to chromosome translocations that drive overexpression of a gene, to gene amplification events that create an overabundance of the encoded mRNA and protein product (see Fig. 8-3).

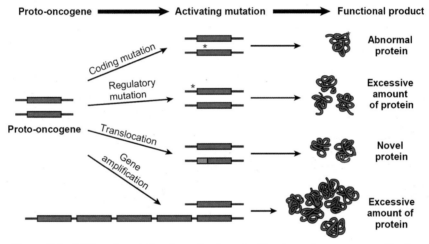

Figure 8-3 Different mutational mechanisms leading to proto-oncogene activation

These include a single point mutation leading to an amino acid change that alters protein function, mutations or translocations that increase expression of an oncogene, a chromosome translocation that produces a novel product with oncogenic properties, and gene amplification leading to excessive amounts of the gene product.

The second, and more common, category of driver genes includes tumor suppressor genes (TSGs), mutations in which cause a loss of expression of proteins necessary to control the development of cancers. To drive oncogenesis, loss of function of a TSG typically requires mutations at both alleles. There are many ways that a cell can lose the function of TSG alleles. Loss-of-function mechanisms can range from missense, nonsense, or frame-shift mutations to gene deletions or loss of a part or even an entire chromosome. Loss of function of TSGs can also result from epigenomic transcriptional silencing due to altered chromatin conformation or promoter methylation, or from translational silencing by miRNAs or disturbances in other components of the translational machinery.

8.2.5 Cellular Heterogeneity Within Individual Tumors

The accumulation of driver gene mutations does not occur synchronously, in lockstep, in every cell of a tumor. To the contrary, cancer evolves along multiple lineages within a tumor, as chance mutational and epigenetic events in different cells activate proto-oncogenes and cripple the machinery for maintaining genome integrity, leading to more genetic changes in a vicious cycle of more mutations and worsening growth control. The lineages that experience an enhancement of growth, survival, invasion, and distant spread will come to predominate as the cancer evolves and progresses. In this way, the original clone of neoplastic cells evolves and gives rise to multiple sublineages, each carrying a set of mutations and epigenomic alterations that are different from but overlap with what is carried in other sublineages. The profile of mutations and epigenomic changes can differ between the primary and its metastases, between different metastases, and even between the cells of the original tumor or within a single metastasis. A paradigm for the development of cancer, as illustrated in Figure 8-4, provides a useful conceptual framework for considering the role of genomic and epigenomic changes in the evolution of cancer, a point we emphasize throughout this chapter. It is a general model that applies to all cancers.

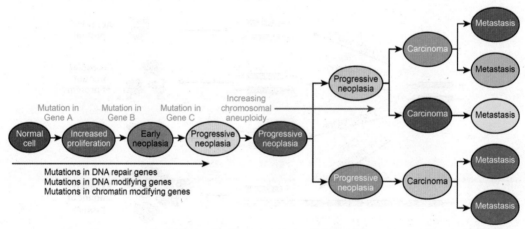

Figure 8-4 Stages in the evolution of cancer

Increasing degrees of abnormality are associated with sequential loss of tumor suppressor genes from several chromosomes and activation of proto-oncogenes, with or without a concomitant defect in DNA repair. Multiple lineages, carrying different mutations and epigenomic profiles, occur within the primary tumor itself, between the primary and metastases and between different metastases.

Although the focus of this chapter is on genomic and epigenomic changes within the tumor, the surrounding normal tissue also plays an important role by providing the blood supply that nourishes the tumor, by permitting cancer cells to escape from the tumor and metastasize, and by shielding the tumor from immune attack. Thus cancer is a complex process, both within the tumor and between the tumor and the normal tissues that surround it.

8.3 Cancer in Families

Although essentially all individuals are at risk for some cancer at some point during their lives, many forms of cancer have a higher incidence in relatives of patients than in the general population. In some cases, this increased incidence is due primarily to inheritance of a single mutant gene with high penetrance. Among these syndromes, we currently know of approximately 100 different genes in which deleterious mutations increase the risk for cancer many-fold higher than in the general population. There are also many dozens of additional genetic disorders that are not usually considered to be hereditary cancer syndromes and yet include some increased predisposition to cancer (for example, the 10- to 20-fold increased lifetime risk for leukemia in Down syndrome). These clear examples notwithstanding, it is important to emphasize that not all families with an apparently increased incidence of cancer can be explained by known mendelian or clearly recognized genetic disorders. These families likely represent the effects of both shared environment and one or more genetic variants that increase susceptibility and are therefore classified as multifactorial, with complex inheritance.

Although individuals with a hereditary cancer syndrome represent probably less than 5% of all patients with cancer, identification of a genetic basis for their disease has great importance both for clinical management of these families and for understanding cancer in general. Firstly, the relatives of individuals with strong hereditary predispositions, which are most often due to mutations in a single gene, can be offered testing and counseling to provide appropriate reassurance or more intensive monitoring and therapy, depending on the results of testing. Secondly, as is the case with many common diseases, understanding the hereditary forms of the disease provides crucial insights into disease mechanisms that go far beyond the rare hereditary forms themselves. These general concepts are illustrated in the examples discussed in the sections that follow.

8.3.1 Activated Oncogenes in Hereditary Cancer Syndromes

Multiple Endocrine Adenomatosis, Type 2

The type A variant of **multiple endocrine adenomatosis**, type 2 (MEN2) is an autosomal dominant disorder characterized by a high incidence of medullary carcinoma of the thyroid that is often but not always associated with pheochromocytoma, benign parathyroid adenomas, or both. Patients with the rarer type B variant, termed MEN2B, have, in addition to the tumors seen in patients with MEN2A, thickening of nerves and the development of benign neural tumors, known as **neuromas**, on the mucosal surface of the mouth and lips and along the gastrointestinal tract.

The mutations responsible for MEN2 are in the RET gene. Individuals who inherit an activating mutation in RET have a greater than 60% chance of developing a particular type of thyroid carcinoma (medullary), although more sensitive tests, such as blood tests for thyrocalcitonin or urinary catecholamines synthesized by pheochromocytomas, are abnormal in well above 90% of heterozygotes for MEN2.

RET encodes a cell-surface protein that contains an extracellular domain that can bind signaling molecules and a cytoplasmic tyrosine kinase domain. Tyrosine kinases are a class of enzymes that phosphorylate tyrosines in proteins. Tyrosine phosphorylation initiates a signaling cascade of changes in protein-protein and DNA-protein interactions and in the enzymatic activity of many proteins (see Fig. 8-5). Normally, tyrosine kinase receptors must bind specific signaling molecules in order to undergo the conformational change that makes them enzymatically active and able to phosphorylate other cellular proteins. The mutations in RET that cause MEN2A increase its kinase activity even in the absence of its ligand (a state referred to as constitutive activation).

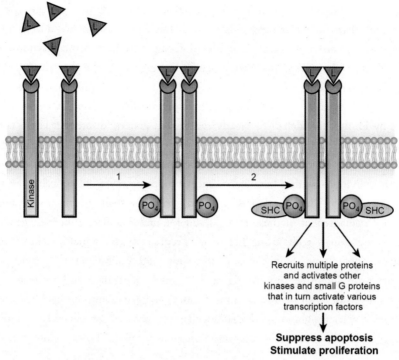

Figure 8-5 Schematic diagram of the function of the Ret receptor, the product of the *RET* proto-oncogene

Upon binding of a ligand (L), such as glial-derived growth factor or neurturin, to the extracellular domain, the protein dimerizes and activates its intracellular kinase domain to autophosphorylate specific tyrosine residues. These then bind the SHC adaptor protein, which sets off multiple cascades of complex protein interactions involving other serine-threonine and phosphatidylinositol kinases and small G proteins, which in turn activate other proteins, ultimately activating certain transcription factors that suppress apoptosis and stimulate cellular proliferation. Mutations in RET that result in type A variant of multiple endocrine adenomatosis, type 2 (MEN2A) cause inappropriate dimerization and activation of its own intrinsic kinase without ligand binding.

The *RET* gene is expressed in many tissues of the body and is required for normal embryonic development of autonomic ganglia and kidney. It is unclear why germline activating mutations in this proto-oncogene result in a particular cancer of distinct histological types restricted to specific tissues, whereas other tissues in which the oncogene is expressed do not develop tumors. Interestingly, RET is the same gene implicated in Hirschsprung disease, although those mutations are usually loss-of-function, not activating, mutations. There are, however, some families in which the same mutation in RET can act as an activated oncogene in some tissues (such as thyroid) and cause MEN2A, while not having sufficient function in other tissues, such as the developing enteric neurons of the gastrointestinal tract, resulting in Hirschsprung disease. Thus even the identical mutation can have different effects on different tissues.

8.3.2 The Two-Hit Theory of Tumor Suppressor Gene Inactivation in Cancer

As introduced earlier, whereas the proteins encoded by proto-oncogenes promote cancer when activated or overexpressed, mutations in TSGs contribute to malignancy by a different mechanism, the loss of function of both alleles of the gene. The products of many TSGs have now been isolated and characterized, some of which are presented in Table 8-2.

Table 8-2 Selected Tumor Suppressor Genes

| Gene | Gene Product and Possible Function | Disorders in Which the Gene Is Affected | |
		Familial	Sporadic
RB1	p110 Cell cycle regulation	Retinoblastoma	Retinoblastoma, small cell lung carcinomas, breast cancer
TP53	p53 Cell cycle	Li-Fraumeni syndrome	Lung cancer, breast cancer, many others
APC	regulation APC Multiple roles in regulating proliferation and cell adhesion	Familial adenomatous polyposis	Colorectal cancer
VHL	VHL Forms part of a cytoplasmic destruction complex with APC that normally inhibits induction of blood vessel growth when oxygen is present	von Hippel-Lindau syndrome	Clear cell renal carcinoma
BRCA1, BRCA2	BRCA1, BRCA2 Chromosome repair in response to double-stranded DNA breaks	Familial breast and ovarian cancer	Breast cancer, ovarian cancer
MLH1, MSH2	MLH1, MSH2 Repair nucleotide mismatches between strands of DNA	Lynch syndrome	Colorectal cancer

The existence of TSG mutations leading to cancer was proposed some five decades ago to explain why certain tumors can occur in either hereditary or sporadic forms (see Fig. 8-6). It was suggested that the hereditary form of the childhood cancer **retinoblastoma** might be initiated when a cell in a person heterozygous for a germline mutation in the retinoblastoma TSG, required to prevent the development of the cancer, undergoes a second, somatic event that inactivates the other retinoblastoma gene allele. As a consequence of this second somatic event, the cell loses function of both alleles, giving rise to a tumor. In the sporadic form of retinoblastoma, both alleles are also inactivated, but in this case, the inactivation results from two somatic events occurring in the same cell.

This so-called two-hit model is now widely accepted as the explanation for many hereditary cancers in addition to retinoblastoma, including **familial polyposis coli**, **familial breast cancer**, **neurofibromatosis type 1** (**NF1**), **Lynch syndrome**, and **Li-Fraumeni syndrome**.

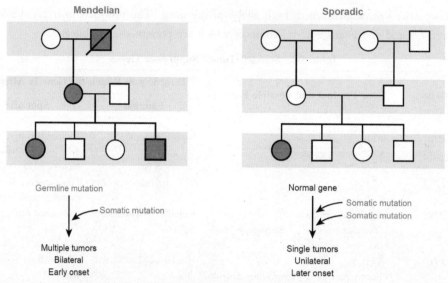

Mendelian

Sporadic

Germline mutation

Somatic mutation

Multiple tumors
Bilateral
Early onset

Normal gene

Somatic mutation
Somatic mutation

Single tumors
Unilateral
Later onset

**Figure 8-6   Comparison of mendelian and sporadic forms of cancers such as retinoblastoma
and familial polyposis of the colon**

8. 3. 3   Tumor Suppressor Genes in Autosomal Dominant Cancer Syndromes

(1) Retinoblastoma

Retinoblastoma is the prototype of diseases caused by mutation in a TSG and is a rare malignant tumor of the retina in infants, with an incidence of approximately 1 in 20,000 births (see Fig. 8-7). Diagnosis of a retinoblastoma must usually be followed by removal of the affected eye, although smaller tumors, diagnosed at an early stage, can be treated by local therapy so that vision can be preserved.

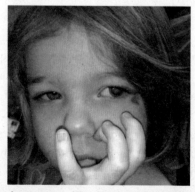

**Figure 8-7   Retinoblastoma in a young girl, showing as a white reflex in the affected left eye
when light reflects directly off the tumor surface**

Approximately 40% of cases of retinoblastoma are of the heritable form, in which the child (as just discussed and as represented generally by the family shown in Figure 8-6) inherits one mutant allele at the retinoblastoma locus (RB1) through the germline from either a heterozygous parent or, more rarely, from a parent with germline mosaicism for an RB1 mutation. In these children, retinal cells, which like all the other cells of the body are already carrying one inherited defective RB1 allele, suffer a somatic mutation or other alteration in the remaining normal allele, leading to loss of both copies of the RB1 gene and initiating development of a tumor in each of those cells (see Fig. 8-8).

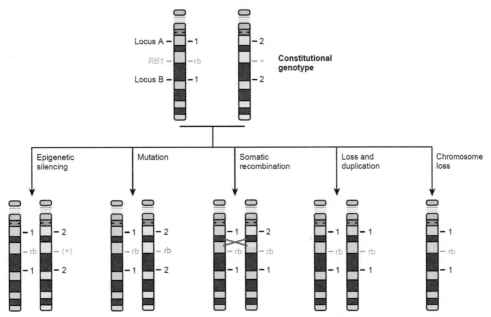

Figure 8-8   Chromosomal mechanisms that could lead to loss of heterozygosity for DNA markers at or near a tumor suppressor gene in an individual heterozygous for an inherited germline mutation

The figure depicts the events that constitute the "second hit" that leads to retinoblastoma with loss of heterozygosity (LOH). Local events such as mutation, gene conversion, or transcriptional silencing by promoter methylation, however, could cause loss of function of both RB1 genes without producing LOH. +, normal allele, rb, the mutant allele.

The disorder appears to be inherited as a dominant trait because the large number of primordial retinoblasts and their rapid rate of proliferation make it very likely that a somatic mutation will occur as a second hit in one or more of the more than 10^6 retinoblasts already carrying an inherited RB1 mutation. Because the chance of a second hit is so great, it occurs frequently in more than one cell, and thus heterozygotes for the disorder often have tumors arising at multiple sites, such as **multifocal tumors** in one eye, in both eyes (**bilateral retinoblastoma**), or in both eyes, as well as in the pineal gland (referred to as "trilateral" retinoblastoma). It is worth emphasizing, however, that the occurrence of a second hit is a matter of chance and does not occur 100% of the time. The penetrance of retinoblastoma therefore, although greater than 90%, is not complete.

The other 60% of cases of retinoblastoma are sporadic. In these cases, both RB1 alleles in a single retinal cell have been mutated or inactivated independently by chance, and the child does not carry an RB1 mutation inherited through the germline. Because two hits in the same cell is a statistically rare event, there is usually only a single clonal tumor, and the retinoblastoma is found at one location (unifocal) in one eye only. Unilateral tumor is no guarantee that the child does not have the heritable form of retinoblastoma, however, because 15% of patients with the heritable type develop a tumor in only one eye. Another difference between hereditary and sporadic tumors is that the average age at onset of the sporadic form is in early childhood, later than in infants with the heritable form (see Fig. 8-6), reflecting the longer time needed on average for two mutations, rather than one, to occur.

In a small percentage of patients with retinoblastoma, the mutation responsible is a cytogenetically detectable deletion or translocation of the portion of chromosome 13 that contains the RB1 gene. Such chromosomal changes, if they also disrupt genes adjacent to RB1, may lead to dysmorphic features in addition to retinoblastoma.

① Nature of the Second Hit

Typically, for retinoblastoma as well as for the other hereditary cancer syndromes, the first hit is an inherited mutation, that is, a change in the DNA sequence. The second hit, however, can be caused by a variety of genetic, epigenetic, or genomic mechanisms (see Fig. 8-8). Although it is most often a somatic mutation, loss of function without mutation, such as occurs with epigenetic silencing, has also been observed in some cancer cells. Although a number of mechanisms have been documented, the common theme is loss of function of RB1. The RB1 gene product, p110 Rb1, is a phosphoprotein that normally regulates entry of the cell into the S phase of the cell cycle. Thus loss of the RB1 gene and/or absence of the normal RB1 gene product (by whatever mechanism) deprives cells of an important checkpoint and allows uncontrolled proliferation (see Table 8-2).

② Loss of Heterozygosity

In addition to mutations and epigenetic silencing, a novel genomic mechanism was uncovered when geneticists made an unusual but highly significant discovery when they compared DNA polymorphisms at the RB1 locus in DNA from normal cells to those in the retinoblastoma tumor from the same patient. Individuals with retinoblastoma who were heterozygous at polymorphic loci flanking the RB1 locus in normal tissues (see Fig. 8-8) had tumors that contained alleles from only one of their two chromosome 13 homologues, revealing a **loss of heterozygosity** (**LOH**) in tumor DNA in and around the RB1 locus. Furthermore, in familial cases, the retained chromosome 13 markers were the ones inherited from the affected parent, that is, the chromosome with the abnormal RB1 allele. Thus, in these cases, LOH represents the second hit of the remaining allele. LOH may occur by interstitial deletion, but there are other mechanisms as well, such as mitotic recombination or monosomy 13 due to nondisjunction (see Fig. 8-8).

LOH is the most common mutational mechanism by which the function of the remaining normal RB1 allele is disrupted in heterozygotes, although each of the mechanisms shown in Figure 8-8 have been documented in different patients. LOH is a feature of tumors in a number of cancers, both heritable and sporadic, and is often considered evidence for the existence of a TSG in the region of LOH.

(2) Familial Breast Cancer due to Mutations in BRCA1 and BRCA2

Breast cancer is common. Among all cases of this disease, a small proportion ($\approx 3\%$ to 5%) appears to be due to a highly penetrant dominantly inherited mendelian predisposition that increases the risk for female breast cancer 4-fold to 7-fold over the 12% lifetime risk observed in the general female population. In these families, one often sees features characteristic of hereditary (as opposed to sporadic) cancer; multiple affected individuals in a family, earlier age at onset, frequent multifocal, bilateral disease or second independent primary breast tumor, and second primary cancers in other tissues such as ovary and prostate.

Although a number of genes in which mutations cause highly penetrant mendelian forms of breast cancer have been discovered from family studies, the two genes responsible for the majority of all hereditary breast cancers are BRCA1 and BRCA2. Together, these two TSGs account for approximately one half and one third, respectively, of autosomal dominant familial breast cancer. Numerous mutant alleles of both genes have now been catalogued. Mutations in BRCA1 and BRCA2 are also associated with a significant increase in the risk for ovarian and fallopian duct cancer in female heterozygotes. Moreover, mutations in BRCA2 and, to a lesser extent, BRCA1, also account for 10% to 20% of all male breast cancer and increase the risk for male breast cancer 10- to 60-fold over the 0.1% lifetime risk observed among males in the general population (see Table 8-3).

Table 8-3   Lifetime Cancer Risks in Carriers of BRCA1 or BRCA2 Mutations Compared to the General Population

Cancer Type	General Population Risk	Cancer Risk When Mutation Present	
		*BRCA*1	*BRCA*2
Breast in females	12%	50% ~80%	40% ~70%
Second primary breast in females	3.5% within 5 yr	27% within 5 yr	12% within 5 yr
	Up to 11%		40% ~50% at 20 yr
Ovarian	1% ~2%	24% ~40%	11% ~18%
Male breast	0.1%	1% ~2%	5% ~10%
Prostate	15% (N. European origin)	<30%	<39%
	18% (African Americans)		
Pancreatic (both sexes)	0.5%	1% ~3%	2% ~7%

The gene products of BRCA1 and BRCA2 are nuclear proteins contained within the same multiprotein complex. This complex has been implicated in the cellular response to double-stranded DNA breaks, such as occur normally during homologous recombination or abnormally as a result of damage to DNA. As might be expected for any TSG, tumor tissue from heterozygotes for BRCA1 and BRCA2 mutations frequently demonstrates LOH with loss of the normal allele.

Penetrance of BRCA1 and BRCA2 Mutations

Presymptomatic detection of women at risk for development of breast cancer as a result of any of these susceptibility genes relies on detecting clearly pathogenic mutations by gene sequencing. For the purposes of patient management and counseling, it would be helpful to know the lifetime risk for development of breast cancer in individuals, whether male or female, carrying particular mutations in the BRCA1 and BRCA2 genes, compared with the risk in the general male or female population (see Table 8-3). Initial studies showed a greater than 80% risk for breast cancer by the age of 70 years in women heterozygous for deleterious BRCA1 mutations, with a somewhat lower estimate for BRCA2 mutation carriers. These estimates relied on estimates of the risk for development of cancer in female relatives within families ascertained because breast cancer had already occurred many times in family members. That is, families in which the particular BRCA1 or BRCA2 mutation was highly penetrant.

When similar risk estimates were made from population-based studies, however, in which women carrying BRCA1 and BRCA2 mutations were not selected because they were members of families in which many cases of breast cancer had already developed, the risk estimates were lower and ranged from 40% to 50% by the age of 70 years. The discrepancy between the penetrance of mutant alleles in families with multiple occurrences of breast cancer and the penetrance seen in women identified by population screening and not by family history suggests that other genetic or environmental factors must play a role in the ultimate penetrance of BRCA1 and BRCA2 mutations in women heterozygous for these mutations.

In addition to mutations in BRCA1 and BRCA2, mutations in other genes can also cause autosomal dominantly inherited breast cancer syndromes, albeit less commonly. These syndromes, which include **the Li-Fraumeni**, **hereditary diffuse gastric cancer**, **Peutz-Jeghers**, and **Cowden syndromes**, demonstrate lifetime breast cancer risks that approach those seen in carriers of BRCA1 or BRCA2 mutations, as well as risks for other forms of cancer such as sarcomas, brain tumors, and carcinomas of the stomach, thyroid, and small intestine.

Clinicians faced with a family with multiple affected individuals with breast cancer often look for distinguishing signs in the patient and in the family history to help guide the choice of which genes to analyze. However, the rapid decline in the cost of gene or even genome-wide sequencing has allowed the development of gene panels in which a dozen or more candidate genes can be accurately and simultaneously tested for mutations, often at a cost that is equivalent or even less than what was charged previously to analyze just one or two genes.

(3) Hereditary Colon Cancer

Colorectal cancer, a malignancy of the epithelial cells of the colon and rectum, is one of the most common forms of cancer. It affects approximately 1.3 million individuals worldwide per year (150,000 of whom are in the United States) and is responsible for approximately 10% to 15% of all cancer. Most cases are sporadic, but a small proportion of colon cancer cases are familial, among which are two autosomal dominant conditions: **familial adenomatous polyposis (FAP)** and **Lynch syndrome (LS)**, along with their variants.

① Familial Adenomatous Polyposis

FAP and its subvariant, Gardner syndrome, together have an incidence of approximately 1 per 10,000. In FAP heterozygotes, benign adenomatous polyps numbering in the many hundreds develop in the colon during the first two decades of life. In almost all cases, one or more of the polyps becomes malignant. Surgical removal of the colon (colectomy) prevents the development of malignancy. Because this disorder is inherited as an autosomal dominant trait, relatives of affected persons must be examined periodically by colonoscopy. FAP is caused by loss-of-function mutations in a TSG known as the APC gene (so-named because the condition used to be called adenomatous polyposis coli). Gardner syndrome is also due to mutations in APC and is therefore allelic to FAP. Patients with Gardner syndrome have, in addition to the adenomatous polyps with malignant transformation seen in FAP, other extracolonic anomalies, including osteomas of the jaw and desmoids, which are tumors arising in the muscle of the abdominal wall. Although the relatives of an individual affected with Gardner syndrome who also carry the same APC mutation tend to also show the extracolonic manifestations of Gardner syndrome, the same mutation in unrelated individuals has been found to cause only FAP in one individual and Gardner syndrome in another. Thus whether or not an individual has FAP or Gardner syndrome is not simply due to which mutation is present in the APC gene but is likely affected by genetic variation elsewhere in the genome.

② **Lynch Syndrome**

Approximately 2% to 4% of cases of colon cancer are attributable to LS. LS is characterized by autosomal dominant inheritance of colon cancer in association with a small number of adenomatous polyps that begin during early adulthood. The number of polyps is generally quite small, in contrast to the hundreds to thousands of adenomatous polyps seen with FAP. Nonetheless, the polyps in LS have high potential to undergo malignant transformation. Heterozygotes for the most commonly mutated LS gene have an approximately 80% lifetime risk for development of cancer of the colon. Female heterozygotes have a somewhat smaller risk (approximately 70%) but also have an approximately 40% risk for endometrial cancer. There are also additional risks of 10% to 20% for cancer of the biliary or urinary tract and the ovary. Sebaceous gland tumors of the skin (**Muir-Torre syndrome**) may be the first presenting sign in LS. Thus the presence of such tumors in a patient should raise suspicion of a possible hereditary colon cancer syndrome.

LS results from loss-of-function mutations in one of four distinct but related DNA repair genes (MLH1, MSH2, MSH6, and PMS2) that encode **mismatch repair** proteins. Although all four of these genes have been implicated in LS in different families, MLH1 and MSH2 are together responsible for the vast majority of LS, whereas the others have been found in only a few patients and are often associated with a lesser degree of mismatch repair deficiency and lower penetrance. Like the BRCA1 and BRCA2 genes, the LS mismatch repair genes are TSGs involved in maintaining the integrity of the genome. Unlike BRCA1 and BRCA2, however, the LS genes are not involved in double-stranded DNA break repair. Instead, their role is to repair incorrect DNA base pairing (i.e., pairing other than A with T or C with G) that can arise during DNA replication.

At the cellular level, the most striking phenotype of cells lacking mismatch repair proteins is an enormous increase in both point mutations and mutations occurring during replication of simple DNA repeats, such as a segment containing a string of the same base, for example $(A)_n$, or a microsatellite, such as $(TG)_n$. Microsatellites are believed to be particularly vulnerable to mismatch because slippage of the strand being synthesized on the template strand can occur more readily when a short tandem repeat is being synthesized. Such instability, referred to as the **microsatellite instability-positive** (**MSI**+) phenotype, occurs at two orders of magnitude higher frequency in cells lacking both copies of a mismatch repair gene. The MSI+ phenotype is easily seen in DNA as three, four, or even more alleles of a microsatellite polymorphism in a single individual's tumor DNA (see Fig. 8-9). It is estimated that cells lacking both copies of a mismatch repair gene may carry 100,000 mutations within simple repeats throughout the genome.

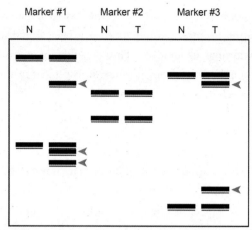

Figure 8-9   Gel electrophoresis of three different microsatellite polymorphic markers in normal (N) and tumor (T) samples from a patient with a mutation in MSH2 and microsatellite instability

Although marker #2 shows no difference between normal and tumor tissues, genotyping at markers #1 and #3 reveals extra alleles (*blue arrows*) , some smaller, some larger, than the alleles present in normal tissue.

Because of the increase in mutation rate in these classes of sequence, loss of function of mismatch repair genes will lead to somatic mutations in other driver genes. Two such driver genes have been isolated and characterized. The first is *APC*, whose normal function and role in FAP were described previously. The second is the gene *TGFBR2*, in which mutations also cause an autosomal dominant hereditary colon cancer syndrome. *TGFBR2* encodes transforming growth factor β receptor II , a serine-threonine kinase that inhibits intestinal cell division. *TGFBR2*, is particularly vulnerable to mutation when mismatch repair proteins are lost because it contains a stretch of 10 adenines encoding three lysines within its coding sequence; deletion of one or more of these As results in a frameshift and loss-of-function mutation. LS is an excellent example of how a gene, like *MLH*1, which has a global effect on mutation rate throughout the genome, can be a driver gene through its effect on other genes, such as *TGFBR2*, that are more specifically involved in driving the development of a cancer.

8. 3. 4   Mutations in Tumor Suppressor Genes Causing Autosomal Recessive Pediatric Cancer Syndromes

As expected from the important role that DNA replication and repair enzymes play in mutation surveillance and prevention, inherited defects that alter the function of repair enzymes can lead to a dramatic increase in the frequency of mutations of all types, including those that lead to cancer.

Mutations in the LS mismatch repair genes are frequent enough in the population for there to be rare individuals with two germline mutations in one of the LS genes. Although much rarer than autosomal dominant forms of LS just discussed, this condition, known as **constitutional mismatch repair syndrome**, results in a markedly elevated risk for many cancers during childhood, including colorectal and small bowel cancer, as well as some cancers not associated with LS, such as leukemia in infancy and various types of brain tumors in childhood.

Several other well-known autosomal recessive disorders, including **xeroderma** pigmentosum, **ataxia-telangiectasia**, **Fanconi anemia**, and **Bloom syndrome**, are also due to loss of function of proteins required for normal DNA repair or replication. Patients with these rare conditions have a high frequency of chromosome and gene mutations and, as a result, a markedly increased risk for various types of cancer, particularly leukemia or, in the case of xeroderma pigmentosum, skin cancers in sun-exposed areas. Clinically, radiography must be used with extreme caution, if at all, in patients with ataxia-telangiectasia, Fanconi anemia, and Bloom syndrome, and exposure to sunlight must be avoided in patients with xeroderma pigmentosum.

Although these syndromes are rare autosomal recessive disorders, heterozygotes for these gene defects are much more common and appear to be at increased risk for malignant neoplasia. For example, Fanconi anemia, in which homozygotes have a number of congenital anomalies, bone marrow failure, leukemia, and squamous cell carcinoma of the head and neck, is a **chromosome instability syndrome** resulting from mutations of at least 18 different loci involved in DNA and chromosome repair. In the aggregate, Fanconi anemia has a population frequency of approximately 1 to 5 per million, which translates to a carrier frequency of approximately 1 to 2 per 500. One of these Fanconi anemia loci turns out to be the known hereditary cancer gene *BRCA2*. Others include *BRIP*1, *PALB*2, and *RAD*51*C*, which are known to increase susceptibility to breast cancer in heterozygotes. Similarly, female heterozygotes for certain ataxia-telangiectasia mutations have overall a 2-fold increased risk for breast cancer compared with controls and a 5-fold higher risk for breast cancer before the age of 50 years. Thus heterozygotes for these chromosome instability syndromes constitute a sizeable pool of individuals at increased risk for cancer.

8.3.5 Testing for Germline Mutations Causing Hereditary Cancer

As introduced earlier, although some sporadic cancers will be truly sporadic and due entirely to somatic mutation(s), others likely reflect a predisposition to a specific cancer due to familial variants in one or more genes. This raises the possibility of using genetic testing or even whole-genome sequencing to screen for germline mutations that might inform risk estimates for members of the general population or for families with insufficient family history to implicate a hereditary cancer syndrome. Here we illustrate the issues involved in the case of two common neoplasias, breast cancer and colorectal cancer.

(1) BRCA1 and BRCA2 Testing

Identification of a germline mutation in *BRCA*1 or *BRCA*2 in a patient with breast cancer is of obvious importance for genetic counseling and cancer risk management for the patient's children, siblings, and other relatives, who may or may not be at increased risk. Such testing is, of course, also important for the patient's own management. For instance, in addition to removal of the cancer, a woman found to carry a *BRCA*1 mutation might also choose to have a prophylactic mastectomy on the unaffected breast or a bilateral oophorectomy simultaneously to minimize the number of separate surgeries and anesthesia exposures. Finding a mutation in the proband or a first-degree relative would also allow mutation-specific testing in the rest of the family.

Importantly, however, the fraction of all female breast cancer patients whose disease is caused by a germline mutation in either the *BRCA*1 or *BRCA*2 gene is small, with estimates that vary between 1% and 3% in populations unselected for family history of breast or ovarian cancer, or for age at onset of the disease. Male breast cancer is 100 times less common than female breast cancer, but when it occurs, the frequency of germline mutations in hereditary breast cancer genes, particularly *BRCA2*, is 16%.

Until quite recently, the cost of mutation analysis in *BRCA1* and *BRCA2* was used to justify limiting gene sequencing to those patients most likely to be carrying a mutation, such as all male breast cancer patients and all women younger than 50 years with breast cancer, women with bilateral breast cancer, or women with first- and second-degree relatives with ovarian cancer or breast cancer. However, as the cost of sequencing falls, and large gene panels of breast cancer susceptibility genes, including *BRCA1* and *BRCA2*, can now be analyzed for less than it cost previously to sequence just *BRCA1* and *BRCA2* alone, the guidelines of just a few years ago will inevitably undergo reevaluation.

(2) Colorectal Cancer Germline Mutation Testing

Only 4% of patients with colon cancer, not selected for a family history of cancer, carry a mutation in one of the four mismatch repair genes *MLH1*, *MSH2*, *MSH6*, and *PMS2* causing LS. An even smaller fraction contain *APC* mutations causing FAP. As with breast cancer, geneticists need to balance the cost and yield of sequencing hereditary colorectal cancer genes in every patient with colon cancer against the obvious importance of finding such a mutation for the patient and his or her family.

For LS, clinical factors such as the presence of multiple polyps, an early age at onset (before the age of 50 years), the location of the tumor in more proximal portions of the colon, the presence of a second tumor or history of colorectal cancer, a family history of colorectal or other cancers (particularly endometrial cancer), and cancer in relatives younger than 50 years of age, all boost the probability that a patient with colon cancer is carrying a mutation in a mismatch repair gene. Molecular studies of the tumor tissue, to look for evidence of the MSI+ phenotype or evidence of absent MSH2 and/or MSH6 protein by antibody staining in the tumor, also increase the probability that an individual patient with colorectal cancer carries a germline mismatch repair mutation. Unfortunately, loss of MLH1 protein staining in tumors due to promoter methylation is a frequent epigenetic finding in sporadic colon cancers and is therefore much less predictive of a germline LS mutation.

Combining clinical and molecular criteria allows the identification of a subset of all colorectal cancer patients in whom the probability of finding a mismatch repair mutation is much greater than 4%. These patients are clearly the most cost-effective group in which sequencing could be recommended. However, as with all such attempts at cost-effectiveness, limiting the number of patients studied to increase the yield of patients with positive sequencing inevitably results in missing a sizeable minority (20%) of patients with germline mismatch repair mutations. Again, the cost of mutation analysis must be reevaluated as the technology gets less expensive.

For FAP, the presence of hundreds of adenomatous polyps developing at an early age, multiple sebaceous adenomas, or the extracolonic signs of Gardner syndrome are sufficient to trigger germline testing for an *APC* mutation. There are, however, certain *APC* mutations that result in many fewer polyps and no extracolonic features (referred to as "attenuated FAP").

Attenuated FAP can be confused clinically with LS, but the tumors generally lack mismatch repair defects or microsatellite instability.

8.4   Familial Occurrence of Cancer

Cancer can also show increased incidence in families without fitting a clear-cut mendelian pattern. For example, it is estimated that as many as 20% of all breast cancer cases occurring in families that lack a clear, highly penetrant mendelian disorder nonetheless have a significant genetic contribution, as revealed by twin and family studies. The observed increase in cancer risk when relatives are affected may be due to mutations in a single gene but with penetrance that is sufficiently reduced to obscure any mendelian inheritance pattern. For example, in breast cancer, mutations in a gene such as *PALB2* can increase lifetime risk for breast cancer to approximately 25% by age 55 and approximately 40% by age 85. A lack of obvious breast cancer risk in men with *PALB2* mutations further obscures the inheritance pattern, although there is a significant increased risk for pancreatic cancer in men with these reduced penetrance alleles. Mutations in *BRIP1* and *RAD51C* have similar effects.

The bulk of familial cancer is, however, likely to be a complex disorder caused by both genetic and shared environmental factors. The degree of complex familial cancer risk can be assessed by epidemiological studies that compare how often the disease occurs in relatives versus the general population. The age-specific incidence of many forms of cancer in family members of probands is increased over the incidence of the same cancer in an age-matched cohort in the general population (see Fig. 8-10). This increased risk has been observed in individuals whose first-degree relatives (parent or sibling) are affected by a wide variety of different cancers, with an even greater increase in incidence when an individual's parent and sibling are both affected. For example, population-based epidemiological studies have shown that approximately 5% of all individuals in North America and Western Europe will develop colorectal cancer in their lifetime, but the lifetime risk for colorectal cancer is increased 2-fold to 3-fold over the average population risk if one first-degree relative is affected.

In agreement with the likely complex inheritance of cancers, genome-wide association studies have identified more than 150 mostly common variants associated with a variety of cancers. Prostate cancer, in particular, shows multiple associations with single nucleotide polymorphisms located in the intergenic or intronic regions of over a dozen loci. Unfortunately, odds ratios for most of these associations are all less than 2.0, and most are less than 1.3, therefore accounting for at most 20% of the observed familial risk for prostate cancer. Overall, then, although the role of inherited variants in the genome is clear, we cannot yet explain in detail the increased familial tendencies of most cancers. Whether common variants do not capture all of the risk or there are unrecognized environmental exposures in common between family members remain nonexclusive possibilities.

8.5   Sporadic Cancer

Previously, we introduced the concept of activation of oncogenes by a variety of mutational mechanisms. Here, we explore these mechanisms and their effects in greater detail, particularly in the context of sporadic cancers.

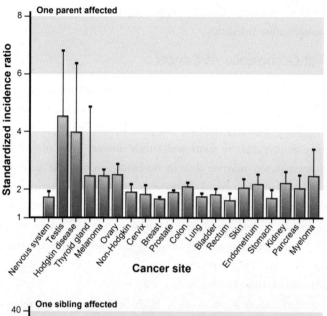

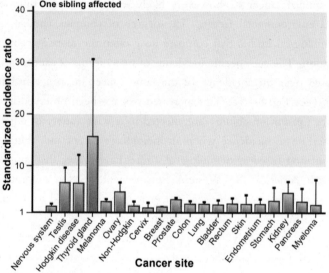

Figure 8-10　Standardized incidence ratios (SIRs) for cancers at various sites in first-degree relatives (child or sibling) of an affected person

A SIR is similar to the relative risk ratio (λ_r) that is based on prevalence of disease, except SIR is the ratio of the incidence of cases of cancer in relatives divided by the number expected from the incidence in an age-matched group in the general population. Error bars reflect 95% confidence limits on the SIRs.

(From HEMMINKI K, SUNDQUIST J, BERMEJO J L. Familial risks for cancer as the basis for evidence-based clinical referral and counseling[J]. The oncologist, 2008,13(3):239-247.)

8.5.1　Activation of Oncogenes by Point Mutation

Many mutated oncogenes were first identified by molecular studies of cell lines derived from sporadic cancers. One of the first activated oncogenes discovered was a mutant *RAS* gene derived from a bladder carcinoma cell line. *RAS* encodes one of a large family of small guanosine triphosphate (GTP)-binding proteins (so-called **G proteins**) that serve as molecular "on-off" switches to activate or inhibit downstream molecules. Remarkably, the activated oncogene and its normal counterpart proto-oncogene differed at only a single nucleotide. The alteration led to synthesis of an abnormal Ras protein that was able to signal continuously, thus stimulating cell division and changing it into a tumor. *RAS* point mutations are now known in many tumors, and the *RAS* genes have been shown experimentally to be the mutational target of known carcinogens, a finding that supports a role for mutated *RAS* genes in the development of many cancers.

To date, nearly 50 human proto-oncogenes have been identified as driver mutations in sporadic cancer. Only a few of these proto-oncogenes have also been found to be inherited in a hereditary cancer syndrome.

8.5.2 Activation of Oncogenes by Chromosome Translocation

As pointed out previously, oncogene activation is not always the result of a DNA mutation. In some instances, a proto-oncogene is activated by a subchromosomal mutation, typically a translocation. More than 40 oncogenic chromosome translocations have been described to date, primarily in sporadic leukemias and lymphomas but also in a few rare connective tissue sarcomas. Although originally detected only by cytogenetic analysis, such chromosome alterations can be detected now by whole-genome sequence analysis, even using cell-free DNA in plasma samples from cancer patients.

In some cases, translocation breakpoints lie within the introns of two genes, thereby fusing two genes into one abnormal gene that encodes a chimeric protein with novel oncogenic properties. The best-known example is the translocation between chromosomes 9 and 22, the so-called Philadelphia chromosome that is seen in **chronic myelogenous leukemia** (**CML**) (see Fig. 8-11). The translocation moves the proto-oncogene *ABL*1, a tyrosine kinase, from its normal position on chromosome 9q to a gene of unknown function, *BCR*, on chromosome 22q. The translocation results in the synthesis of a novel, chimeric protein, **BCR-ABL1**, containing a portion of the normal Abl protein with increased tyrosine kinase activity. The enhanced tyrosine kinase activity of the novel protein encoded by the chimeric gene is the primary event causing the chronic leukemia. New, highly effective drug therapies for CML, such as imatinib, have been developed, based on inhibition of this tyrosine kinase activity.

In other cases, a translocation activates an oncogene by placing it downstream of a strong, constitutive promoter belonging to a different gene. Burkitt lymphoma is a B-cell tumor in which the *MYC* proto-oncogene is translocated from its normal chromosomal position at 8q24 to a position distal to the immunoglobulin heavy chain locus at 14q32 or the immunoglobulin light chain genes on chromosomes 22 and 2. The function of the Myc protein is still not entirely known, but it appears to be a transcription factor with powerful effects on the expression of a number of genes involved in cellular proliferation, as well as on telomerase expression. The translocation brings enhancer or other transcriptional activating sequences, normally associated with the immunoglobulin genes, near to the *MYC* gene (see Table 8-4). These translocations allow unregulated *MYC* expression, resulting in uncontrolled cell division.

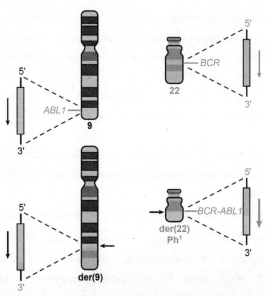

Figure 8-11　The Philadelphia chromosome translocation, t(9;22)(q34;q11)

The Philadelphia chromosome (Ph1) is the derivative chromosome 22, which has exchanged part of its long arm for a segment of material from chromosome 9q that contains the *ABL*1 oncogene. Formation of the chimeric *BCR-ABL*1 gene on the Ph1 chromosome is the critical genetic event in the development of chronic myelogenous leukemia.

Table 8-4　Characteristic Chromosome Translocations in Selected Human Malignant Neoplasms

Neoplasm	Chromosome Translocation	Percentage of Cases	Proto-oncogene Affected
Burkitt lymphoma	t(8;14)(q24;q32)	80	*MYC*
	t(8;22)(q24;q11)	15	
	t(2;8)(q11;q24)	5	
Chronic myelogenous leukemia	t(9;22)(q34;q11)	90~95	*BCR-ABL*1
Acute lymphocytic leukemia	t(9;22)(q34;q11)	10~15	*BCR-ABL*1
Acute lymphoblastic leukemia	t(1;19)(q23;p13)	3~6	*TCF3-PBX*1
Acute promyelocytic leukemia	t(15;17)(q22;q11)	≈95	*RARA-PML*
Chronic lymphocytic leukemia	t(11;14)(q13;q32)	10~30	*BCL*1
Follicular lymphoma	t(14;18)(q32;q21)	≈100	*BCL*2

8.5.3　Telomerase as an Oncogene

Another type of oncogene is the gene-encoding **telomerase**, a reverse transcriptase that is required to synthesize the hexamer repeat, TTAGGG, a component of telomeres at the ends of chromosomes. Telomerase is needed because, during normal semiconservative replication of DNA, DNA polymerase can only add nucleotides to the 3′end of DNA and cannot complete the synthesis of a growing strand all the way out to the very end of that strand on the chromosome arm. Thus, in the absence of a specific mechanism to allow replication of telomeres, the end of each chromosome arm would shorten each and every cell division.

In human germline cells and embryonic cells, telomeres contain approximately 15 kb of the telomeric repeat. As cells differentiate, telomerase activity declines in all somatic tissues. As telomerase function is lost, telomeres shorten, with a loss of approximately 35 bp of telomeric repeat DNA with each cell division. After hundreds of cell divisions, the chromosome ends become damaged, leading cells to stop dividing and to enter G_0 of the cell cycle. The cells will ultimately undergo apoptosis and die.

In contrast, in highly proliferative cells of tissues such as bone marrow, telomerase expression persists, allowing self-renewal. Similarly, telomerase persistence is observed in many tumors, which permits tumor cells to proliferate indefinitely. In some cases, telomerase activity results from chromosome or genome mutations that directly up-regulate the telomerase gene. In others, telomerase may be only one of many genes whose expression is altered by a transforming oncogene, such as *MYC*.

8.5.4 Loss of Tumor Suppressor Gene in Sporadic Cancer

TP53 and RB1 in Sporadic Cancers

Although Li-Fraumeni syndrome, caused by a dominantly inherited germline mutation in the *TP53* gene, is a rare familial syndrome, somatic mutation causing a loss of function of both alleles of *TP53* is one of the most common genetic alterations seen in sporadic cancer (see Table 8-2). Mutations of *TP53*, deletion of the segment of chromosome 17p that includes *TP53*, or loss of the entire chromosome 17 is frequently and repeatedly seen in a wide range of sporadic cancers. These include breast, ovarian, bladder, cervical, esophageal, colorectal, skin, and lung carcinomas; glioblastoma of the brain; osteogenic sarcoma; and hepatocellular carcinoma.

The retinoblastoma gene *RB1* is also frequently mutated in many sporadic cancers, including breast cancer. For example, 13q14 LOH in human breast cancers is associated with loss of *RB1* mRNA in the tumor tissues. In still other cancers, the *RB1* gene is intact and its mRNA appears to be at or near normal levels, yet the RB1 protein is deficient. This anomaly has now been explained by the recognition that *RB1* can be down-regulated in association with overexpression of the oncomir *miR-106a*, which targets *RB1* mRNA and blocks its translation.

8.6 Cytogenetic Changes in Cancer

➢ Aneuploidy and Aneusomy

Cytogenetic changes are hallmarks of cancer, whether sporadic or familial, particularly in later and more malignant or invasive stages of tumor development. Cytogenetic alterations suggest that a critical element of cancer progression includes defects in genes involved in maintaining chromosome stability and integrity and ensuring accurate mitotic segregation.

Initially, most of the cytogenetic studies of tumor progression were carried out in leukemias because the tumor cells were amenable to being cultured and karyotyped by standard methods. For example, when CML, with the 9;22 Philadelphia chromosome, evolves from the typically indolent chronic phase to a severe, life-threatening blast crisis, there may be several additional cytogenetic abnormalities, including numerical or structural changes, such as a second copy of the 9;22 translocation chromosome or an isochromosome for 17q. In advanced stages of other forms of leukemia, other translocations are common. In contrast, a vast array of chromosomal abnormalities are seen in most solid tumors. Cytogenetic abnormalities found repeatedly in a specific type of cancer are likely to be driver chromosome mutations involved in the initiation or progression of the malignant neoplasm. A current focus of cancer research is to develop a comprehensive cytogenetic and genomic definition of these abnormalities, many of which result in enhanced proto-oncogene expression or the loss of TSG alleles. Whole-genome sequencing is replacing cytogenetic analysis in many instances, because it provides a level of sensitivity and precision well beyond detection of cytologically visible genome changes.

Gene Amplification

In addition to translocations and other rearrangements, another cytogenetic aberration seen in many cancers is **gene amplification**, a phenomenon in which many additional copies of a segment of the genome are present in the cell (see Fig. 8-3). Gene amplification is common in many cancers, including neuroblastoma, squamous cell carcinoma of the head and neck, colorectal cancer, and malignant glioblastomas of the brain. Amplified segments of DNA are readily detected by comparative genome hybridization or whole-genome sequencing and appear as two types of cytogenetic change in routine chromosome analysis: **double minutes** (very small accessory chromosomes) and **homogeneously staining regions** that do not band normally and contain multiple, amplified copies of a particular DNA segment. How and why double minutes and homogeneously staining regions develop are poorly understood, but amplified regions are known to include extra copies of proto-oncogenes such as the genes encoding Myc, Ras, and epithelial growth factor receptor, which stimulate cell growth, block apoptosis, or both. For example, amplification of the *MYCN* proto-oncogene encoding N-Myc is an important clinical indicator of prognosis in the childhood cancer **neuroblastoma**. *MYCN* is amplified more than 200-fold in 40% of advanced stages of neuroblastoma. Despite aggressive treatment, only 30% of patients with advanced disease survive 3 years. In contrast, *MYCN* amplification is found in only 4% of early-stage neuroblastoma, and the 3-year survival is 90%. Amplification of genes encoding the targets of chemotherapeutic agents has also been implicated as a mechanism for the development of drug resistance in patients previously treated with chemotherapy.

8.7 Applying Genomics to Individualize Cancer Therapy

Genomics is already having a major impact on diagnostic precision and optimization of therapy in cancer. In this section, we describe how one such approach, **gene expression profiling**, is used to guide diagnosis and treatment.

8.7.1 Gene Expression Profiling and Clustering to Create Signatures

Comparative hybridization techniques can be used to measure simultaneously the level of mRNA expression of some or all of the estimated 20,000 protein-coding genes in any human tissue sample. A measurement of mRNA expression in a sample of tissue constitutes a **gene expression profile** specific to that tissue. Figure 8-12 depicts a hypothetical, idealized situation of eight samples, four from each of two types of tumor, A and B, profiled for 100 different genes. The expression profile derived from expression arrays for this simple example is already substantial, consisting of 800 expression values. In a real expression profiling experiment, however, hundreds of samples may be analyzed for the expression of all human genes, producing a massive data set of millions of expression values. Organizing the data and analyzing them to extract key information are challenging problems that have inspired the development of sophisticated statistical and bioinformatic tools. Using such tools, one can organize the data to find groups of genes whose expression seems to correlate, that is, increase or decrease together, between and among the samples. Grouping genes by their patterns of expression across samples is termed **clustering**.

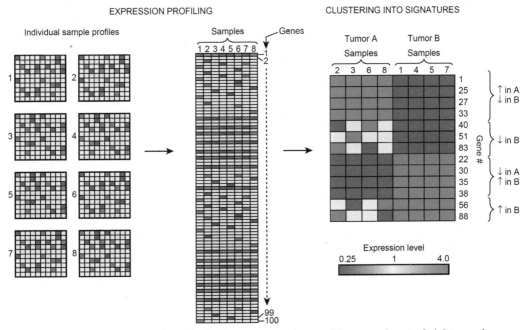

Figure 8-12   Schematic of an idealized gene expression profiling experiment of eight samples and 100 genes

Left, Individual arrays of gene sequences spotted on glass or silicon chips are used for comparative hybridization of eight different samples relative to a common standard. *Red* indicates decreased expression compared with control, *green* indicates increased expression, and *yellow* is unchanged expression. (In this schematic, *red*, *yellow*, and *green* represent decreased, equal or increased expression, whereas a real experiment would provide a continuous quantitative reading with shades of *red* and *green*.) *Center*, All 800 expression measurements are organized so that the relative expression for each gene, 1 through 100, is put in order vertically in a column under the number of each sample. *Right*, Clustering into signatures involves only those 13 genes that showed correlation across subsets of samples. Some genes have reciprocal (high versus low) expression in the two tumors; others show a correlated increase or decrease in one tumor and not the other.

Clusters of gene expression can then be tested to determine if any correlate with particular characteristics of the samples of interest. For example, profiling might indicate that a cluster of genes with a correlated expression profile is found more frequently in samples from tumor A than from tumor B, whereas another cluster of genes with a correlated expression profile is more frequent in samples derived from tumor B than from tumor A. Clusters of genes whose expression correlates with each other and with a particular set of samples constitute a so-called **expression signature** characteristic of those samples. In the hypothetical profiles in Figure 8-12, certain genes have a correlated expression that serves as a signature for tumor A; tumor B has a signature derived from the correlated expression of a different subset of these 100 genes.

Application of Gene Signatures

The application of gene expression profiles to characterize tumors is useful in a number of ways.

- Firstly, it increases our ability to discriminate between different tumors in ways that complement the standard criteria applied by pathologists to characterize tumors, such as histological appearance, cytogenetic markers, and expression of specific marker proteins. Once distinguishing signatures for different tumor types (e.g., tumor A versus tumor B) are defined using known samples, the expression pattern of unknown tumor samples can then be compared with the expression signatures for tumor A and tumor B and classified as A-like, B-like, or neither, depending on how well their expression profiles match the signatures of A and B. Pathologists have used expression profiling to make difficult distinctions between tumors that require very different management approaches. These include distinguishing large B-cell lymphoma from Burkitt lymphoma, differentiating primary lung cancers from squamous cell carcinomas of the head and neck metastatic to lung, and identifying the tissue of origin of a cryptic primary tumor whose metastasis gives too little information to allow its classification.

- Secondly, different signatures may be found to correlate with known clinical outcomes, such as prognosis, response to therapy, or any other outcome of interest. If validated, such signatures can be applied prospectively to help guide therapy in newly diagnosed patients.

- Thirdly, for basic research, clustering may reveal previously unsuspected connections of functional importance among genes involved in a disease process.

8.7.2 Gene Expression Profiling in Cancer Prognosis

Choosing the appropriate therapy for most cancers is difficult for patients and their physicians alike, because recurrence is common and difficult to predict. Better characterization of each patient's cancer as to recurrence risk and metastatic potential would clearly be beneficial for deciding between more or less aggressive courses of surgery and/or chemotherapy. For example, in breast cancer, although presence of the estrogen and progesterone receptors, amplification of the human epidermal growth factor receptor 2 (HER2) oncogene, and absence of metastatic tumor in lymph nodes found on dissection of axillary lymphatics are strong predictors of better response to therapy and prognosis, they are still imprecise. Expression profiling (see Fig. 8-13) is opening up a promising new avenue for clinical decision making in the management of breast cancer, as well as in other cancers, including lymphoma, prostate cancer, and metastatic adenocarcinomas of diverse tissue origins (lung, breast, colorectal, uterine, and ovarian).

Gene expression profiling of various sets of genes is clinically available for use in the management of breast, colon, and ovarian cancer; which genes and how many are included in the profile depends on the tumor type and vendor. Although the clinical utility and cost-effectiveness continue to be debated, there is a general consensus that combinations of clinical and gene expression data in patients newly diagnosed with cancer will provide better prospective estimates of prognosis and improved guidance of therapy. It is hoped that by improving the accuracy of prognosis with tumor expression profiling, oncologists can choose to forgo more vigorous and expensive chemotherapies in patients who do not need and/or will not benefit from them.

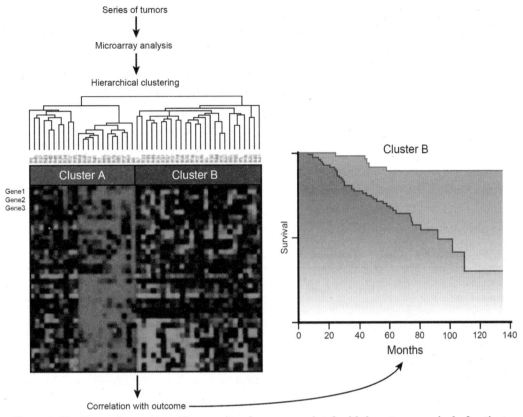

Figure 8-13　Expression patterns for a series of genes correlated with long-term survival of patients

Expression patterns for a series of genes (along the vertical axis at *left*) for series of patient tumors, with the tumors arranged along the horizontal axis at *top* so that tumors with more similar expression patterns are grouped more closely together. The tumors appear to generally cluster into two groups, which are then correlated with long-term survival.

(From REIS-FILHO J S, PUSZTAI L. Gene expression profiling in breast cancer: Classification, prognostication, and prediction[J]. The lancet, 2011,378(9805):1812-1823.)

The fact that the prognosis of practically every single patient could be associated with a particular combination of clinical features, genome sequence, and expression signatures underscores a crucial point about cancer: each person's cancer is a unique disorder. The genomic and gene expression heterogeneity among patients who all carry the same cancer diagnosis should not be surprising. Every patient is unique in the genetic variants he or she carries, including those variants that will affect how the cancer develops and the body responds to it. Moreover, the clonal evolution of a cancer implies that chance mutational and epigenetic events will likely occur in different and unique combinations in every patient's particular cancer.

8.7.3　Targeted Cancer Therapy

Until recently, most nonsurgical cancer treatment relied on cytotoxic agents, such as chemotherapeutic agents or radiation, designed to preferentially kill tumor cells while attempting to spare normal tissues. Despite tremendous successes in curing such diseases as childhood acute lymphocytic leukemia and Hodgkin lymphoma, most cancer patients in whom complete removal of the tumor with surgery is no longer possible receive remission, not cure, of their disease, usually at the cost of substantial toxicity from cytotoxic agents. The discovery of specific driver genes and their mutations in cancers has opened a new avenue for precisely targeted, less toxic treatments. Activated oncogenes are tempting targets for cancer therapy through direct blockade of their aberrant function. This can include blocking an activated cell surface receptor by monoclonal antibodies, or targeted inhibition of intracellular constitutive kinase activity with drugs designed to specifically inhibit their enzymatic activities.

The proof of principle for this approach was established with the development of imatinib, a highly effective inhibitor of a number of tyrosine kinases, including the ABL1 kinase in CML. Prolonged remissions of this disease have been seen, in some cases with apparently indefinite postponement of the transformation into a virulent acute leukemia (blast crisis) that so often meant the end of a CML patient's life. Additional kinase inhibitors have been developed to target other activated oncogene driver genes in a variety of tumor types (see Table 8-5).

Table 8-5 Cancer Treatments Targeted to Specific Activated Driver Oncogenes

Tumor Type	Driver Gene and Mutation	Representative FDA-Approved Targeted Therapeutic	Mechanism of Action
Breast cancer	Amplified HER2	Trastuzumab	Anti-HER2 monoclonal antibody
Non-small cell lung cancer	Activated EGFR	Gefitinib	Tyrosine kinase inhibitor
Chronic myelogenous leukemia and gastrointestinal stromal tumor	Activated receptor tyrosine kinases Abl, KIT, and PDGF	Imatinib, nilotinib, and dasatinib	Tyrosine kinase inhibitor
Non-small cell lung cancer	Translocated ALK	Crizotinib	Tyrosine kinase inhibitor
Melanoma	Activated MEK	Trametinib	Serine-threonine kinase inhibitor
Melanoma	Activated BRAF kinase	Vemurafenib	Serine-threonine kinase inhibitor

Note: ALK, Anaplastic lymphoma kinase; EGFR, epidermal growth factor receptor; FDA, U.S. Food and Drug Administration; HER2, human epidermal growth factor receptor 2; MEK, mitogen-activated extracellular signal-regulated kinase; PDGF, platelet-derived growth factor.

The initial results with targeted therapies, although very promising in some cases, have not led to permanent cures in most patients because tumors develop resistance to the targeted therapy. The outgrowth of resistant tumors is not surprising. First, as previously discussed, cancer cells are highly mutable, and their genomes undergo recurrent mutation. Even if only a small minority of cells acquire resistance through either mutation of the targeted oncogene itself, or through a compensatory mutation elsewhere, the tumor can progress even in the face of oncogene inhibition. Newer compounds that can overcome drug resistance are being developed and used in clinical trials. Ultimately, combination therapy that targets different driver genes may be required, based on the idea that a tumor cell is less likely to develop resistance in multiple unrelated pathways targeted by a combination of agents.

Review Points:

1. The evidences of monoclonal origin hypothesis, such as X chromosome evidence and the same mutation of genes which are involved in cancer.

2. Oncogenes.

Proto-oncogenes: To promote cell division, if mutate are activated improperly.

Onco-genes: Proto-oncogenes mutate into oncogenes, which are activated improperly.

Virus oncogenes: Discovery process of virus oncogenes and relationship between virus oncogenes and cell oncogenes.

Cell-oncogenes: Key genes are responsible for cell proliferation. Its expression and activity is controlled by cell accurately.

Cell-oncogenes in signal pathway: To introduce the cell proliferation signal pathway, in which cell-oncogenes take functions.

The pattern of proto-oncogenes mutate into cell-oncogenes, such as point mutations, amplification, viruses insertion, etc.

Tumor suppressive gene: Negative regulation during cell division; The functions and mutations of RB gene and P53 gene.

Introduce the two hits theory and multistep oncogenesis theory.

Study Questions:

1. A patient with retinoblastoma has a single tumor in one eye; the other eye is free of tumors. What steps would you take to try to determine whether this is sporadic or heritable retinoblastoma? What genetic counseling would you provide? What information should the parents have before a subsequent pregnancy?

2. Discuss possible reasons why colorectal cancer is an adult cancer, whereas retinoblastoma affects children.

3. Many tumor types are characterized by the presence of an isochromosome for the long arm of chromosome 17. Provide a possible explanation for this finding.

4. Wanda, whose sister has premenopausal bilateral breast cancer, has a greater risk for developing breast cancer herself than Wilma, whose sister has premenopausal breast cancer in only one breast. Both Wanda and Wilma, however, have a greater risk than does Winnie, who has a completely negative family history. Discuss the role of molecular testing in these women. What would their breast cancer risks be if a pathogenic BRCA1 or BRCA2 mutation were found in the affected relative? What if no mutations were found?

5. Propose a theory for why so few hereditary cancer syndromes, inherited as autosomal dominant diseases, are caused by activated oncogenes, whereas so many are caused by germline mutations in a tumor suppressor gene (TSG).

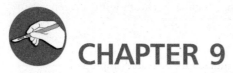

CHAPTER 9
Genetic Variation in Individuals and Populations: Mutation and Polymorphism

Purpose and Requirement:

Students must make sure the sorts of mutation which is the nature of genetically determined differences among individuals. And the Hardy-Weinberg equilibrium law also should be understood that the applications of the law are in the estimation of gene frequency, genotype frequency, relative mating harmful effect and genetic hypothesis test.

The study of genetic and genomic variation is the conceptual cornerstone for genetics in medicine and for the broader field of human genetics. During the course of evolution, the steady influx of new nucleotide variation has ensured a high degree of genetic diversity and individuality, and this theme extends through all fields in human and medical genetics. Genetic diversity may manifest as differences in the organization of the genome, as nucleotide changes in the genome sequence, as variation in the copy number of large segments of genomic DNA, as alterations in the structure or amount of proteins found in various tissues, or as any of these in the context of clinical disease.

This chapter is one of several in which we explore the nature of genetically determined differences among individuals. The sequence of nuclear DNA is approximately 99.5% identical between any two unrelated humans. Yet it is precisely the small fraction of DNA sequence difference among individuals that is responsible for the genetically determined variability that is evident both in one's daily existence and in clinical medicine. Many DNA sequence differences have little or no effect on outward appearance, whereas other differences are directly responsible for causing disease. Between these two extremes is the variation responsible for genetically determined variability in anatomy, physiology, dietary intolerances, susceptibility to infection, predisposition to cancer, therapeutic responses or adverse reactions to medications, and perhaps even variability in various personality traits, athletic aptitude, and artistic talent.

One of the important concepts of human and medical genetics is that diseases with a clearly inherited component are only the most obvious and often the most extreme manifestation of genetic differences, one end of a continuum of variation that extends from rare deleterious variants that cause illness, through more common variants that can increase susceptibility to disease, to the most common variation in the population that is of uncertain relevance with respect to disease.

9.1 The Nature of Genetic Variation

As described in Chapter 2, a segment of DNA occupying a particular position or location on a chromosome is a **locus** (plural **loci**). A locus may be large, such as a segment of DNA that contains many genes, such as the major histocompatibility complex locus involved in the response of the immune system to foreign substances. It may be a single gene, such as the β-globin locus. Or it may even be just a single base in the genome, as in the case of a single nucleotide variant. Alternative versions of the DNA sequence at a locus are called **alleles**. For many genes, there is a single prevailing allele, usually present in more than half of the individuals in a population, that geneticists call the **wild-type** or common allele. (In lay parlance, this is sometimes referred to as the "normal" allele. However, because genetic variation is itself very much "normal", the existence of different alleles in "normal" individuals is commonplace. Thus one should avoid using "normal" to designate the most common allele.) The other versions of the gene are **variant** (or **mutant**) alleles that differ from the wild-type allele because of the presence of a **mutation**, a permanent change in the nucleotide sequence or arrangement of DNA. Note that the terms mutation and mutant refer to DNA, but not to the human beings who carry mutant alleles. The terms denote a change in sequence but otherwise do not carry any connotation with respect to the function or fitness of that change.

The frequency of different variants can vary widely in different populations around the globe. If there are two or more relatively common alleles (defined by convention as having an allele frequency $> 1\%$) at a locus in a population, that locus is said to exhibit **polymorphism** (literally "many forms") in that population. Most variant alleles, however, are not frequent enough in a population to be considered polymorphisms. Some are so rare as to be found in only a single family and are known as "**private**" **alleles**.

9.1.1 The Concept of Mutation

In this chapter, we begin by exploring the nature of **mutation**, ranging from the change of a single nucleotide to alterations of an entire chromosome. To recognize a change means that there has to be a "gold standard", compared to which the variant shows a difference. There is no single individual whose genome sequence could serve as such a standard for the human species, and thus one arbitrarily designates the most common sequence or arrangement in a population at any one position in the genome as the so-called reference sequence. As more and more genomes from individuals around the globe are sampled (and thus as more and more variation is detected among the currently 7 billion genomes that make up our species), this reference genome is subject to constant evaluation and change. Indeed, a number of international collaborations share and update data on the nature and frequency of DNA variation in different populations in the context of the reference human genome sequence and make the data available through publicly accessible databases that serve as essential resources for scientists, physicians, and other health care professionals (see Table 9-1).

Table 9-1 Useful Databases of Information on Human Genetic Diversity

Description	URL
The **Human Genome Project**, completed in 2003, was an international collaboration to sequence and map the genome of our species. The draft sequence of the genome was released in 2001, and the "essentially complete" reference genome assembly was published in 2004	http://www.genome.gov/10001772 http://igenome.ucs.edu/cgi-bin/heGareway http://www.ensembl.org/Homo_sapiensi/Info/Index
The **Single Nucleotide Polymorphism Database (dbSNP) and the Structural Variation Database (dbVar)** are databases of small-scale and large-scale variations, including single nucleotide variants, microsatellites, indels, and CNVs	http://www.ncbi.nlm.nih.gov/snp/ http://www.ncbi.nlm.mih.gov/dbvat/
The 1,000 **Genomes Project** is sequencing the genomes of a large number of individuals to provide a comprehensive resource on genetic variation in our species. All data are publicly available	www.1000genomes.org
The **Human Gene Mutation Database** is a comprehensive collection of germline mutations associated with or causing human inherited disease (currently including over 120,000 mutations in 4,400 genes)	www.hgnd.org
The **Database b Cenomic Variants** is a curated catalogue of structural variation in the human genome. As of 2012, the database contains over 400,000 entries, including over 200,000 CNVs, 1,000 inversions, and 34,000 indels	http://dgv.tcag.ca
The Japanese Sing/Siuclcotide Polymorphisms Database (**JSNP Database**) reports SNPs discovered as part of the Millennium Genome Project	http://snp.ims.u-tokyo.ac.jp/

Note: CNV, Copy number variant; SNP, single nucleotide polymorphism.

(From GINSBURG G S, WILLARD H F. Preface [M]//Genomic and Personalized Medicine. Amsterdam: Elsevier, 2013:xi‒xii.)

Mutations are sometimes classified by the size of the altered DNA sequence and, at other times, by the functional effect of the mutation on gene expression. Although classification by size is somewhat arbitrary, it can be helpful conceptually to distinguish among mutations at three different levels:

- Mutations that leave chromosomes intact but change the number of chromosomes in a cell (**chromosome mutations**).
- Mutations that change only a portion of a chromosome and might involve a change in the copy number of a subchromosomal segment or a structural rearrangement involving parts of one or more chromosomes (**regional** or **subchromosomal mutations**).
- Alterations of the sequence of DNA, involving the substitution, deletion, or insertion of DNA, ranging from a single nucleotide up to an arbitrarily set limit of approximately 100 kb (**gene** or **DNA mutations**).

The functional consequences of DNA mutations, even those that change a single base pair, run the gamut from being completely innocuous to causing serious illness, all depending on the precise location, nature, and size of the mutation. For example, even a mutation within a coding exon of a gene may have no effect on how a gene is expressed if the change does not alter the primary amino acid sequence of the polypeptide product. Even if it does, the resulting change in the encoded amino acid sequence may not alter the functional properties of the protein. Not all mutations, therefore, are manifest in an individual.

9.1.2 The Concept of Genetic Polymorphism

The DNA sequence of a given region of the genome is remarkably similar among chromosomes carried by many different individuals from around the world. In fact, any randomly chosen segment of human DNA approximately 1,000 bp in length contains, on average, only one base pair that is different between the two homologous chromosomes inherited from that individual's parents (assuming the parents are unrelated). However, across all human populations, many tens of millions of single nucleotide differences and over a million more complex variants have been identified and catalogued. Because of limited sampling, these figures are likely to underestimate the true extent of genetic diversity in our species. Many populations around the globe have yet to be studied, and, even in the populations that have been studied, the number of individuals examined is too small to reveal most variants with minor allele frequencies below 1% to 2%. Thus, as more people are included in variant discovery projects, additional (and rarer) variants will certainly be uncovered.

Whether a variant is formally considered a polymorphism or not depends entirely on whether its frequency in a population exceeds 1% of the alleles in that population, and not on what kind of mutation caused it, how large a segment of the genome is involved, or whether it has a demonstrable effect on the individual. The location of a variant with respect to a gene also does not determine whether the variant is a polymorphism. Although most sequence polymorphisms are located between genes or within introns and are inconsequential to the functioning of any gene, others may be located in the coding sequence of genes themselves and result in different protein variants that may lead in turn to distinctive differences in human populations. Still others are in regulatory regions and may also have important effects on transcription or RNA stability.

One might expect that deleterious mutations that cause rare monogenic diseases are likely to be too rare to achieve the frequency necessary to be considered a polymorphism. Although it is true that the alleles responsible for most clearly inherited clinical conditions are rare, some alleles that have a profound effect on health—such as alleles of genes encoding enzymes that metabolize drugs (for example, sensitivity to abacavir in some individuals infected with human immunodeficiency virus [HIV]), or the sickle cell mutation in African and African American populations—are relatively common. Nonetheless, these are exceptions, and, as more and more genetic variation is discovered and catalogued, it is clear that the vast majority of variants in the genome, whether common or rare, reflect differences in DNA sequence that have no known significance to health.

Polymorphisms are key elements for the study of human and medical genetics. The ability to distinguish different inherited forms of a gene or different segments of the genome provides critical tools for a wide array of applications, both in research and in clinical practice.

9.2 Inherited Variation and Polymorphism in DNA

The original Human Genome Project and the subsequent study of now many thousands of individuals worldwide have provided a vast amount of DNA sequence information. With this information in hand, one can begin to characterize the types and frequencies of polymorphic variation found in the human genome and to generate catalogues of human DNA sequence diversity around the globe. DNA polymorphisms can be classified according to how the DNA sequence varies between the different alleles (see Table 9-2 and Figs. 9-1 and 9-2).

Table 9-2   Common Variation in the Human Genome

Type of Variation	Size Range (approx.)	Basis for the Polymorphism	Number of Alleles
Single nucleotide polymorphisms	1 bp	Substitution of one or another base pair at a particular location in the genome	Usually 2
Insertion/deletions (indels)	1 bp to >100 bp	*Simple*: Presence or absence of a short segment of DNA 100~1,000 bp in length *Microsatellites*: Generally, a 2-, 3-, or 4-nucleotide unit repeated in tandem 5~25 times	*Simple*: 2 *Microsatellites*: typically 5 or more
Copy number variants	10 kb to >1 Mb	Typically the presence or absence of 200-bp to 1.5-Mb segments of DNA, although tandem duplication of 2, 3, 4, or more copies can also occur	2 or more
Inversions	Few bp to >1 Mb	A DNA segment present in either of two orientations with respect to the surrounding DNA	2

Note: bp, Base pair; kb, kilobase pair; Mb, megabase pair.

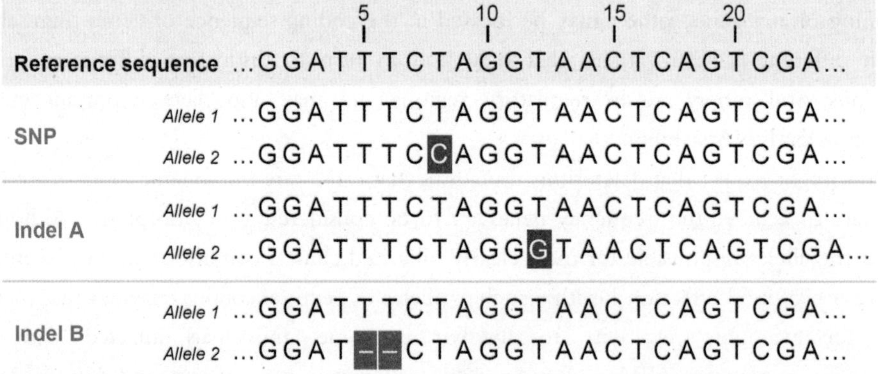

Figure 9-1   Three polymorphisms in genomic DNA from the segment of the human genome
The reference sequence is shown at the top. The single nucleotide polymorphism (SNP) at position 8 has two alleles, one with a T (corresponding to the reference sequence) and one with a C. There are two indels in this region. At indel A, allele 2 has an insertion of a G between positions 11 and 12 in the reference sequence (allele 1). At indel B, allele 2 has a 2 bp deletion of positions 5 and 6 in the reference sequence.

9.2.1 Single Nucleotide Polymorphisms

The simplest and most common of all polymorphisms are **single nucleotide polymorphisms**

(**SNPs**). A locus characterized by a SNP usually has only two alleles, corresponding to the two different bases occupying that particular location in the genome (see Fig. 9-1). As mentioned previously, SNPs are common and are observed on average once every 1,000 bp in the genome. However, the distribution of SNPs is uneven around the genome. Many more SNPs are found in noncoding parts of the genome, in introns and in sequences that are some distance from known genes. Nonetheless, there is still a significant number of SNPs that do occur in genes and other known functional elements in the genome. For the set of protein-coding genes, over 100,000 exonic SNPs have been documented to date. Approximately half of these do not alter the predicted amino acid sequence of the encoded protein and are thus termed **synonymous**, whereas the other half do alter the amino acid sequence and are said to be **nonsynonymous**. Other SNPs introduce or change a stop codon, and yet others alter a known splice site. Such SNPs are candidates to have significant functional consequences.

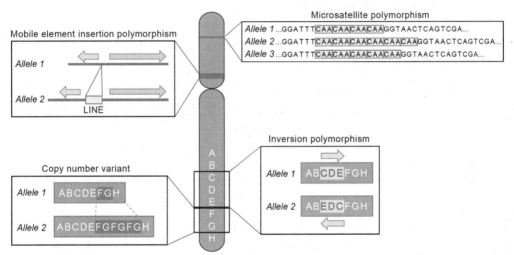

Figure 9-2 Examples of polymorphism in the human genome larger than SNPs

Clockwise from upper right: The microsatellite locus has three alleles, with four, five, or six copies of a CAA trinucleotide repeat. The inversion polymorphism has two alleles corresponding to the two orientations (indicated by the *arrows*) of the genomic segment shown in green. Such inversions can involve regions up to many megabases of DNA. Copy number variants involve deletion or duplication of hundreds of kilobase pairs to over a megabase of genomic DNA. In the example shown, allele 1 contains a single copy, whereas allele 2 contains three copies of the chromosomal segment containing the F and G genes. Other possible alleles with zero, two, four, or more copies of F and G are not shown. The mobile element insertion polymorphism has two alleles, one with and one without insertion of an approximately 6 kb LINE repeated retroelement. The insertion of the mobile element changes the spacing between the two genes and may alter gene expression in the region.

The significance for health of the vast majority of SNPs is unknown and is the subject of ongoing research. The fact that SNPs are common does not mean that they are without effect on health or longevity. What it does mean is that any effect of common SNPs is likely to involve a relatively subtle altering of disease susceptibility rather than a direct cause of serious illness.

9.2.2 Insertion-Deletion Polymorphisms

A second class of polymorphism is the result of variations caused by **insertion** or **deletion** (**in/dels** or simply **indels**) of anywhere from a single base pair up to approximately 1,000 bp, although larger indels have been documented as well. Over a million indels have been described, numbering in the hundreds of thousands in any one individual's genome. Approximately half of all indels are referred to as "simple" because they have only two alleles—that is, the presence or absence of the inserted or deleted segment (see Fig. 9-1).

(1) Microsatellite Polymorphisms

Other indels, however, are multiallelic due to variable numbers of the segment of DNA that is inserted in tandem at a particular location, thereby constituting what is referred to as a **microsatellite**. They consist of stretches of DNA composed of units of two, three, or four nucleotides, such as TGTGTG, CAACAACAA, or AAATAAATAAAT, repeated between one and a few dozen times at a particular site in the genome (see Fig. 9-2). The different alleles in a microsatellite polymorphism are the result of differing numbers of repeated nucleotide units contained within any one microsatellite and are therefore sometimes also referred to as **short tandem repeat (STR) polymorphisms**. A microsatellite locus often has many alleles (repeat lengths) that can be rapidly evaluated by standard laboratory procedures to distinguish different individuals and to infer familial relationships (see Fig. 9-3). Many tens of thousands of microsatellite polymorphic loci are known throughout the human genome.

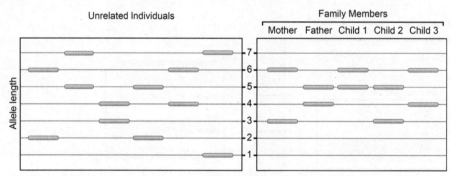

Figure 9-3   A schematic of a hypothetical microsatellite marker in human DNA

The different-sized alleles (numbered 1 to 7) correspond to fragments of genomic DNA containing different numbers of copies of a microsatellite repeat, and their relative lengths are determined by separating them by gel electrophoresis. The shortest allele (allele 1) migrates toward the bottom of the gel, whereas the longest allele (allele 7) remains closest to the top. *Left*, For this multiallelic microsatellite, each of the six unrelated individuals has two different alleles. *Right*, Within a family, the inheritance of alleles can be followed from each parent to each of the three children.

Microsatellites are a particularly useful group of indels. Determining the alleles at multiple microsatellite loci is currently the method of choice for **DNA fingerprinting** used for identity testing. For example, the Federal Bureau of Investigation (FBI) in the United States currently uses the collection of alleles at 13 such loci for its DNA fingerprinting panel. Two individuals (other than monozygotic twins) are so unlikely to have exactly the same alleles at all 13 loci that the panel will allow definitive determination of whether two samples came from the same individual. The information is stored in the FBI's Combined DNA Index System (CODIS), which has grown as of December 2014 to include over 11,548,700 offender profiles, 1,300,000 arrestee profiles, and 601,600 forensic profiles (material obtained at crime scenes). Many states and the U. S. Department of Defense have similar databases of DNA fingerprints, as do corresponding units in other countries.

(2) Mobile Element Insertion Polymorphisms

Nearly half of the human genome consists of families of repetitive elements that are dispersed around the genome. Although most of the copies of these repeats are stationary, some of them are mobile and contribute to human genetic diversity through the process of **retrotransposition**, a process that involves transcription into an RNA, reverse transcription into a DNA sequence, and insertion (i.e., transposition) into another site in the genome. The two most common mobile element families are the Alu and LINE families of repeats, and nearly 10,000 mobile element insertion polymorphisms have been described in different populations. Each polymorphic locus consists of two alleles, one with and one without the inserted mobile element (see Fig. 9-2). Mobile element polymorphisms are found on all human chromosomes. Although most are found in nongenic regions of the genome, a small proportion of them are found within genes. At least 5,000 of these polymorphic loci have an insertion frequency of greater than 10% in various populations.

9.2.3　Copy Number Variants

Another important type of human polymorphism includes **copy number variants** (**CNVs**). CNVs are conceptually related to indels and microsatellites but consist of variation in the number of copies of larger segments of the genome, ranging in size from 1,000 bp to many hundreds of kilobase pairs. Variants larger than 500 kb are found in 5% to 10% of individuals in the general population, whereas variants encompassing more than 1 Mb are found in 1% to 2%. The largest CNVs are sometimes found in regions of the genome characterized by repeated blocks of homologous sequences called **segmental duplications** (or **segdups**).

Smaller CNVs in particular may have only two alleles (i.e., the presence or absence of a segment), similar to indels in that regard. Larger CNVs tend to have multiple alleles due to the presence of different numbers of copies of a segment of DNA in tandem (see Fig. 9-2). In terms of genome diversity between individuals, the amount of DNA involved in CNVs vastly exceeds the amount that differs because of SNPs. The content of any two human genomes can differ by as much as 50 to 100 Mb because of copy number differences at CNV loci.

Notably, the variable segment at many CNV loci can include one to as many as several dozen genes, and thus CNVs are frequently implicated in traits that involve altered gene dosage. When a CNV is frequent enough to be polymorphic, it represents a background of common variation that must be understood if alterations in copy number observed in patients are to be interpreted properly. As with all DNA polymorphism, the significance of different CNV alleles in health and disease susceptibility is the subject of intensive investigation.

9.2.4　Inversion Polymorphisms

A final group of polymorphisms to be discussed is inversions, which differ in size from a few base pairs to large regions of the genome (up to several megabase pairs) that can be present in either of two orientations in the genomes of different individuals (see Fig. 9-2). Most inversions are characterized by regions of sequence homology at the edges of the inverted segment, implicating a process of homologous recombination in the origin of the inversions. In their balanced form, inversions, regardless of orientation, do not involve a gain or loss of DNA, and the inversion polymorphisms (with two alleles corresponding to the two orientations) can achieve substantial frequencies in the general population. However, anomalous recombination can result in the duplication or deletion of DNA located between the regions of homology, associated with clinical disorders.

9.3 The Origin and Frequency of Different Types of Mutations

Along the spectrum of diversity from rare variants to more common polymorphisms, the different kinds of mutations arise in the context of such fundamental processes of cell division as DNA replication, DNA repair, DNA recombination, and chromosome segregation in mitosis or meiosis. The **frequency of mutations per locus per cell division** is a basic measure of how error prone these processes are, which is of fundamental importance for genome biology and evolution. However, of greatest importance to medical geneticists is the **frequency of mutations per disease locus per generation**, rather than the overall mutation rate across the genome per cell division. Measuring disease-causing mutation rates can be difficult, however, because many mutations cause early embryonic lethality before the mutation can be recognized in a fetus or newborn, or because some people with a disease-causing mutation may manifest the condition only late in life or may never show signs of the disease. Despite these limitations, we have made great progress is determining the overall frequency—sometimes referred to as the **genetic load**—of all mutations affecting the human species.

The major types of mutation briefly introduced earlier occur at appreciable frequencies in many different cells in the body. In the practice of genetics, we are principally concerned with inherited genome variation. However, all such variation had to originate as a new (*de novo*) change occurring in germ cells. At that point, such a variant would be quite rare in the population (occurring just once), and its ultimate frequency in the population over time depends on chance and on the principles of inheritance and population genetics. Although the original mutation would have occurred only in the DNA of cells in the **germline**, anyone who inherits that mutation would then carry it as a constitutional mutation in all the cells of the body.

In contrast, **somatic mutations** occur throughout the body but cannot be transmitted to the next generation. Given the rate of mutation, one would predict that, in fact, every cell in an individual has a slightly different version of his or her genome, depending on the number of cell divisions that have occurred since conception to the time of sample acquisition. In highly proliferative tissues, such as intestinal epithelial cells or hematopoietic cells, such genomic heterogeneity is particularly likely to be apparent. However, most such mutations are not typically detected, because, in clinical testing, one usually sequences DNA from collections of many millions of cells. In such a collection, the most prevalent base at any position in the genome will be the one present at conception, and rare somatic mutations will be largely invisible and unascertained. Such mutations can be of clinical importance, however, in disorders caused by mutation in only a subset of cells in certain tissues, leading to somatic mosaicism.

The major exception to the expectation that somatic mutations will be typically undetected within any multicell DNA sample is in cancer, in which the mutational basis for the origins of cancer and the clonal nature of tumor evolution drives certain somatic changes to be present in essentially all the cells of a tumor. Indeed, 1,000 to 10,000 somatic mutations (and sometimes many more) are readily found in the genomes of most adult cancers, with mutation frequencies and patterns specific to different cancer types.

9.3.1　Chromosome Mutations

Mutations that produce a change in chromosome number because of chromosome missegregation are among the most common mutations seen in humans, with a rate of one mutation per 25 to 50 meiotic cell divisions. This estimate is clearly a minimal one because the developmental consequences of many such events are likely so severe that the resulting fetuses are aborted spontaneously shortly after conception without being detected.

9.3.2　Regional Mutations

Mutations affecting the structure or regional organization of chromosomes can arise in a number of different ways. Duplications, deletions, and inversions of a segment of a single chromosome are predominantly the result of homologous recombination between DNA segments with high sequence homology located at more than one site in a region of a chromosome. Not all structural mutations are the result of homologous recombination, however. Others, such as chromosome translocations and some inversions, can occur at the sites of spontaneous double-stranded DNA breaks. Once breakage occurs at two places anywhere in the genome, the two broken ends can be joined together even without any obvious homology in the sequence between the two ends (a process termed nonhomologous end-joining repair).

9.3.3　Gene Mutations

Gene or DNA mutations, including base pair substitutions, insertions, and deletions (see Fig. 9-4), can originate by either of two basic mechanisms: errors introduced during DNA replication or mutations arising from a failure to properly repair DNA after damage. Many such mutations are spontaneous, arising during the normal (but imperfect) processes of DNA replication and repair, whereas others are induced by physical or chemical agents called **mutagens**.

(1) DNA Replication Errors

The process of DNA replication is typically highly accurate. The majority of replication errors (i.e., inserting a base other than the complementary base that would restore the base pair at that position in the double helix) are rapidly removed from the DNA and corrected by a series of DNA repair enzymes that first recognize which strand in the newly synthesized double helix contains the incorrect base and then replace it with the proper complementary base, a process termed **DNA proofreading**. DNA replication needs to be a remarkably accurate process. Otherwise, the burden of mutation on the organism and the species would be intolerable. The enzyme DNA polymerase faithfully duplicates the two strands of the double helix based on strict base-pairing rules (A pairs with T, C with G) but introduces one error every 10 million bp. Additional proofreading then corrects more than 99.9% of these errors of DNA replication. Thus the overall mutation rate per base as a result of replication errors is a remarkably low 1×10^{-10} per cell division—fewer than one mutation per genome per cell division.

(2) Repair of DNA Damage

It is estimated that, in addition to replication errors, between 10,000 and 1 million nucleotides are damaged per human cell per day by spontaneous chemical processes such as depurination, demethylation, or deamination; by reaction with chemical mutagens (natural or otherwise) in the environment; and by exposure to ultraviolet or ionizing radiation. Some but not all of this damage is repaired. Even if the damage is recognized and excised, the repair machinery may create mutations by introducing incorrect bases. Thus, in contrast to replication-related DNA changes, which are usually corrected through proofreading mechanisms, nucleotide changes introduced by DNA damage and repair often result in permanent mutations.

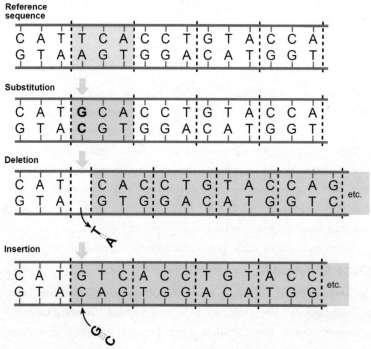

Figure 9-4   Examples of mutations in a portion of a hypothetical gene with five codons shown (delimited by the *dotted lines*)

The first base pair of the second codon in the reference sequence (shaded in *blue*) is mutated by a base substitution, deletion, or insertion. The base substitution of a G for the T at this position leads to a codon change (shaded in *green*) and, assuming that the upper strand is the sense or coding strand, a predicted nonsynonymous change from a serine to an alanine in the encoded protein; all other codons remain unchanged. Both the single base pair deletion and insertion lead to a frameshift mutation in which the translational reading frame is altered for all subsequent codons (shaded in *green*), until a termination codon is reached.

A particularly common spontaneous mutation is the substitution of T for C (or A for G on the other strand). The explanation for this observation comes from considering the major form of epigenetic modification in the human genome, DNA methylation. Spontaneous deamination of 5-methylcytosine to thymidine (compare the structures of cytosine and thymine) in the CpG doublet gives rise to C to T or G to A mutations (depending on which strand the 5-methylcytosine is deaminated). Such spontaneous mutations may not be recognized by the DNA repair machinery and thus become established in the genome after the next round of DNA replication. More than 30% of all single nucleotide substitutions are of this type, and they occur at a rate 25 times greater than those of any other single nucleotide mutations. Thus the CpG doublet represents a true "hot spot" for mutation in the human genome.

(3) Overall Rate of DNA Mutations

Although the rate of DNA mutations at specific loci has been estimated using a variety of approaches over the past 50 years, the overall impact of replication and repair errors on the occurrence of new mutations throughout the genome can now be determined directly by **whole-genome sequencing** of trios consisting of a child and both parents, looking for new mutations in the child that are not present in the genome sequence of either parent. The overall rate of new mutations averaged between maternal and paternal gametes is approximately 1.2×10^{-8} mutations per base pair per generation. Thus every person is likely to receive approximately 75 new mutations in his or her genome from one or the other parent. This rate, however, varies from gene to gene around the genome and perhaps from population to population or even individual to individual. Overall, this rate, combined with considerations of population growth and dynamics, predicts that there must be an enormous number of relatively new (and thus very rare) mutations in the current worldwide population of 7 billion individuals.

As might be predicted, the vast majority of these mutations will be single nucleotide changes in noncoding portions of the genome and will probably have little or no functional significance. Nonetheless, at the level of populations, the potential collective impact of these new mutations on genes of medical importance should not be overlooked. In the United States, for example, with over 4 million live births each year, approximately 6 million new mutations will occur in coding sequences. Thus, even for a single protein-coding gene of average size, we can anticipate several hundred newborns each year with a new mutation in the coding sequence of that gene.

Conceptually similar studies have determined the rate of mutations in CNVs, where the generation of a new length variant depends on recombination, rather than on errors in DNA synthesis to generate a new base pair. The measured rate of formation of new CNVs ($\approx 1.2 \times 10^{-2}$ per locus per generation) is orders of magnitude higher than that of base substitutions.

(4) Rate of Disease-Causing Gene Mutations

The most direct way of estimating the rate of disease-causing mutations per locus per generation is to measure the incidence of new cases of a genetic disease that is not present in either parent and is caused by a single mutation that causes a condition that is clearly recognizable in all neonates who carry that mutation. **Achondroplasia**, a condition of reduced bone growth leading to short stature, is a condition that meets these requirements. In one study, seven achondroplastic children were born in a series of 242,257 consecutive births. All seven were born to parents of normal stature, and, because achondroplasia always manifests when a mutation is present, all were considered to represent new mutations. The new mutation rate at this locus can be calculated to be seven new mutations in a total of $2 \times 242,257$ copies of the relevant gene, or approximately 1.4×10^{-5} disease-causing mutations per locus per generation. This high mutation rate is particularly striking because it has been found that virtually all cases of achondroplasia are due to the identical mutation, a G to A mutation that changes a glycine codon to an arginine in the encoded protein.

The rate of gene mutations that cause disease has been estimated for a number of other disorders in which the occurrence of a new mutation was determined by the appearance of a detectable disease (see Table 9-3). The measured rates for these and other disorders vary over a 1,000-fold range, from 10^{-4} to 10^{-7} mutations per locus per generation. The basis for these differences may be related to some or all of the following: the size of different genes; the fraction of all mutations in that gene that will lead to the disease; the age and sex of the parent in whom the mutation occurred; the mutational mechanism; and the presence or absence of mutational hot spots in the gene. Indeed, the high rate of the particular site-specific mutation in achondroplasia may be partially explained by the fact that the mutation on the other strand is a C to T change in a position that undergoes CpG methylation and is a hot spot for mutation by deamination, as discussed earlier.

Table 9-3   Estimates of Mutation Rates for Selected Human Disease Genes

Disease	Locus (Protein)	Mutation Rate*
Achondroplasia	*FGFR3* (fibroblast growth factor receptor 3)	1.4×10^{-5}
Aniridia	*PAX6* (Pax6)	$(2.9 \sim 5) \times 10^{-6}$
Duchenne muscular dystrophy	*DMD* (dystrophin)	$(3.5 \sim 10.5) \times 10^{-5}$
Hemophilia A	*F8* (factor VIII)	$(3.2 \sim 5.7) \times 10^{-5}$
Hemophilia B	*F9* (factor IX)	$(2 \sim 3) \times 10^{-6}$
Neurofibromatosis, type 1	*NF1* (neurofibromin)	$(4 \sim 10) \times 10^{-5}$
Polycystic kidney disease, type 1	*PKD1* (polycystin)	$(6.5 \sim 12) \times 10^{-5}$
Retinoblastoma	*RB1* (Rb1)	$(5 \sim 12) \times 10^{-6}$

Note: * Expressed as mutations per locus per generation.

Notwithstanding this range of rates among different genes, the median gene mutation rate is approximately 1×10^{-6}. Given that there are at least 5,000 genes in the human genome in which mutations are currently known to cause a discernible disease or other trait, approximately 1 in 200 persons is likely to receive a new mutation in a known disease-associated gene from one or the other parent.

9.4 Types of Mutations and Their Consequences

In this section, we consider the nature of different mutations and their effect on the genes involved. Each type of mutation discussed here is illustrated by one or more disease examples. Notably, the specific mutation found in almost all cases of achondroplasia is the exception rather than the rule, and the mutations that underlie a single genetic disease are more typically heterogeneous among a group of affected individuals. Different cases of a particular disorder will therefore usually be caused by different underlying mutations (see Table 9-4).

Table 9-4   Types of Mutation in Human Genetic Disease

Type of Mutation	Percentage of Disease-Causing Mutations
Nucleotide Substitutions	
• Missense mutations (amino acid substitutions)	50%
• Nonsense mutations (premature stop codons)	10%
• RNA processing mutations (destroy consensus splice sites, cap sites, and polyadenylation sites or create cryptic sites)	10%
• Splice-site mutations leading to frameshift mutations and premature stop codons	10%
• long-range regulatory mutations	Rare

Continued

Type of Mutation	Percentage of Disease-Causing Mutations
Deletions and Insertions	
• Addition or deletions of a small number of bases	25%
• larger gene deletions, inversions, fusions, and duplications (may be mediated by DNA sequence homology either within or between DNA strands)	5%
• Insertion of a LINE or *Alu* element (disrupting transcription or interrupting the coding sequence)	Rare
• Dynamic mutations (expansion of trinucleotide or tetranucleotide repeat sequences)	Rare

9.4.1   Nucleotide Substitutions

(1) Missense Mutations

A single nucleotide substitution (or **point mutation**) in a gene sequence, such as that observed in the example of achondroplasia just described, can alter the code in a triplet of bases and cause the nonsynonymous replacement of one amino acid by another in the gene product (the example in Fig. 9-4). Such mutations are called **missense mutations** because they alter the coding (or "sense") strand of the gene to specify a different amino acid. Although not all missense mutations lead to an observable change in the function of the protein, the resulting protein may fail to work properly, may be unstable and rapidly degraded, or may fail to localize in its proper intracellular position. In many disorders, such as **β-thalassemia**, most of the mutations detected in different patients are missense mutations.

(2) Nonsense Mutations

Point mutations in a DNA sequence that cause the replacement of the normal codon for an amino acid by one of the three termination (or "stop") codons are called **nonsense mutations**. Because translation of messenger RNA (mRNA) ceases when a termination codon is reached, a mutation that converts a coding exon into a termination codon causes translation to stop partway through the coding sequence of the mRNA. The consequences of premature termination mutations are twofold. First, the mRNA carrying a premature mutation is often targeted for rapid degradation (through a cellular process known as **nonsense-mediated mRNA decay**), and no translation is possible. And second, even if the mRNA is stable enough to be translated, the truncated protein is usually so unstable that it is rapidly degraded within the cell.

Whereas some point mutations create a premature termination codon, others may destroy the normal termination codon and thus permit translation to continue until another termination codon in the mRNA is reached further downstream. Such a mutation will lead to an abnormal protein product with additional amino acids at its carboxyl terminus, and may also disrupt regulatory functions normally provided by the 3′ untranslated region downstream from the normal stop codon.

(3) Mutations Affecting RNA Transcription, Processing, and Translation

The normal mechanism by which initial RNA transcripts are made and then converted into mature mRNAs (or final versions of noncoding RNAs) requires a series of modifications, including transcription factor binding, 5′ capping, polyadenylation, and splicing. All of these steps in RNA maturation depend on specific sequences within the RNA. In the case of splicing, two general classes of splicing mutations have been described. For introns to be excised from unprocessed RNA and the exons spliced together to form a mature RNA requires particular nucleotide sequences located at or near the exon-intron (5′donor site) or the intron-exon (3′acceptor site) junctions. Mutations that affect these required bases at either the splice donor or acceptor site interfere with (and in some cases abolish) normal RNA splicing at that site. A second class of splicing mutations involves base substitutions that do not affect the donor or acceptor site sequences themselves but instead create alternative donor or acceptor sites that compete with the normal sites during RNA processing. Thus at least a proportion of the mature mRNA or noncoding RNA in such cases may contain improperly spliced intron sequences.

For protein-coding genes, even if the mRNA is made and is stable, point mutations in the 5′ and 3′-untranslated regions can also contribute to disease by changing mRNA stability or translation efficiency, thereby reducing the amount of protein product that is made.

9.4.2 Deletions, Insertions, and Rearrangements

Mutations can also be caused by the insertion, deletion, or rearrangement of DNA sequences. Some deletions and insertions involve only a few nucleotides and are generally most easily detected by direct sequencing of that part of the genome. In other cases, a substantial segment of a gene or an entire gene is deleted, duplicated, inverted, or translocated to create a novel arrangement of gene sequences. Depending on the exact nature of the deletion, insertion, or rearrangement, a variety of different laboratory approaches can be used to detect the genomic alteration.

Some deletions and insertions affect only a small number of base pairs. When such a mutation occurs in a coding sequence and the number of bases involved is not a multiple of three (i.e., is not an integral number of codons), the reading frame will be altered beginning at the point of the insertion or deletion. The resulting mutations are called **frameshift mutations** (see Fig. 9-4). From the point of the insertion or deletion, a different sequence of codons is thereby generated that encodes incorrect amino acids followed by a termination codon in the shifted frame, typically leading to a functionally altered protein product. In contrast, if the number of base pairs inserted or deleted is a multiple of three, then no frameshift occurs and there will be a simple insertion or deletion of the corresponding amino acids in the otherwise normally translated gene product. Larger insertions or deletions, ranging from approximately 100 to more than 1,000 bp, are typically referred to as "indels", as we saw in the case of polymorphisms earlier. They can affect multiple exons of a gene and cause major disruptions of the coding sequence.

One type of insertion mutation involves insertion of a mobile element, such as those belonging to the LINE family of repetitive DNA. It is estimated that, in any individual, approximately 100 copies of a particular subclass of the LINE family in the genome are capable of movement by **retrotransposition**, introduced earlier. Such movement not only generates genetic diversity in our species (see Fig. 9-2) but can also cause disease by insertional mutagenesis. For example, in some patients with the severe bleeding disorder **hemophilia A**, LINE sequences several kilobase pairs long are found to be inserted into an exon in the factor VIII gene, interrupting the coding sequence and inactivating the gene. LINE insertions throughout the genome are also common in colon cancer, reflecting retrotransposition in somatic cells.

Duplications, deletions, and inversions of a larger segment of a single chromosome are predominantly the result of homologous recombination between DNA segments with high sequence homology (see Fig. 9-5). Disorders arising as a result of such exchanges can be due to a change in the dosage of otherwise wild-type gene products when the homologous segments lie outside the genes themselves. Alternatively, such mutations can lead to a change in the nature of the encoded protein itself when recombination occurs between different genes within a gene family or between genes on different chromosomes. Abnormal pairing and recombination between two similar sequences in opposite orientation on a single strand of DNA leads to inversion. For example, nearly half of all cases of hemophilia A are due to recombination that inverts a number of exons, thereby disrupting gene structure and rendering the gene incapable of encoding a normal gene product (see Fig. 9-5).

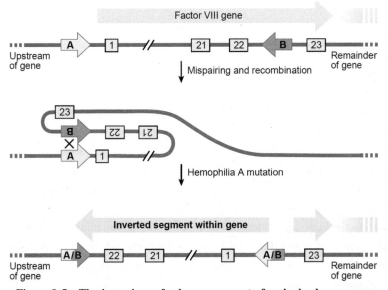

Figure 9-5   The inversions of a larger segment of a single chromosome
Inverted homologous sequences, labeled A and B, located 500 kb apart on the X chromosome, one upstream of the factor VIII gene, the other in an intron between exons 22 and 23 of the gene. Intrachromosomal mispairing and recombination results in inversion of exons 1 through 22 of the gene, thereby disrupting the gene and causing severe hemophilia.

Dynamic Mutations

The mutations in some disorders involve amplification of a simple nucleotide repeat sequence. For example, simple repeats such as $(CCG)_n$, $(CAG)_n$, or $(CCTG)_n$ located in the coding portion of an exon, in an untranslated region of an exon, or even in an intron may expand during gametogenesis, in what is referred to as a **dynamic mutation**, and interfere with normal gene expression or protein function. An expanded repeat in the coding region will generate an abnormal protein product, whereas repeat expansion in the untranslated regions or introns of a gene may interfere with transcription, mRNA processing, or translation. How dynamic mutations occur is not completely understood. They are conceptually similar to microsatellite polymorphisms but expand at a rate much higher than typically seen for microsatellite loci.

In disorders caused by dynamic mutations, marked parent-of-origin effects are well known and appear characteristic of the specific disease and/or the particular simple nucleotide repeat involved. Such differences may be due to fundamental biological differences between oogenesis and spermatogenesis but may also result from selection against gametes carrying certain repeat expansions.

9.5 Variation in Individual Genomes

The most extensive current inventory of the amount and type of variation to be expected in any given genome comes from the direct analysis of individual diploid human genomes. The first of such genome sequences, that of a male individual, was reported in 2007. Now, tens of thousands of individual genomes have been sequenced, some as part of large international research consortia exploring human genetic diversity in health and disease, and others in the context of clinical sequencing to determine the underlying basis of a disorder in particular patients.

What degree of genome variation does one detect in such studies? Individual human genomes typically carry 5 to 10 million SNPs, of which—depending in part on the population—as many as a quarter to a third are novel. This suggests that the number of SNPs described for our species is still incomplete, although presumably the fraction of such novel SNPs will decrease as more and more genomes from more and more populations are sequenced.

Within this variation lie variants with known, likely, or suspected clinical impact. Based on studies to date, each genome carries 50 to 100 variants that have previously been implicated in known inherited conditions. In addition, each genome carries thousands of nonsynonymous SNPs in protein-coding genes around the genome, some of which would be predicted to alter protein function. Each genome also carries approximately 200 to 300 likely loss-of-function mutations, some of which are present at both alleles of genes in that individual. Within the clinical setting, this realization has important implications for the interpretation of genome sequence data from patients, particularly when trying to predict the impact of mutations in genes of currently unknown function.

An interesting and unanticipated aspect of individual genome sequencing is that the reference human genome assembly still lacks considerable amounts of undocumented and unannotated DNA that are discovered in literally every individual genome being sequenced. These "new" sequences are revealed only as additional genomes are sequenced. Thus the complete collection of all human genome sequences to be found in our current population of 7 billion individuals, estimated to be 20 to 40 Mb larger than the extant reference assembly, still remains to be fully elucidated.

As impressive as the current inventory of human genetic diversity is, it is clear that we are still in a mode of discovery. No doubt millions of additional SNPs and other variants remain to be uncovered, as does the degree to which any of them might affect an individual's clinical status in the context of wellness and health care.

➢ Clinical Sequencing Studies

In the context of genomic medicine, a key question is to what extent variation in the sequence and/or expression of one's genome influences the likelihood of disease onset, determines or signals the natural history of disease, and/or provides clues relevant to the management of disease. As just discussed, variation in one's constitutional genome can have a number of different direct or indirect effects on gene function.

Sequencing of entire genomes (so-called **whole-genome sequencing**) or of the subset of genomes that include all of the known coding exons (so-called **whole-exome sequencing**) has been introduced in a number of clinical settings. Both whole-exome and whole-genome sequencing have been used to detect *de novo* mutations (both point mutations and CNVs) in a variety of conditions of complex and/or unknown etiology, including, for example, various neurodevelopmental or neuropsychiatric conditions, such as autism, schizophrenia, epilepsy, or intellectual disability and developmental delay.

Clinical sequencing studies can target either germline or somatic variants. In cancer, especially, various strategies have been used to search for somatic mutations in tumor tissue to identify genes potentially relevant to cancer progression.

9.6   Impact of Mutation and Polymorphism

Although it will be self-evident to students of human genetics that new deleterious mutations or rare variants in the population may have clinical consequences, it may appear less obvious that common polymorphic variants can be medically relevant. For the proportion of polymorphic variation that occurs in the genes themselves, such loci can be studied by examining variation in the proteins encoded by the different alleles. It has long been estimated that any one individual is likely to carry two distinct alleles determining structurally differing polypeptides at approximately 20% of all protein-coding loci. When individuals from different geographic or ethnic groups are compared, an even greater fraction of proteins has been found to exhibit detectable polymorphism. In addition, even when the gene product is identical, the levels of expression of that product may be very different among different individuals, determined by a combination of genetic and epigenetic variation.

Thus a striking degree of biochemical individuality exists within the human species in its makeup of enzymes and other gene products. Furthermore, because the products of many of the encoded biochemical and regulatory pathways interact in functional and physiological networks, one may plausibly conclude that each individual, regardless of his or her state of health, has a unique, genetically determined chemical makeup and thus responds in a unique manner to environmental, dietary, and pharmacological influences. This concept of **chemical individuality**, first put forward over a century ago by Garrod, the remarkably prescient British physician, remains true today. The broad question of what is normal—an essential concept in human biology and in clinical medicine—remains very much an open one when it comes to the human genome.

9.7   Genotypes and Phenotypes in Populations

9.7.1   Allele and Genotype Frequencies in Populations

To illustrate the relationship between allele and genotype frequencies in populations, we begin with an important example of a common autosomal trait governed by a single pair of alleles. Consider the gene *CCR5*, which encodes a cell surface cytokine receptor that serves as an entry point for certain strains of the human immunodeficiency virus (HIV), which causes the **acquired immunodeficiency syndrome** (**AIDS**). A 32-bp deletion in this gene results in an allele (Δ*CCR5*) that encodes a nonfunctional protein due to a frameshift and premature termination. Individuals homozygous for the Δ*CCR5* allele do not express the receptor on the surface of their immune cells and, as a consequence, are resistant to HIV infection. Loss of function of *CCR5* appears to be a benign trait, and its only known phenotypic consequence is resistance to HIV infection. A sampling of 788 individuals from Europe illustrates the distribution of individuals who were homozygous for the wildtype *CCR5* allele, homozygous for the Δ*CCR5* allele, or heterozygous (see Table 9-5).

Table 9-5   Genotype Frequencies for the Wild-Type *CCR5* Allele and the Δ*CCR5* Deletion Allele

Genotype	Number of Individuals	Observed Genotype Frequency	Allele	Derived Allele Frequencies
CCR5/CCR5	647	0.821		
*CCR5/*Δ*CCR5*	134	0.168	*CCR5*	0.906
Δ*CCR5/*Δ*CCR5*	7	0.011	Δ*CCR5*	0.094
Total	788	1.000		

On the basis of the observed genotype frequencies, we can directly determine the allele frequencies by simply counting the alleles. In this context, when we refer to the population frequency of an allele, we are considering a hypothetical **gene pool** as a collection of all the alleles at a particular locus for the entire population. For autosomal loci, the size of the gene pool at one locus is twice the number of individuals in the population because each autosomal genotype consists of two alleles. That is, a Δ*CCR5/*Δ*CCR5* individual has two Δ*CCR5* alleles, and a *CCR5/*Δ*CCR5* individual has one of each. In this example, then, the observed frequency of the *CCR5* allele is:

$$\frac{(2 \times 647) + (1 \times 134)}{788 \times 2} \approx 0.906$$

Similarly, one can calculate the frequency of the Δ*CCR5* allele as 0.094, by adding up how many Δ*CCR5* alleles are present [(2×7) + (1×134)] =148 out of a total of 1576 alleles in this sample, resulting in a Δ*CCR5* allele frequency of 148/1576 ≈ 0.094. Alternatively (and more simply), one can subtract the frequency of the normal *CCR5* allele, 0.906, from 1, because the frequencies of the two alleles must add up to 1, resulting in a Δ*CCR5* allele frequency of 0.094.

9.7.2   The Hardy-Weinberg Law

As we have just shown with the *CCR5* example, we can use a sample of individuals with known genotypes in a population to derive estimates of the allele frequencies by simply counting the alleles in individuals with each genotype. How about the converse? Can we calculate the proportion of the population with various genotypes once we know the allele frequencies? Deriving genotype frequencies from allele frequencies is not as straightforward as counting because we actually do not know in advance how the alleles are distributed among homozygotes and heterozygotes. If a population meets certain assumptions, however, there is a simple mathematical equation for calculating genotype frequencies from allele frequencies. This equation is known as the Hardy-Weinberg law. This law, the cornerstone of population genetics, was named for Godfrey Hardy, an English mathematician, and Wilhelm Weinberg, a German physician, who independently formulated it in 1908.

The Hardy-Weinberg law has two critical components. The first is that under certain ideal conditions, a simple relationship exists between allele frequencies and genotype frequencies in a population. Suppose p is the frequency of allele A, and q is the frequency of allele a in the gene pool. Assume alleles combine into genotypes randomly; that is, mating in the population is completely at random with respect to the genotypes at this locus. The chance that two A alleles will pair up to give the AA genotype is then $p2$; the chance that two a alleles will come together to give the aa genotype is $q2$; and the chance of having one A and one a pair, resulting in the Aa genotype, is $2pq$ (the factor 2 comes from the fact that the A allele could be inherited from the mother and the a allele from the father, or vice versa). The Hardy-Weinberg law states that the frequency of the three genotypes AA, Aa, and aa is given by the terms of the binomial expansion of $(p+q)^2 = p^2 + 2pq + q^2$. This law applies to all autosomal loci and to the X chromosome in females, but not to X-linked loci in males who have only a single X chromosome.

The law can be adapted for genes with more than two alleles. For example, if a locus has three alleles, with frequencies p, q, and r, the genotypic distribution can be determined from $(p+q+r)^2$. In general terms, the genotype frequencies for any known number of alleles a_n with allele frequencies p_1, p_2, $\cdots p_n$ can be derived from the terms of the expansion of $(p_1+p_2+\cdots p_n)^2$.

A second component of the Hardy-Weinberg law is that if allele frequencies do not change from generation to generation, the proportion of the genotypes will not change either. That is, the population genotype frequencies from generation to generation will remain constant, at equilibrium, if the allele frequencies p and q remain constant. More specifically, when there is random mating in a population that is at equilibrium and genotypes AA, Aa, and aa are present in the proportions $p^2 : 2pq : q^2$, then genotype frequencies in the next generation will remain in the same relative proportions, $p^2 : 2pq : q^2$. Proof of this equilibrium is shown in Table 9-6. It is important to note that Hardy-Weinberg equilibrium does not specify any particular values for p and q; whatever allele frequencies happen to be present in the population will result in genotype frequencies of $p^2 : 2pq : q^2$, and these relative genotype frequencies will remain constant from generation to generation as long as the allele frequencies remain constant and the other conditions are met.

Applying the Hardy-Weinberg formula to the $CCR5$ example given earlier, with relative frequencies of the two alleles in the population of 0.906 (for the wild-type allele $CCR5$) and 0.094 (for $\Delta CCR5$), then the Hardy-Weinberg law states that the relative proportions of the three combinations of alleles (genotypes) are $p^2 = 0.906 \times 0.906 \approx 0.821$ (for an individual having two wild-type $CCR5$ alleles), $q^2 = 0.094 \times 0.094 \approx 0.009$ (for two $\Delta CCR5$ alleles), and $2pq = (0.906 \times 0.094) + (0.094 \times 0.906) \approx 0.170$ (for one $CCR5$ and one $\Delta CCR5$ allele). When these genotype frequencies, which were calculated by the Hardy-Weinberg law, are applied to a population of 788 individuals, the derived numbers of people with the three different genotypes (647 : 134 : 7) are, in fact, identical to the actual observed numbers in Table 9-5. As long as the assumptions of the Hardy-Weinberg law are met in a population, we would expect these genotype frequencies (0. 821 : 0. 170 : 0. 009) to remain constant generation after generation in that population.

Table 9-6 Frequencies of Mating Types and Offspring for a Population in Hardy-Weinberg Equilibrium With Parental Genotypes in the Proportion $p^2 : 2pq : q^2$

Types of Matings			Offspring		
Mother	Father	Frequency	AA	Aa	aa
AA	AA	$p^2 \times p^2 = p^4$	p^4		
AA	Aa	$p^2 \times 2pq = 2p^3 q$	$1/2(2p^3 q)$	$1/2(2p^3 q)$	
Aa	AA	$2pq \times p^2 = 2p^3 q$	$1/2(2p^3 q)$	$1/2(2p^3 q)$	
AA	aa	$p^2 \times q^2 = p^2 q^2$		$p^2 q^2$	
aa	AA	$q^2 \times p^2 = p^2 q^2$		$p^2 q^2$	
Aa	Aa	$2pq \times 2pq = 4p^2 q^2$	$1/4(4p^2 q^2)$	$1/2(4p^2 q^2)$	$1/4(4p^2 q^2)$
Aa	aa	$2pq \times q^2 = 2pq^3$		$1/2(2pq^3)$	$1/2(2pq^3)$
aa	Aa	$q^2 \times 2pq = 2pq^3$		$1/2(2pq^3)$	$1/2(2pq^3)$
aa	aa	$q^2 \times q^2 = q^4$			q^4

Note: Sum of AA offspring$= p^4 + p^3 q + p^3 q + p^2 q^2 = p^2(p^2 + 2pq + q^2) = p^2(p+q)^2 = p^2$. (Remember that $p+q=1$.)
Sum of Aa offspring$= p^3 q + p^3 q + p^2 q^2 + p^2 q^2 + 2p^2 q^2 + pq^3 + pq^3 = 2pq(p^2 + 2pq + q^2) = 2pq(p+q)^2 = 2pq$.
Sum of aa offspring$= p^2 q^2 + pq^3 + pq^3 + q^4 = q^2(p^2 + 2pq + q^2) = q^2(p+q)^2 = q^2$.

9.7.3 The Hardy-Weinberg Law in Autosomal Recessive Disease

The major practical application of the Hardy-Weinberg law in medical genetics is in genetic counseling for autosomal recessive disorders. For a disease such as **phenylketonuria** (**PKU**), there are hundreds of different mutant alleles with frequencies that vary among different population groups defined by geography and/or ethnicity. Affected individuals can be homozygotes for the same mutant allele but, more often than not, are compound heterozygotes for different mutant alleles. For many disorders, however, it is convenient to consider all disease-causing alleles together and treat them as a single mutant allele, with frequency q, even when there is significant allelic heterogeneity in disease-causing alleles. Similarly, the combined frequency of all wild-type or normal alleles, p, is given by $1 - q$.

Suppose we would like to know the frequency of all disease-causing PKU alleles in a population for use in genetic counseling, for example, to inform couples of their risk for having a child with PKU. If we were to attempt to determine the frequency of disease-causing PKU alleles directly from genotype frequencies, as we did in the earlier example of the $\Delta CCR5$ allele, we would need to know the frequency of heterozygotes in the population, a frequency that cannot be measured directly because of the recessive nature of PKU; heterozygotes are asymptomatic silent carriers, and their frequency in the population (i. e., $2pq$) cannot be reliably determined directly from phenotype.

However, the frequency of affected homozygotes/compound heterozygotes for disease-causing alleles in the population (i.e., q^2) can be determined directly, by counting the number of babies with PKU born over a given period of time and identified through newborn screening programs, divided by the total number of babies screened during that same period of time. Now, using the Hardy-Weinberg law, we can calculate the mutant allele frequency (q) from the observed frequency of homozygotes/compound heterozygotes alone (q^2), thereby providing an estimate ($2pq$) of the frequency of heterozygotes for use in genetic counseling.

To illustrate this example further, consider a population in Ireland, where the frequency of PKU is approximately 1 per 4500. If we group all disease-causing alleles together and treat them as a single allele with frequency q, then the frequency of affected individuals $q^2 = 1/4,500$. From this, we calculate $q = 0.015$, and thus $2pq = 0.029$. The carrier frequency for all disease-causing alleles lumped together in the Irish population is therefore approximately 3%. For an individual known to be a carrier of PKU through the birth of an affected child in the family, there would then be an approximately 3% chance that he or she would find a new mate of Irish ethnicity who would also be a carrier, and this estimate could be used to provide genetic counseling. Note, however, that this estimate applies only to the population in question. If the new mate was not from Ireland, but from Finland, where the frequency of PKU is much lower (≈ 1 per $200,000$), his or her chance of being a carrier would be only 0.6%.

In this example, we lumped all PKU-causing alleles together for the purpose of estimating q. For other disorders, however, such as hemoglobin disorders, different mutant alleles can lead to very different diseases, and therefore it would make no sense to group all mutant alleles together, even when the same locus is involved. Instead, the frequency of alleles leading to different phenotypes (such as sickle cell anemia and β-thalassemia in the case of different mutant alleles at the β-globin locus) is calculated separately.

9.7.4   The Hardy-Weinberg Law in X-Linked Disease

For X-linked genes, there are three female genotypes but only two possible male genotypes. To illustrate gene frequencies and genotype frequencies when the gene of interest is X-linked, we use the trait known as X-linked **red-green color blindness**, which is caused by mutations in the series of visual pigment genes on the X chromosome. We use color blindness as an example because, as far as we know, it is not a deleterious trait (except for possible difficulties with traffic lights), and color blind persons are not subject to selection. As discussed later, allowing for the effect of selection complicates estimates of gene frequencies.

In this example, we use the symbol *cb* for all the mutant color blindness alleles and the symbol $+$ for the wild-type allele, with frequencies q and p, respectively (see Table 9-7). The frequencies of the two alleles can be determined directly from the incidence of the corresponding phenotypes in males by simply counting the alleles. Because females have two X chromosomes, their genotypes are distributed like autosomal genotypes, but because color blindness alleles are recessive, the normal homozygotes and heterozygotes are typically not distinguishable. As shown in Table 9-7, the frequency of color blindness in females is much lower than that in males. Less than 1% of females are color blind, but nearly 15% are carriers of a mutant color blindness allele and have a 50% chance of having a color blind son with each male pregnancy.

Table 9-7 X-Linked Genes and Genotype Frequencies (Color Blindness)

Sex	Genotype	Phenotype	Incidence (Approximate)
Male	X^+	Normal color vision	$p=0.92$
	X^{cb}	Color blind	$q=0.08$
Female	X^+/X^+	Normal (homozygote)	$p^2=(0.92)^2=0.8464$
	X^+/X^{cb}	Normal (heterozygote)	$2pq=2\times0.92\times0.08=0.1472$
		Normal (combined)	$p^2+2pq=0.9936$
	X^{cb}/X^{cb}	Color blind	$q^2=(0.08)^2=0.0064$

9.8 Factors That Disturb Hardy-Weinberg Equilibrium

Underlying the Hardy-Weinberg law and its use are a number of assumptions, not all of which can be met (or reasonably inferred to be met) by all populations. The first is that the population under study is large and that mating is random. However, a very small population in which random events can radically alter an allele frequency may not meet this first assumption. This first assumption is also breached when the population contains subgroups whose members choose to marry within their own subgroup rather than the population at large. The second assumption is that allele frequencies do not change significantly over time. This requires that there is no migration in or out of the population by groups whose allele frequencies at a locus of interest are radically different from the allele frequencies in the population as a whole. Similarly, selection for or against particular alleles, or the addition of new alleles to the gene pool due to mutations, will break the assumptions of the Hardy-Weinberg law.

9.8.1 The Hardy-Weinberg Law in X-Linked Disease

In practice, some of these violations are more damaging than others to the application of the law to human populations. As shown in the sections that follow, violating the assumption of random mating can cause large deviations from the frequency of individuals homozygous for an autosomal recessive condition that we might expect from population allele frequencies. What's more, changes in allele frequency due to mutation, selection, or migration usually cause more minor and subtle deviations from Hardy-Weinberg equilibrium. Finally, when Hardy-Weinberg equilibrium does not hold for a particular disease allele at a particular locus, it may be instructive to investigate why the allele and its associated genotypes are not in equilibrium because this may provide clues about the pathogenesis of the condition or point to historical events that have affected the frequency of alleles in different population groups over time.

9.8.2 Exceptions to Large Populations With Random Mating

As introduced earlier, the principle of random mating is that for any locus, an individual of a given genotype has a purely random probability of mating with an individual of any other genotype, the proportions being determined only by the relative frequencies of the different genotypes in the population. One's choice of mate, however, may not be at random. In human populations, nonrandom mating may occur because of three distinct but related phenomena: **stratification**, **assortative mating**, and **consanguinity**.

(1) Stratification

Stratification describes a population in which there are a number of subgroups that have—

for a variety of historical, cultural, or religious reasons—remained relatively genetically separate during modern times. Worldwide, there are numerous stratified populations. For example, the United States population is stratified into many subgroups, including whites of northern or southern European ancestry, African Americans, and numerous Native American, Asian, and Hispanic groups. Similarly stratified populations exist in other parts of the world as well, either currently or in the recent past, such as Sunni and Shia Muslims, Orthodox Jews, French-speaking Canadians, or different castes in India. When mate selection in a population is restricted for any reason to members of one particular subgroup, and that subgroup happens to have a variant allele with a higher frequency than in the population as a whole, the result will be an apparent excess of homozygotes in the overall population beyond what one would predict from allele frequencies in the population as a whole if there were truly random mating.

To illustrate this point, suppose a population contains a minority group, constituting 10% of the population, in which a mutant allele for an autosomal recessive disease has a frequency $q_{min} = 0.05$ and the wild-type allele has frequency $p_{min} = 0.95$. In the remaining majority 90% of the population, the mutant allele is nearly absent (i.e., q_{maj} is ≈ 0 and $p_{maj} = 1$). An example of just such a situation is the African American population of the United States and the mutant allele at the β-globin locus responsible for **sickle cell disease**. The overall frequency of the disease allele in the total population, q_{pop}, is therefore equal to $0.1 \times 0.05 = 0.005$, and, simply applying the Hardy-Weinberg law, the frequency of the disease in the population as a whole would be predicted to be $q_{pop}^2 = (0.005)^2 = 2.5 \times 10^{-5}$ if mating were perfectly random throughout the entire population. If, however, individuals belonging to the minority group were to mate exclusively with other members of that same minority group (an extreme situation that does not apply in reality), then the frequency of affected individuals in the minority group would be $(q_{min}^2) = (0.05)^2 = 0.0025$. Because the minority group is one tenth of the entire population, the frequency of disease in the total population is $0.0025/10 = 2.5 \times 10^{-4}$, or 10-fold higher than the calculated $q_{pop}^2 = 2.5 \times 10^{-5}$ obtained by naively applying the Hardy-Weinberg law to the population as a whole without consideration of stratification.

By way of comparison, stratification has no effect on the frequency of autosomal dominant disease and would have only a minor effect on the frequency of X-linked disease by increasing the small number of females homozygous for the mutant allele.

(2) Assortative Mating

Assortative mating is the choice of a mate because the mate possesses some particular trait. Assortative mating is usually positive. That is, people tend to choose mates who resemble themselves (e.g., in native language, intelligence, stature, skin color, musical talent, or athletic ability). To the extent that the characteristic shared by the partners is genetically determined, the overall genetic effect of positive assortative mating is an increase in the proportion of the homozygous genotypes at the expense of the heterozygous genotype.

A clinically important aspect of assortative mating is the tendency to choose partners with similar medical problems, such as congenital deafness or blindness or exceptionally short stature. In such a case, the expectations of Hardy-Weinberg equilibrium do not apply because the genotype of the mate at the disease locus is not determined by the allele frequencies found in the general population. For example, consider **achondroplasia**, an autosomal dominant form of skeletal dysplasia with a population incidence of 1 per 15,000 to 1 per 40,000 live births. Offspring homozygous for the achondroplasia mutation have a severe, lethal form of skeletal dysplasia that is almost never seen unless both parents have achondroplasia and are thus heterozygous for the mutation. This would be highly unlikely to occur by chance, except for assortative mating among those with achondroplasia.

When mates have autosomal recessive disorders caused by the same mutation or by allelic mutations in the same gene, all of their offspring will also have the disease. Importantly, however, not all cases of blindness, deafness, or short stature have the same genetic basis. Many families have been described, for example, in which two parents with albinism have had children with normal pigmentation, or two deaf parents have had hearing children, because of locus heterogeneity. Even if there is locus heterogeneity with assortative mating, however, the chance that two individuals are carrying mutations in the same disease locus is increased over what it would be under true random mating, and therefore the risk for the disorder in their offspring is also increased. Although the long-term population effect of this kind of positive assortative mating on disease gene frequencies is insignificant, a specific family may find itself at very high genetic risk that would not be predicted from strict application of the Hardy-Weinberg law.

(3) Consanguinity and Inbreeding

Consanguinity, like stratification and positive assortative mating, brings about an increase in the frequency of autosomal recessive disease by increasing the frequency with which carriers of an autosomal recessive disorder mate. Unlike the disorders in stratified populations, in which each subgroup is likely to have a high frequency of a few alleles, the kinds of recessive disorders seen in the offspring of related parents may be very rare and unusual in the population as a whole because consanguineous mating allows an uncommon allele inherited from a heterozygous common ancestor to become homozygous. A similar phenomenon is seen in **genetic isolates**, small populations derived from a limited number of common ancestors who tended to mate only among themselves. Mating between two apparently "unrelated" individuals in a genetic isolate may have the same risk for certain recessive conditions as that observed in consanguineous marriages because the individuals are both carriers by inheritance from common ancestors of the isolate, a phenomenon known as **inbreeding**.

For example, among Ashkenazi Jews in North America, mutant alleles for Tay-Sachs disease (GM2 gangliosidosis), are relatively more common than in other ethnic groups. The frequency of Tay-Sachs disease is 100 times higher in Ashkenazi Jews (1 per 3,600) than in most other populations (1 per 360,000). Thus the Tay-Sachs carrier frequency among Ashkenazi Jews is approximately 1 in 30 ($q^2=1/3,600$, $q=1/60$, $2pq=1/30$) as compared to a carrier frequency of approximately 1 in 300 in non-Ashkenazi individuals.

9.8.3 Exceptions to Constant Allele Frequencies

(1) Effect of Mutation

We have shown that nonrandom mating can substantially upset the relative frequency of various genotypes predicted by the Hardy-Weinberg law, even within the time of a single generation. In contrast, changes in allele frequency due to selection or mutation usually occur slowly, in small increments, and cause much less deviation from Hardy-Weinberg equilibrium, at least for recessive diseases.

The rates of new mutations are generally well below the frequency of heterozygotes for autosomal recessive diseases; the addition of new mutant alleles to the gene pool thus has little effect in the short term on allele frequencies for such diseases. In addition, most deleterious recessive alleles are hidden in asymptomatic heterozygotes and thus are not subject to selection. As a consequence, selection is not likely to have major short-term effects on the allele frequency of these recessive alleles. Therefore, to a first approximation, Hardy-Weinberg equilibrium may apply even for alleles that cause severe autosomal recessive disease.

Importantly, however, for dominant or X-linked disease, mutation and selection do perturb allele frequencies from what would be expected under Hardy-Weinberg equilibrium, by substantially reducing or increasing certain genotypes.

(2) Selection and Fitness

Here we examine the concept of **fitness**, the chief factor that determines whether a mutation is eliminated immediately, becomes stable in the population, or even becomes, over time, the predominant allele at the locus concerned. The frequency of an allele in a population at any given time represents a balance between the rate at which mutant alleles appear through mutation and the effects of selection. If either the mutation rate or the effectiveness of selection is altered, the allele frequency is expected to change.

Whether an allele is transmitted to the succeeding generation depends on its fitness, f, which is a measure of the number of offspring of affected persons who survive to reproductive age, compared with an appropriate control group. If a mutant allele is just as likely as the normal allele to be represented in the next generation, f equals 1. If an allele causes death or sterility, selection acts against it completely, and f equals 0. Values between 0 and 1 indicate transmission of the mutation, but at a rate that is less than that of individuals who do not carry the mutant allele.

A related parameter is the **coefficient of selection**, s, which is a measure of the loss of fitness and is defined as $1-f$, that is, the proportion of mutant alleles that are not passed on and are therefore lost as a result of selection. In the genetic sense, a mutation that prevents reproduction by an adult is just as "lethal" as one that causes a very early miscarriage of an embryo, because in neither case is the mutation transmitted to the next generation. Fitness is thus the outcome of the joint effects of survival and fertility. When a genetic disorder limits reproduction so severely that the fitness is zero (i.e., $s=1$), it is thus referred to as a **genetic lethal**. In the biological sense, fitness has no connotation of superior endowment except in a single respect: comparative ability to contribute alleles to the next generation.

① Selection in Recessive Disease

Selection against harmful recessive mutations has far less effect on the population frequency of the mutant allele than does selection against dominant mutations because only a small proportion of the genes are present in homozygotes and are therefore exposed to selective forces. Even if there were complete selection against homozygotes ($f=0$), as in many lethal autosomal recessive conditions, it would take many generations to reduce the gene frequency appreciably because most of the mutant alleles are carried by heterozygotes with normal fitness. For example, the frequency of mutant alleles causing Tay-Sachs disease, q, can be as high as 1.5%

in Ashkenazi Jewish populations. Given this value of q, we can estimate that approximately 3% of such populations ($2 \times p \times q$) are heterozygous and carry one mutant allele, whereas only 1 individual per 3,600 (q^2) is a homozygote with two mutant alleles. The proportion of all mutant alleles found in homozygotes in such a population is thus given by:

$$\frac{2 \times 0.00028}{(2 \times 0.00028) + (1 \times 0.03)} \approx 0.0183$$

Thus, less than 2% of all the mutant alleles in the population are in affected homozygotes and would therefore be exposed to selection in the absence of effective treatment.

Reduction or removal of selection against an autosomal recessive disorder by successful medical treatment (e.g., as in the case of PKU would have just as slow an effect on increasing the gene frequency over many generations. Thus as long as mating is random, genotypes in autosomal recessive diseases can be considered to be in Hardy-Weinberg equilibrium, despite selection against homozygotes for the recessive allele. Thus the mathematical relationship between genotype and allele frequencies described in the Hardy-Weinberg law holds for most practical purposes in recessive disease.

② **Selection in Dominant Disorders**

In contrast to recessive mutant alleles, dominant mutant alleles are exposed directly to selection. Consequently, the effects of selection and mutation are more obvious and can be more readily measured for dominant traits. A genetic lethal dominant allele, if fully penetrant, will be exposed to selection in heterozygotes, thus removing all alleles responsible for the disorder in a single generation. Several human diseases are thought or known to be autosomal dominant traits with zero or near-zero fitness and thus always result from new rather than inherited autosomal dominant mutations (see Table 9-8), a point of great significance for genetic counseling. In some, the genes and specific mutant alleles are known, and family studies show new mutations in the affected individuals that were not inherited from the parents. In other conditions, the genes are not known, but a paternal age effect has been seen, suggesting (but not proving) that a de novo mutation in the paternal germline is a possible cause of the disorder. The implication for genetic counseling is that the parents of a child with an autosomal dominant but genetically lethal condition will typically have a very low risk for recurrence in subsequent pregnancies because the condition would generally require another independent mutation to recur. A caveat to keep in mind, however, is the possibility of germline mosaicism.

Table 9-8 Examples of Disorders Occurring as Sporadic Conditions due to New Mutations With Zero Fitness

Disorder	Description
Atelosteogenesis	Early lethal form of short-limbed skeletal dysplasia
Cornelia de Lange syndrome	Intellectual disability, micromelia, synophrys, and other abnormalities; can be caused by mutation in the NIPBL gene
Osteogenesisimperfecta, type II	Perinatal lethal type, with a defect in type I collagen (COL1A1, COL1A2)
Thanatophoric dys-plasia	Early lethal form of skeletal dysplasia due to de novo mutations in the FGFR3 gene

③ Mutation and Selection Balance in Dominant Disease

If a dominant disease is deleterious but not lethal, affected persons may reproduce but will nevertheless contribute fewer than the average number of offspring to the next generation. That is, their fitness, f, will be reduced. Such a mutation will be lost through selection at a rate proportional to the reduced fitness of heterozygotes. The frequency of the mutant alleles responsible for the disease in the population therefore represents a balance between loss of mutant alleles through the effects of selection and gain of mutant alleles through recurrent mutation. A stable allele frequency will be reached at whatever level balances the two opposing forces: one (selection) that removes mutant alleles from the gene pool and one (de novo mutation) that adds new ones back. The mutation rate per generation, μ, at a disease locus must be sufficient to account for that fraction of all the mutant alleles (allele frequency q) that are lost by selection from each generation. Thus,

$$\mu = sq$$

As an illustration of this relationship, in achondroplasia, the fitness of affected patients is not zero, but they have only approximately one fifth as many children as people of normal stature in the population. Thus their average fitness, f, is 0.20, and the coefficient of selection, s, is $1-f$, or 0.80. In the subsequent generation, then, only 20% of current achondroplasia alleles are passed on from the current generation to the next. Because the frequency of achondroplasia appears stable from generation to generation, new mutations must be responsible for replacing the 80% of mutant genes in the population lost through selection.

If the fitness of affected persons suddenly improved (e.g., because of medical advances), the observed incidence of the disease in the population would be predicted to increase and reach a new equilibrium. **Retinoblastoma** and other dominant embryonic tumors with childhood onset are examples of conditions that now have a greatly improved prognosis, with a predicted consequence of increased disease frequency in the population. Allele frequency, mutation rate, and fitness are related. Thus, if any two of these three characteristics are known, the third can be estimated.

④ Mutation and Selection Balance in X-Linked Recessive Mutations

For those X-linked phenotypes of medical interest that are recessive, or nearly so, selection occurs in hemizygous males and not in heterozygous females, except for the small proportion of females who are manifesting heterozygotes with reduced fitness. In this brief discussion, however, we assume that heterozygous females have normal fitness.

Because males have one X chromosome and females two, the pool of X-linked alleles in the entire population's gene pool is partitioned at any given time, with one third of mutant alleles present in males and two thirds in females. As we saw in the case of autosomal dominant mutations, mutant alleles lost through selection must be replaced by recurrent new mutations to maintain the observed disease incidence. If the incidence of a serious X-linked disease is not changing and selection is operating against (and only against) hemizygous males, the mutation rate, μ, must equal the coefficient of selection, s (i.e., the proportion of mutant alleles that are not passed on), times q, the allele frequency, adjusted by a factor of 3 because selection is operating only on the third of the mutant alleles in the population that are present in males at any time. Thus,

$$\mu = sq/3$$

For an X-linked genetic lethal disease, $s = 1$, and one third of all copies of the mutant gene responsible are lost from each generation and must, in a stable equilibrium, be replaced by de novo mutations. Therefore, in such disorders, one third of all persons who have X-linked lethal disorders are predicted to carry a new mutation, and their genetically normal mothers have a low risk for having subsequent children with the same disorder (again, assuming the absence of germline mosaicism). The remaining two thirds of the mothers of individuals with an X-linked lethal disorder would be carriers, with a 50% risk for having another affected son. However, the prediction that two thirds of the mothers of individuals with an X-linked lethal disorder are carriers of a disease-causing mutation is based on the assumption that mutation rates in males and in females are equal. It can be shown that if the mutation rate in males is much greater than in females, then the chance of a new mutation in the egg is very low, and most of the mothers of affected children will be carriers, having inherited the mutation as a new mutation from their unaffected fathers and then passing it on to their affected children.

In less severe disorders, such as **hemophilia A**, the proportion of affected individuals representing new mutations is less than one third (currently approximately 15%). Because the treatment of hemophilia is improving rapidly, the total frequency of mutant alleles can be expected to rise relatively rapidly and to reach a new equilibrium. Assuming (as seems reasonable) that the mutation rate at this locus stays the same over time, the proportion of hemophiliacs who result from a new mutation will decrease, but the overall incidence of the disease will increase. Such a change would have significant implications for genetic counseling for this disorder.

(3) Genetic Drift

Chance events can have a much greater effect on allele frequencies in a small population than in a large one. For example, when a new mutation occurs in a small population, its frequency is represented by only one copy among all the copies of that gene in the population. Random effects of environment or other chance occurrences that are independent of the genotype (i.e., events that occur for reasons unrelated to whether an individual is carrying the mutant allele) can produce significant changes in the frequency of the disease allele when the population is small. Such chance occurrences disrupt Hardy-Weinberg equilibrium and cause the allele frequency to change from one generation to the next. This phenomenon, known as **genetic drift**, can explain how allele frequencies can change as a result of chance. During the next few generations, although the population size of the new group remains small, there may be considerable fluctuation in gene frequency until allele frequencies come to a new equilibrium as the population increases in size. In contrast to **gene flow**, in which allele frequencies change because of the mixing of previously distinct populations, the mechanism of genetic drift is simply chance operating on a small population.

Founder Effect

One special form of genetic drift is referred to as **founder effect**. When a small subpopulation breaks off from a larger population, the gene frequencies in the small population may be different from those of the population from which it originated because the new group contains a small, random sample of the parent group and, by chance, may not have the same gene frequencies as the parent group. If one of the original founders of a new group just happens to carry a relatively rare allele, that allele will have a far higher frequency than it had in the larger group from which the new group was derived.

(4) Migration and Gene Flow

Migration can change allele frequency by the process of **gene flow**, defined as the slow diffusion of genes across a barrier. Gene flow usually involves a large population and a gradual change in gene frequencies. The genes of migrant populations with their own characteristic allele frequencies are gradually merged into the gene pool of the population into which they have migrated, a process referred to as **genetic admixture**. The term migration is used here in the broad sense of crossing a reproductive barrier, which may be racial, ethnic, or cultural and not necessarily geographical and requiring physical movement from one region to another. Some examples of admixture reflect well-known and well-documented events in human history (e.g., the African diaspora from the 15th to the 19th century), whereas others can only be inferred from the genomic study of variation in ancient DNA samples.

Returning to the example of the 32-bp deletion allele of the *CCR*5 cytokine receptor gene, $\Delta CCR5$, the frequency of this allele has been studied in many populations all over the world. The frequency of the $\Delta CCR5$ allele is highest, up to 18%, in parts of northwestern Europe and then declines along a gradient into eastern and southern Europe, falling to a few percent in the Middle East and the Indian subcontinent. The $\Delta CCR5$ allele is virtually absent from Africa and the Far East. The best interpretation of the current geographical distribution of the $\Delta CCR5$ allele is that the mutation originated in northern Europe and then underwent both positive selection and gene flow over long distances.

Review Points:

Introduction: understand the nature of genetically determined differences among individuals.

Mutation is defined as any change in the nucleotide sequence or arrangement of DNA. Mutations can be classified into three categories.

1. Genome mutations: mutations that affect the number of chromosomes in the cell.

2. Chromosome mutations: mutations that alter the structure of individual chromosomes.

3. Gene mutations: mutations that alter individual genes. Types of mutations and their consequences. Nucleotide substitutions include missense mutations, chain termination mutation, RNA processing mutations, deletions and insertions, effects of recombination and dynamic mutations.

The Hardy-Weinberg Law.

If a population meets certain assumptions, however, there is a simple mathematical relationship known as the Hardy-Weinberg law for calculating genotype frequencies from allele frequencies.

Know the assumptions of the Law.

Know the disturb Hardy-Weinberg Equilibrium.

Study Questions:

1. Aniridia is an eye disorder characterized by the complete or partial absence of the iris and is always present when a mutation occurs in the responsible gene. In one population, 41 children diagnosed with aniridia were born to parents of normal vision among 4.5 million births during a period of 40 years. Assuming that these cases were due to new mutations, what is the estimated mutation rate at the aniridia locus? On what assumptions is this estimate based, and why might this estimate be either too high or too low?

2. Which of the following types of polymorphism would be most effective for distinguishing two individuals from the general population: a SNP, a simple indel, or a microsatellite? Explain your reason.

3. Consider two cell lineages that differ from one another by a series of 100 cell divisions. Given the rate of mutation for different types of variation, how different would the genomes of those lineages be?

4. If the allele frequency for Rh-negative is 0.26 in a population, what fraction of first pregnancies would sensitize the mother (assume Hardy-Weinberg equilibrium)? If no prophylaxis were given, what fraction of second pregnancies would be at risk for hemolytic disease of the newborn due to Rh incompatibility?

5. In a population at equilibrium, three genotypes are present in the following proportions: A/A, 0.81; A/a, 0.18; a/a, 0.01.
   a. What are the frequencies of A and a?
   b. What will their frequencies be in the next generation?

6. Which of the following populations is in Hardy-Weinberg equilibrium?
   a. A/A, 0.70; A/a, 0.21; a/a, 0.09.
   b. For the MN blood group polymorphism, with two codominant alleles, M and N: (i) M, 0.33; MN, 0.34; N, 0.33. (ii) 100% MN.
   c. A/A, 0.32; A/a, 0.64; a/a, 0.04.
   d. A/A, 0.64; A/a, 0.32; a/a, 0.04.

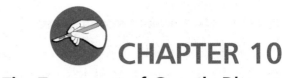

CHAPTER 10
The Treatment of Genetic Disease

Purpose and Requirement:

In this chapter students should understand the purpose of the treatment of genetic disease is to eliminate or ameliorate the effects of the disorder, not only on the patient but also on his or her family. Genetic heterogeneity and treatment should be considered. Treatment strategies and the molecular treatment of disease should also be understood.

The understanding of genetic disease at a molecular level is the foundation of rational therapy. In the coming decades, increasing annotation of the human genome sequence and the catalogue of human genes, as well as gene, RNA, and protein therapy, will have an enormous impact on the treatment of genetic conditions and other disorders. In this chapter, we review established therapies as well as new strategies for treating genetic disease. Our emphasis will be on therapies that reflect the genetic approach to medicine, and our focus is on single-gene diseases, rather than genetically complex disorders.

The objective of treating genetic disease is to eliminate or ameliorate the effects of the disorder, not only on the patient but also on his or her family. The importance of educating the patient is paramount—not only to achieve understanding of the disease and its treatment, but also to ensure compliance with therapy that may be inconvenient and lifelong. The family must be informed about the risk that the disease may occur in other members. Thus genetic counseling is a major component of the management of hereditary disorders and will be dealt with separately in Chapter 11.

For single-gene disorders due to loss-of-function mutations, treatment is directed to replacing the defective protein, improving its function, or minimizing the consequences of its deficiency. Replacement of the defective gene product (RNA or protein) may be achieved by direct administration, cell or organ transplantation, or gene therapy. In principle, gene therapy or gene editing will be the preferred mode of treatment of some and perhaps many single-gene diseases, once these approaches become routinely safe and effective. However, even when copies of a normal gene can be transferred into the patient to effect permanent cure, the family will need ongoing genetic counseling, carrier testing, and prenatal diagnosis, in many cases for several generations.

Recent discoveries promise many more exciting and dramatic therapies for genetic disease. These achievements include the first cures of inherited disorders using gene therapy, the development of novel small molecule therapies that can restore activity to mutant proteins, and the ability to prevent the clinical manifestations of previously lethal disorders, including lysosomal storage diseases, by protein replacement therapy.

10.1 The Current State of Treatment of Genetic Disease

Genetic disease can be treated at any level from the mutant gene to the clinical phenotype (see Fig. 10-1). Treatment at the level of the clinical phenotype includes all the medical or surgical interventions that are not unique to the management of genetic disease. Throughout this chapter, we describe the rationale for treatment at each of these levels. For diseases in which the biochemical or genetic defect is known, the approximate frequency with which the most common strategies are employed is shown in Figure 10-2. The current treatments are not necessarily mutually exclusive, although only gene therapy, gene editing, or cell transplantation can potentially provide cures.

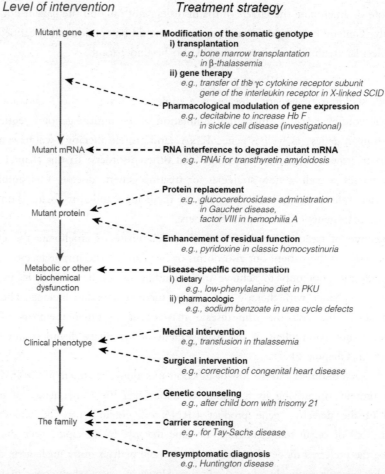

Figure 10-1 The various levels of treatment that are relevant to genetic disease, with the corresponding strategies used at each level

For each level, a disease discussed in the book is given as an example. All the therapies listed are used clinically in many centers, unless indicated otherwise. Hb F, Fetal hemoglobin; mRNA, messenger RNA; PKU, phenylketonuria; RNAi, RNA interference; SCID, severe combined immunodeficiency. (Modified from VALLE D. Genetic disease: an overview of current therapy[J]. Hospital practice, 1987,22(7):167−182.)

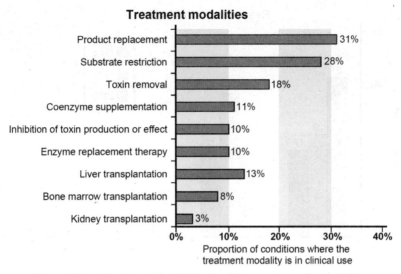

Figure 10-2   Treatment modalities for inborn errors of metabolism

This figure represents the findings of an analysis of the treatment efficacy of 57 inborn errors of metabolism. The total of the nine different approaches used exceeds 100% because more than one treatment can sometimes be used for a given condition.

Although powerful advances are being made, the overall treatment of single-gene diseases is presently deficient. A 25-year longitudinal survey of the effectiveness of treatment of 57 inborn errors of metabolism, reflecting the state of the field up to 2008, is shown in Figure 10-3. Note, however, that inborn errors are a group of diseases for which treatment is advanced, in general, compared to most other types of genetic disorders such as those due, for example, to chromosomal abnormalities, imprinting defects, or copy number variation. An encouraging trend over past decades is that treatment is more likely to be successful if the basic biochemical defect is known. In one study, for example, although treatment increased life span in only 15% of all single-gene diseases studied, life span was improved by approximately 50% in the subset of 57 inborn errors in which the cause was known. Significant improvements were also observed for other phenotypes, including growth, intelligence, and social adaptation. Thus research to elucidate the genetic and biochemical bases of hereditary disease has a major impact on the clinical outcome.

The improving but still unsatisfactory state of treatment of monogenic diseases is due to numerous factors, including the following:
- **Gene not identified or pathogenesis not understood.** Although more than 3,000 genes have been associated with monogenic diseases, the affected gene is still unknown in more than half of these disorders. This fraction will decrease dramatically over the next decade because of the impact of whole-genome and whole-exome sequencing. However, even when the mutant gene in known, knowledge of the pathophysiological mechanism is often inadequate and can lag well behind gene discovery. In phenylketonuria (PKU), for example, despite decades of study, the mechanisms by which the elevation in phenylalanine impairs brain development and function are still poorly understood.

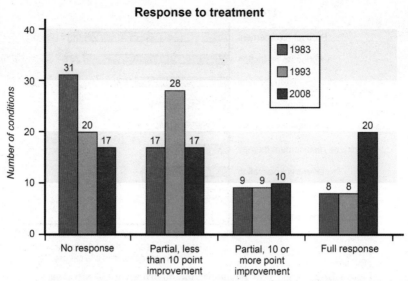

Figure 10-3 **The effect of treatment of 57 genetic diseases in which the affected gene or biochemical function is known and for which sufficient information was available for analysis in 2008**

A quantitative phenotype scoring system was used to evaluate the efficacy of the therapies. The fraction of treatable diseases will have increased to a small extent since this 2008 survey because of the increasing success of enzyme replacement and a few other treatments, including gene therapy.
(From CAMPEAU P M, SCRIVER C R, MITCHELL J J. A 25-year longitudinal analysis of treatment efficacy in inborn errors of metabolism[J]. Molecular genetics and metabolism, 2008,95 (1/2):11−16.)

- **Prediagnostic fetal damage.** Some mutations act early in development or cause irreversible pathological changes before they are diagnosed. These problems can sometimes be anticipated if there is a family history of the genetic disease or if carrier screening identifies couples at risk. In some cases, prenatal treatment is possible (see Table 10-1).

Table 10-1 Examples of Prenatal Medical Treatment of Monogenic Disorders

Disease	Treatment
Biotinidase deficiency	Prenatal biotin administration
Cobalamin-responsive methylmalonic aciduria	Prenatal maternal cobalamin administration
Congenital adrenal hyperplasial	Dexamethasone, a cortisol analogue
Phosphoglycerate dehydrogenase (PGDH) deficiency, a disorder of L-serine synthesis	Prenatal L-serine administration

- **Severe phenotypes are less amenable to intervention.** The initial cases of a disease to be recognized are usually the most severely affected, but they are often less amenable to treatment. In such individuals, the mutation frequently leads to the absence of the encoded protein or to a severely compromised mutant protein with no residual activity. In contrast, when the mutation is less disruptive, the mutant protein may retain some residual function and it may be possible to increase the small amount of function sufficiently to have a therapeutic effect, as described later.

- **The challenge of dominant negative alleles.** For some dominant disorders, the mutant protein interferes with the function of the normal allele. The challenge is to decrease the expression or impact of the mutant allele or its encoded mutant protein specifically, without disrupting expression or function of the normal allele or its normal protein.

10.2 Special Considerations in Treating Genetic Disease

10.2.1 Long-Term Assessment of Treatment is Critical

For treating monogenetic diseases, long-term evaluation of cohorts of treated individuals, often over decades, is critical for several reasons. Firstly, treatment initially judged as successful may eventually be revealed to be imperfect. For example, although well-managed children with PKU have escaped severe retardation and have normal or nearly normal IQs (see later), they often manifest subtle learning disorders and behavioral disturbances that impair their academic performance in later years.

Secondly, successful treatment of the pathological changes in one organ may be followed by unexpected problems in tissues not previously observed to be clinically involved, because the patients typically did not survive long enough for the new phenotype to become evident. Galactosemia, a well-known inborn error of carbohydrate metabolism, illustrates this point. This disorder results from an inability to metabolize galactose, a component of lactose (milk sugar), because of the autosomal recessive deficiency of galactose-1-phosphate uridyltransferase (GALT).

$$\text{Galactose-1-phosphate} \xrightarrow{\text{GALT}} \text{UDP galactose}$$

Affected infants are usually normal at birth but develop gastrointestinal problems, cirrhosis of the liver, and cataracts in the weeks after they are given milk. The pathogenesis is thought to be due to the negative impact of galactose-1-phosphate accumulation on other critical enzymes. If not recognized, galactosemia causes severe intellectual disability and is often fatal. Complete removal of milk from the diet, however, can protect against most of the harmful consequences, although, as with PKU, learning disabilities are now recognized to be common, even in well-treated patients. Moreover, despite conscientious treatment, most females with galactosemia have ovarian failure that appears to result from continued galactose toxicity.

Another example is provided by hereditary retinoblastoma due to germline mutations in the **retinoblastoma (RB1)** gene. Patients successfully treated for the eye tumor in the first years of life are unfortunately at increased risk for development of other independent malignant neoplasms, particularly osteosarcoma, after the first decade of life. Ironically, therefore, treatment that successfully prolongs life provides an opportunity for the manifestation of a previously unrecognized phenotype.

In addition, therapy that is free of side effects in the short term may be associated with serious problems in the long term. For example, clotting factor infusion in hemophilia sometimes results in the formation of antibodies to the infused protein, and blood transfusion in thalassemia invariably produces iron overload, which must then be managed by the administration of iron-chelating agents, such as deferoxamine.

10.2.2 Genetic Heterogeneity and Treatment

The optimal treatment of single-gene defects requires an unusual degree of diagnostic precision. One must often define not only the biochemical abnormality, but also the specific gene that is affected. For example, hyperphenylalaninemia can result from mutations in either the phenylalanine hydroxylase (*PAH*) gene or in one of the genes that encodes the enzymes required for the synthesis of tetrahydrobiopterin (BH4) , the cofactor of the PAH enzyme. The treatment of these two different causes of hyperphenylalaninemia is entirely different.

Allelic heterogeneity may also have critical implications for therapy. Some alleles may produce a protein that is decreased in abundance but has some residual function, so that strategies to increase the expression, function, or stability of such a partially functional mutant protein may correct the biochemical defect. This situation is again illustrated by some patients with hyperphenylalaninemia due to mutations in the *PAH* gene. The mutations in some patients lead to the formation of a mutant PAH enzyme whose activity can be increased by the administration of high doses of the BH4 cofactor. Of course, if a patient carries two alleles with no residual function, nothing will be gained by increasing the abundance of the mutant protein. One of the most striking examples of the importance of knowing the specific mutant allele in a patient with a genetic disease is exemplified by cystic fibrosis (CF). The drug ivacaftor (Kalydeco) is presently approved for treating CF patients carrying any one of only nine of the many hundreds of *CFTR* missense alleles.

10.3 Treatment by the Manipulation of Metabolism

Presently, the most successful disease-specific approach to the treatment of genetic disease is directed at the metabolic abnormality in inborn errors of metabolism. The principal strategies used to manipulate metabolism in the treatment of this group of diseases are listed in Table 10-2.

Table 10-2 Treatment of Genetic Disease by Metabolic Manipulation

Type of Metabolic Intervention	Substance or Technique	Disease
Avoidance	Antimalarial drugs Isoniazid	G6PD deficiency Slow acetylators
Dietary restriction	Phenylalanine Galactose	PKU Galactosemia
Replacement	Thyroxine Biotin	Monogenic forms of congenital hypothyroidism Biotinidase deficiency
Diversion	Sodium benzoate	Urea cycle disorders
	Drugs that sequester bile acids in the intestine (e.g., colesevelam)	Familial hypercholesterolemia heterozygotes
Enzyme inhibition	Statins	Familial hypercholesterolemia heterozygotes
Receptor antagonism	Losartan (investigational)	Marfan syndrome
Depletion	LDL apheresis (direct removal of LDL from plasma)	Familial hypercholesterolemia homozygotes

Note: G6PD, Glucose-6-phosphate dehydrogenase; LDL, low-density lipoprotein; PKU, phenylketonuria.

10.3.1 Substrate Reduction

As illustrated by the damaging effects of hyperphenylalaninemia in PKU, enzyme deficiencies may lead to substrate accumulation, with pathophysiological consequences. Strategies to prevent the accumulation of the offending substrate have been one of the most effective methods of treating genetic disease. The most common approach is to reduce the dietary intake of the substrate or of a precursor of it, and presently several dozen disorders—most involving amino acid catabolic pathways—are managed in this way. The drawback is that severe lifelong restriction of dietary protein intake is often necessary, requiring strict adherence to an artificial diet that is onerous for the family as well as for the patient. Nutrients such as 20 essential amino acids cannot be withheld entirely, however. Their intake must be sufficient for anabolic needs such as protein synthesis.

A diet restricted in phenylalanine largely circumvents the neurological damage in classic PKU. Phenylketonuric children are normal at birth because the maternal enzyme protects them during prenatal life. Treatment is most effective if begun promptly after diagnosis by newborn screening. Without treatment, irreversible developmental delay occurs, the degree of intellectual deficit being directly related to the delay in commencing the low-phenylalanine diet. It is now recommended that patients with PKU remain on a low-phenylalanine diet for life because neurological and behavioral abnormalities develop in many (although perhaps not all) patients if the diet is stopped. However, even PKU patients who have been effectively treated throughout life may have neuropsychological deficits (e. g., impaired conceptual, visual-spatial, and language skills), despite their having normal intelligence as measured by IQ tests. Nonetheless, treatment produces results vastly superior to the severe developmental delay that occurs without treatment. Continued phenylalanine restriction is particularly important in women with PKU during pregnancy to prevent prenatal damage to the fetus, even though the fetus is highly unlikely to be affected by PKU.

10.3.2   Replacement

The provision of essential metabolites, cofactors, or hormones whose deficiency is due to a genetic disease is simple in concept and often simple in application. Some of the most successfully treated single-gene defects belong to this category. A prime example is provided by **congenital hypothyroidism**, of which 10% to 15% of cases are monogenic in origin. Monogenic congenital hypothyroidism can result from mutations in any one of numerous genes encoding proteins required for the development of the thyroid gland or the biosynthesis or metabolism of thyroxine. Because congenital hypothyroidism from all causes is common (approximately 1 in 4,000 neonates), neonatal screening is conducted in many countries so that thyroxine administration may be initiated soon after birth to prevent the severe intellectual defects that are otherwise inevitable.

10.3.3   Diversion

Diversion therapy is the enhanced use of alternative metabolic pathways to reduce the concentration of a harmful metabolite. A major use of this strategy is in the treatment of the **urea cycle disorders** (see Fig. 10-4). The function of the urea cycle is to convert ammonia, which is neurotoxic, to urea, a benign end product of protein catabolism excreted in urine. If the cycle is disrupted by an enzyme defect such as **ornithine transcarbamylase deficiency**, the consequent hyperammonemia can be only partially controlled by dietary protein restriction.

Blood ammonia levels can be reduced to normal, however, by the diversion of ammonia to metabolic pathways that are normally of minor significance, leading to the synthesis of harmless compounds. Thus, the administration to hyperammonemic patients of large quantities of sodium benzoate forces the ligation of ammonia with glycine to form hippurate, which is excreted in urine (see Fig. 10-4). Glycine synthesis is thereby increased, and for each mole of glycine formed, one mole of ammonia is consumed.

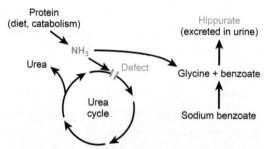

Figure 10-4   The strategy of metabolite diversion

In this example, ammonia cannot be removed by the urea cycle because of a genetic defect of a urea cycle enzyme. The administration of sodium benzoate diverts ammonia to glycine synthesis, and the nitrogen moiety is subsequently excreted as hippurate.

A comparable approach is used to reduce cholesterol levels in heterozygotes for **familial hypercholesterolemia**. If bile acids are sequestered in the intestine by the oral administration of a compound such as colesevelam and then excreted in feces rather than being reabsorbed, bile acid synthesis from cholesterol increases (see Fig. 10-5). The reduction in hepatic cholesterol levels leads to increased production of low-density lipoprotein (LDL) receptors from their single normal LDL receptor gene, increased hepatic uptake of LDL-bound cholesterol, and lower levels of plasma LDL cholesterol. This treatment significantly reduces plasma cholesterol levels because 70% of all LDL receptor uptake of cholesterol occurs in the liver. An important general principle is illustrated by this example: autosomal dominant diseases may sometimes be treated by increasing the expression of the normal allele.

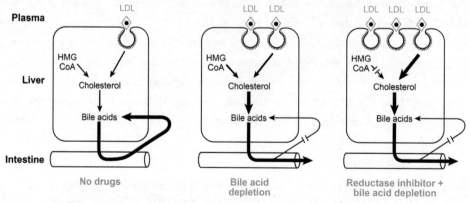

Figure 10-5   A comparable approach for reducing cholesterol levels

Rationale for the combined use of a reagent that sequesters bile acids, such as colesevelam, together with an inhibitor of 3-hydroxy-3-methylglutaryl coenzyme A reductase (HMG CoA reductase) in the treatment of familial hypercholesterolemia heterozygotes. LDL, Low-density lipoprotein.

(From BROWN M S, GOLDSTEIN J L. A receptor-mediated pathway for cholesterol homeostasis [J]. Science, 1986,232(4746):34−47.)

10.3.4   Enzyme Inhibition

The pharmacological inhibition of enzymes is sometimes used to reduce the impact of metabolic abnormalities in treating inborn errors. This principle is also illustrated by the treatment of heterozygotes of familial hypercholesterolemia. If a statin, a class of drugs that are powerful inhibitors of 3-hydroxy-3-methylglutaryl coenzyme A reductase, or HMG CoA reductase (the rate-limiting enzyme of cholesterol synthesis), is used to decrease hepatic de novo cholesterol synthesis in these patients, the liver compensates by increasing the synthesis of LDL receptors from the remaining intact LDL receptor allele. The increase in LDL receptors typically lowers plasma LDL cholesterol levels by 40% to 60% in familial hypercholesterolemia heterozygotes. Used together with colesevelam, the effect is synergistic, and even greater decreases can be achieved (see Fig. 10-5).

10.3.5   Receptor Antagonism

In some instances, the pathophysiology of an inherited disease results from the increased and inappropriate activation of a biochemical or signaling pathway. In such cases, one therapeutic approach is to antagonize critical steps in the pathway. A powerful example is provided by an investigational treatment of an autosomal dominant connective tissue disorder, **Marfan syndrome**. The disease results from mutations in the gene that encodes fibrillin 1, an important structural component of the extracellular matrix. The syndrome is characterized by many connective tissue abnormalities, such as aortic aneurysm, pulmonary emphysema, and eye-lens dislocation (see Fig. 10-6).

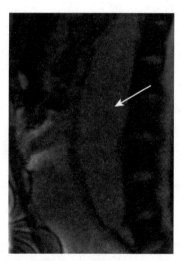

Figure 10-6   Magnetic resonance image (MRI) of the abdominal aorta of a 29-year-old pregnant woman with Marfan syndrome

The massive dilatation of the abdominal aorta is indicated by the *arrow*.

(From GOYA M, ALVAREZ M, TEIXIDO-TURA G, et al. Abdominal aortic dilatation during pregnancy in Marfan syndrome[J]. Revista española de cardiología (english edition), 2012,65(3): 288–289.)

Unexpectedly, the pathophysiology of Marfan syndrome is only partially explained by the impact of the reduction in fibrillin-1 microfibrils on the structure of the extracellular matrix.

Rather, it has been found that a major function of microfibrils is to regulate signaling by the transforming growth factor β (TGF-β), by binding TGF-β to the large latent protein complex of TGF-β. The decreased abundance of microfibrils in Marfan syndrome leads to an increase in the local abundance of unbound TGF-β and in local activation of TGF-β signaling. This increased TGF-β signaling has been suggested to underlie the pathogenesis of many of the phenotypes of Marfan syndrome, particularly the progressive dilation of the aortic root, and aortic aneurysm and dissection, the major cause of death in this disorder. Moreover, a recently recognized group of other vasculopathies, such as nonsyndromic forms of thoracic aortic aneurysm, has also proved to be driven by altered TGF-β signaling.

Angiotensin II signaling is known to increase TGF-β activity and the angiotensin II type 1 receptor antagonist, losartan, a widely used antihypertensive agent, has been shown to attenuate TGF-β signaling by decreasing the transcription of genes encoding TGF-β ligands, receptor subunits, and activators. Treatment with losartan has been found to decrease substantially the rate of aortic root dilation in initial clinical trials of Marfan syndrome patients, an effect that appears to be largely due to decreased TGF-β signaling.

The novel use of a U.S. Food and Drug Administration (FDA) approved drug, losartan, to treat a rare inherited disease, Marfan syndrome, is likely to represent a paradigm that will be repeated regularly in the future, as small molecule chemical screens to identify compounds with therapeutic potential—often including the thousands of FDA approved drugs—are undertaken to identify safe, effective treatments for other uncommon genetic disorders.

10.3.6 Depletion

Genetic diseases characterized by the accumulation of a harmful compound are sometimes treated by direct removal of the compound from the body. This principle is illustrated by the treatment of homozygous familial hypercholesterolemia. In this instance, for patients whose LDL levels cannot be lowered by other approaches, a procedure called apheresis is used to remove LDL from the circulation. Whole blood is removed from the patient, LDL is removed from plasma by any one of several methods, and the plasma and blood cells are returned to the patient. The use of phlebotomy to alleviate the iron accumulation of **hereditary hemochromatosis** provides another example of depletion therapy.

10.4 Treatment to Increase the Function of the Affected Gene or Protein

The growth in knowledge of the molecular pathophysiology of monogenic diseases has been accompanied by a small but promising increase in therapies that—at the level of DNA, RNA, or protein—increase the function of the gene affected by the mutation.

Some of the novel treatments have led to striking improvement in the lives of affected individuals, an outcome that, until recently, would have seemed fanciful. An overview of the molecular treatment of single-gene diseases is presented in Figure 10-7. These molecular therapies represent one facet of the important paradigm embraced by the concept of **personalized** or **precision medicine**. The term precision medicine is a general one used to describe the diagnosis, prevention, and treatment of a disease—tailored to individual patients—based on a profound understanding of the mechanisms that underlie its etiology and pathogenesis.

The Molecular Treatment of Genetic Disease

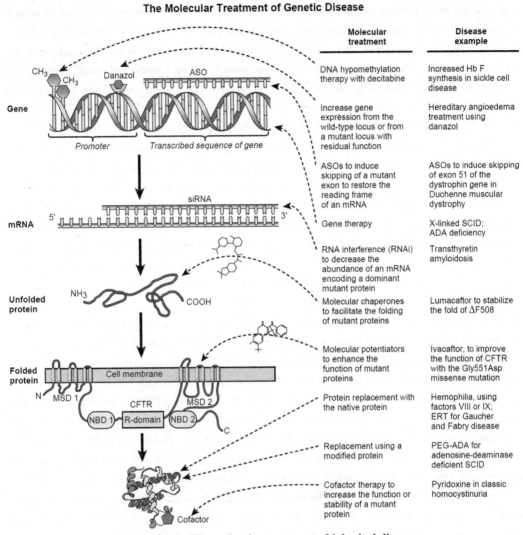

Molecular treatment	Disease example
DNA hypomethylation therapy with decitabine	Increased Hb F synthesis in sickle cell disease
Increase gene expression from the wild-type locus or from a mutant locus with residual function	Hereditary angioedema treatment using danazol
ASOs to induce skipping of a mutant exon to restore the reading frame of an mRNA	ASOs to induce skipping of exon 51 of the dystrophin gene in Duchenne muscular dystrophy
Gene therapy	X-linked SCID; ADA deficiency
RNA interference (RNAi) to decrease the abundance of an mRNA encoding a dominant mutant protein	Transthyretin amyloidosis
Molecular chaperones to facilitate the folding of mutant proteins	Lumacaftor to stabilize the fold of ΔF508
Molecular potentiators to enhance the function of mutant proteins	Ivacaftor, to improve the function of CFTR with the Gly551Asp missense mutation
Protein replacement with the native protein	Hemophilia, using factors VIII or IX; ERT for Gaucher and Fabry disease
Replacement using a modified protein	PEG-ADA for adenosine-deaminase deficient SCID
Cofactor therapy to increase the function or stability of a mutant protein	Pyridoxine in classic homocystinuria

Figure 10-7   The molecular treatment of inherited disease

Each molecular therapy is discussed in the text. ADA, Adenosine deaminase; ASO, antisense oligonucleotide; ERT, enzyme replacement therapy; Hb F, fetal hemoglobin; mRNA, messenger RNA; MSD, membrane-spanning domain; NBD, nucleotide-binding domain; PEG, polyethylene glycol; SCID, severe combined immunodeficiency; siRNA, small interfering RNA.

10.4.1 Treatment at the Level of the Protein

In many situations, if a mutant protein product is made, it may be possible to increase its function. For example, the stability or function of a mutant protein with some residual function may be further increased. With enzymopathies, the improvement in function obtained by this approach is usually very small, on the order of a few percent, but this increment is often all that is required to restore biochemical homeostasis.

(1) Enhancement of Mutant Protein Function With Small Molecule Therapy

Small molecules are compounds with molecular weights in the few hundreds to thousands. They include vitamins, nonpeptide hormones, and indeed most drugs, whether synthesized by organic chemists or isolated from nature. A new strategy for identifying potential drugs is to use high-throughput screening of chemical compound libraries, often containing tens of thousands of known chemicals, against a drug target, such as the protein whose function is disrupted by a mutation. As we will discuss, two drugs that are now FDA approved for the treatment of some patients with CF, and another that is investigational, were discovered using such high-throughput screens. Progress in the development of these drugs represents a new frontier with great potential for the treatment of genetic disease.

① Small Molecule Therapy to Allow Skipping over Nonsense Codons

Nonsense mutations account for 11% of defects in the human genome. Approximately 9% of all *CFTR* alleles are nonsense mutations, and approximately 50% of Ashkenazi Jewish patients with CF carry at least one *CFTR* allele with a premature stop codon (e.g., Arg553Stop). A potentially ideal therapeutic approach (other than gene therapy) for patients with a nonsense mutation would be a safe drug that encourages the translational apparatus to misread the stop codon by a transfer RNA (tRNA) that is near-cognate to the stop codon tRNA. If the amino acid thereby inserted into the polypeptide by that tRNA still produces a functional protein, the activity of the protein would be restored. An event of this type, for example, would convert the *CFTR* Arg553Stop mutation to 553Tyr, a substitution that generates a CFTR peptide with nearly normal properties. High-throughput chemical screens for a drug of this type identified ataluren (PTC124), and evidence suggests that it is most effective in allowing read-through of TGA nonsense codons. Moreover, studies in model organisms have firmly demonstrated that it can correct the mutant phenotype of some nonsense mutations. Ataluren has not been established to be clinically effective, but a Phase Ⅲ clinical trial in CF patients carrying at least one nonsense mutation showed a promising trend toward statistically significant improvement in lung function, and a follow-up trial is underway. Even if ataluren proves ineffective in humans, thousands of other small molecules are being examined in laboratories around the world to identify novel nontoxic compounds that facilitate the skipping of nonsense codons, not only for the treatment of CF but also for Duchenne muscular dystrophy patients carrying nonsense codons, as well as other diseases. Safe, effective drugs of this type will have a major impact on the treatment of inherited disease.

② Small Molecules to Correct the Folding of Mutant Membrane Proteins: Pharmacological Chaperones

Some mutations in membrane proteins may disrupt their ability to fold, pass through the endoplasmic reticulum, and be trafficked to the plasma membrane. These mutant proteins are recognized by the cellular protein quality control machinery, trapped in the endoplasmic reticulum, and prematurely degraded by the proteosome. The ΔF508 deletion of the CFTR protein—which constitutes 65% of all CF mutations worldwide—is perhaps the best-known example of a mutation that impairs trafficking of a membrane protein. If the folding/trafficking defect could be overcome to increase the abundance of CFTR channels at the apical surface of the cell by 20% to 25%, it is thought that a clinical benefit would be obtained, because once the ΔF508 CFTR protein reaches the cell surface, it is an effective Cl⁻ channel.

Small molecule screens to identify compounds that can serve as a chaperone to prevent misfolding and correct the ΔF508 CFTR trafficking defect in in vitro assay systems have identified lumacaftor (VX-809) as an effective, although incomplete, corrector of this specific

CFTR mutant polypeptide (see Fig. 10-7). Lumacaftor interacts directly with the mutant CFTR to stabilize its three-dimensional structure, specifically correcting the underlying trafficking defect and enhancing Cl⁻ transport. Although monotherapy with lumacaftor had no clinical benefits, a recently completed Phase Ⅲ clinical trial using lumacaftor together with another small molecule, ivacaftor (VX-770), discussed later, showed significant improvements in lung function in homozygous ΔF508 *CFTR* patients. This finding is notable because it is the first treatment shown to have a favorable impact on the primary biochemical defect in patients carrying the most common *CFTR* allele, ΔF508. Ongoing studies of the long-term effectiveness and safety of the lumacaftor-ivacaftor combination therapy are in progress. Irrespective of their success, this example is a milestone in medical genetics, because it establishes the principle that molecular chaperones can have clinical benefits in the treatment of monogenic disease.

③ **Small Molecules to Increase the Function of Correctly Trafficked Mutant Membrane Proteins**

Amino acid substitutions in membrane proteins may not disrupt the trafficking of the mutant polypeptide to the plasma membrane, but rather interfere with its function at the cell surface. Small molecule screens for new treatments for CF have also led this area of drug discovery. Screens for so-called potentiators—molecules that could enhance the function of mutant CFTR proteins that are correctly positioned at the cell surface—identified ivacaftor (VX-770), which improves the Cl⁻ transport of some mutant CFTR proteins, such as the Gly551Asp CFTR missense mutation that inactivates anion transport. This allele is carried by 4% to 5% of all CF patients. In one clinical trial, patients carrying at least one Gly551Asp allele experienced a significant improvement in lung function (see Fig. 10-8), weight gain, respiratory symptoms, and a decline in sweat Cl⁻. Ivacaftor is presently FDA approved for the

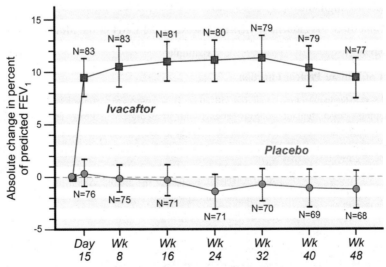

Figure 10-8   The effect of ivacaftor (Kalydeco) on lung function of cystic fibrosis patients carrying at least one Gly551Asp CFTR allele

The figure shows the absolute mean change from baseline in the percent of predicted forced expiratory volume in 1 second (FEV1) through week 48 of a clinical trial. N refers to the number of subjects studied at each time point during the trial.

treatment of eight other CFTR missense mutations, and more alleles will certainly be added to this group. Although fewer than 200 CF patients in the United States have one of these eight alleles, the allele-specific indications for ivacaftor treatment highlight both the benefits and dilemmas of personalized medicine for genetic disease: effective drugs can be discovered, but they may be effective only in a relatively small numbers of individuals. Moreover, at present ivacaftor is extremely expensive, costing approximately \$300,000 per year.

④ **Small Molecules to Enhance the Function of Mutant Enzymes: Vitamin-Responsive Inborn Errors of Metabolism**

The biochemical abnormalities of a number of inherited metabolic diseases may respond, sometimes dramatically, to the administration of large amounts of the vitamin cofactor of the enzyme impaired by the mutation (see Table 10-3). In fact, the vitamin-responsive inborn errors are among the most successfully treated of all genetic diseases. The vitamins used are remarkably nontoxic, generally allowing the safe administration of amounts 100 to 500 times greater than those required for normal nutrition. In **homocystinuria** due to cystathionine synthase deficiency, for example, approximately 50% of patients respond to the administration of high doses of pyridoxine (vitamin B6, the precursor of pyridoxal phosphate, the cofactor for the enzyme), an example—as we saw earlier in the case of BH4 administration in PKU—of cofactor responsiveness in a metabolic disease. In most of these responsive patients, homocystine completely disappears from the plasma, even though the increase in hepatic cystathionine synthase activity is usually only a fewfold, from 1.5% to 4.5% of control activity. The increased pyridoxal phosphate concentrations may stabilize the mutant enzyme or overcome reduced affinity of the mutant enzyme for the cofactor (see Fig. 10-9). In any case, vitamin B6 treatment substantially improves the clinical course of the disease in responsive patients. Nonresponsive patients generally carry null alleles and therefore have no residual cystathionine synthase activity to augment.

Table 10-3   Treatment of Genetic Disease at the Level of the Mutant Protein

Strategy	Example	Status
Enhancement of Mutant Protein Function		
Small molecules that facilitate translational "skipping" over mutant stop codons	Ataluren in the 10% of cystic fibrosis patients with nonsense mutations in the CFTR gene	Investigational in CF; confirmatory Phase III clinical trial was begun in 2014
Small molecule "correctors" that increase the trafficking of the mutant protein through the ER to the plasma membrane	Lumacaftor (VX-809) to increase the abundance of the ΔF508 mutant CFTR protein at the apical membrane of epithelial cells in CF patients	Investigational: very promising improvements in lung function in ΔF508 homozygotes, when used in combination with ivacaftor; expensive
Small molecule "potentiators" that increase the function at the cell membrane of correctly trafficked membrane proteins	Ivacaftor (VX-770) used alone to enhance the function of specific mutant CFTR proteins at the epithelial apical membrane	FDA approved for the treatment of CF patients carrying specific alleles; expensive
Vitamin cofactor administration to increase the residual activity of the mutant enzyme	Vitamin B6 for pyridoxine-responsive homocystinuria	Treatment of choice in the 50% of cystathionine synthase patients who are responsive

Continued

Strategy	Example	Status
Protein Augmentation		
Replacement of an extracellular protein	Factor VIII in hemophilia A	Well-established, effective, safe
Extracellular replacement of an intracellular protein	Polyethylene glycol-modified adenosine deaminase (PEG-ADA) in ADA deficiency	Well-established, safe, and effective, but costly; now used principally to stabilize patients before gene therapy or HLA-matched bone marrow transplantation
Replacement of an intracellular protein-cell targeting	β-glucocerebrosidase in non-neuronal Gaucher disease	Established; biochemically and clinically effective; expensive

Note: ADA, Adenosine deaminase; CF, cystic fibrosis; ER, endoplasmic reticulum; FDA, U.S. Food and Drug Administration; HLA, human leukocyte antigen; PEG, polyethylene glycol.

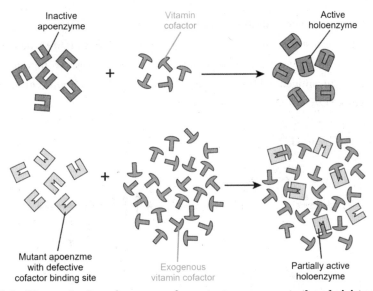

Figure 10-9 The mechanism of response of a mutant apoenzyme to the administration of its cofactor at high doses

Vitamin-responsive enzyme defects are often due to mutations that reduce the normal affinity (*top*) of the enzyme protein (apoenzyme) for the cofactor needed to activate it. In the presence of the high concentrations of the cofactor that result from the administration of up to 500 times the normal daily requirement, the mutant enzyme acquires a small amount of activity sufficient to restore biochemical normalcy.

(Redrawn from VALLE D. Genetic disease: an overview of current therapy[J]. Hospital practice, 1987,22(7):167-182.)

(2) Protein Augmentation

The principal types of protein augmentation are summarized in Table 10-3. Protein augmentation is a routine therapeutic approach in only a few diseases, all involving proteins whose principal site of action is in the plasma or extracellular fluid. The prime example is the prevention or arrest of bleeding episodes in patients with **hemophilia** by the infusion of plasma fractions enriched for the appropriate factor. The decades of experience with this disease illustrate the problems that can be anticipated as new strategies for replacing other, particularly intracellular, polypeptides are attempted. These problems include the difficulty and cost of procuring sufficient amounts of the protein to treat all patients at the optimal frequency, the need to administer the protein at a frequency consistent with its half-life (only 8 to 10 hours for factor Ⅷ), and the formation of neutralizing antibodies in some patients (5% of classic hemophiliacs).

① Enzyme Replacement Therapy: Extracellular Administration of an Intracellular Enzyme

Adenosine Deaminase Deficiency

Adenosine deaminase (ADA) is a critical enzyme of purine metabolism that catalyzes the deamination of adenosine to inosine and of deoxyadenosine to deoxyinosine (see Fig. 10-10). The pathology of ADA deficiency, an autosomal recessive disease, results entirely from the accumulation of toxic purines, particularly deoxyadenosine, in lymphocytes. A profound failure of both cell-mediated (T-cell) and humoral (B-cell) immunity results, making ADA deficiency one cause of **severe combined immunodeficiency** (**SCID**). Untreated patients die of infection within the first 2 years of life. The long-term treatment of ADA deficiency is rapidly evolving, with gene therapy now a strong alternative to bone marrow transplantation from a fully human leukocyte antigen (HLA) compatible donor. The administration of a modified form of the bovine ADA enzyme, described in the next section, is no longer a first choice for long-term management, but it is an effective stabilizing measure in the short term until these other treatments can be used.

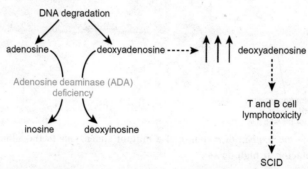

Figure 10-10   Adenosine deaminase (ADA) converts adenosine to inosine and deoxyadenosine to deoxyinosine

In ADA deficiency, deoxyadenosine accumulation in lymphocytes is lymphotoxic, killing the cells by impairing DNA replication and cell division to cause severe combined immunodeficiency (SCID).

Modified Adenosine Deaminase

The infusion of bovine ADA modified by the covalent attachment of an inert polymer, polyethylene glycol (PEG), is superior in several ways to the use of the unmodified ADA enzyme. Firstly, PEG-ADA largely protects the patient from a neutralizing antibody response (which would remove the ADA from plasma). Secondly, the modified enzyme remains in the extracellular fluid where it can degrade toxic purines. Thirdly, the plasma half-life of PEG-ADA is 3 to 6 days, much longer than the half-life of unmodified ADA. Although the near-normalization of purine metabolism obtained with PEG-ADA does not completely correct immune function (most patients remain T lymphopenic), immunoprotection is restored, with dramatic clinical improvement.

The general principles exemplified by the use of PEG-ADA are that proteins can be chemically modified to improve their effectiveness as pharmacological reagents, and an enzyme that is normally located inside the cell can be effective extracellularly if its substrate is in equilibrium with the extracellular fluid and if its product can be taken up by the cells that require it.

② **Enzyme Replacement Therapy: Targeted Augmentation of an Intracellular Enzyme**

Enzyme replacement therapy (ERT) is now established therapy for six lysosomal storage diseases, with clinical trials being conducted for several others. Non-neuronal (type 1) **Gaucher disease** was the first lysosomal storage disease for which ERT was shown to be effective. It is the most prevalent lysosomal storage disorder, affecting up to 1 in 450 Ashkenazi Jews and 1 in 40,000 to 100,000 individuals in other populations. This autosomal recessive condition results from deficiency of β-glucocerebrosidase. Loss of this enzyme activity leads to the accumulation of its substrate, the complex lipid glucocerebroside, in the lysosome, where it is normally degraded. The lysosomal accumulation of glucocerebroside, particularly in the macrophages and monocytes of the reticuloendothelial system, leads to gross enlargement of the liver and spleen. Bone marrow is slowly replaced by lipid-laden macrophages (Gaucher cells), leading to anemia and thrombocytopenia. The bone lesions cause episodic pain, osteonecrosis, and substantial morbidity.

More than 5,000 patients with non-neuronal Gaucher disease have been treated worldwide with β-glucocerebrosidase ERT, with dramatic clinical benefits. The increase in the hemoglobin level of one patient, a response that is representative of the effectiveness of this treatment, is shown in Figure 10-11. Overall, this therapy also reduces the enlargement of liver and spleen, increases the platelet count, accelerates growth, and improves the characteristic skeletal abnormalities and bone density. Early treatment is most effective in preventing irreversible damage to bones and liver.

The success of ERT for non-neuronopathic Gaucher disease provides guidance in the development of enzyme and protein replacement therapy for other lysosomal storage disorders, and perhaps other classes of diseases as well, for several reasons. Firstly, this use of ERT highlights the importance of understanding the biology of the relevant cell types. As demonstrated by I -cell disease, lysosomal hydrolases such as β-glucocerebrosidase contain post-translationally added mannose sugars that target the enzyme to the macrophage through a mannose receptor on the plasma membrane. Once bound, the enzyme is internalized and delivered to the lysosome. Thus, β-glucocerebrosidase ERT in Gaucher disease targets the protein both to a particular relevant cell and to a specific intracellular address, in this case the macrophage and the lysosome, respectively.

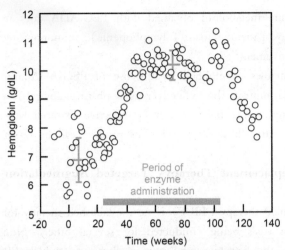

Figure 10-11 **The effect of weekly intravenous infusions of modified glucocerebrosidase on the hemoglobin concentration of a child with non-neuronal (type 1) Gaucher disease**

A review of the response of more than 1,000 patients indicates that this response is representative. Treatment was begun at 4 years of age and continued for 18 months. The therapy was accompanied by an increased platelet count and radiological improvement in the bone abnormalities. The hematological parameters returned to pretreatment levels when the infusions were stopped.

Secondly, the human enzyme can be produced in abundance from cultured cells expressing the glucocerebrosidase gene, a key factor because this treatment, given as twice-monthly infusions, must be continuous. Only approximately 1% to 5% of the normal intracellular enzyme activity is required to correct the biochemical abnormalities in this and other lysosomal storage disorders. Thirdly, the administered β-glucocerebrosidase is not recognized as a foreign antigen because patients with non-neuronal Gaucher disease have small amounts of residual enzyme activity. Unfortunately, however, because β-glucocerebrosidase does not cross the blood-brain barrier, ERT cannot treat the neuronopathic forms of Gaucher disease. Although ERT for any lysosomal disease is very expensive, its success has been a tremendous advance in the treatment of monogenic disorders. It has established the feasibility of directing an intracellular enzyme to its physiologically relevant location to produce clinically significant effects.

10.4.2 Modulation of Gene Expression

Decades ago, the idea that one might treat a genetic disease through the use of drugs that modulate gene expression would have seemed fanciful. Increasing knowledge of the normal and pathological bases of gene expression, however, has made this approach feasible. Indeed, it seems likely that this strategy will become only more widely used as our understanding of gene expression, and how it might be manipulated, increases.

(1) Increasing Gene Expression From the Wild-Type or Mutant Locus

Therapeutic effects can be obtained by increasing the amount of messenger RNA (mRNA) transcribed from the wild-type locus associated with a dominant disease or from the mutant locus, if the mutant protein retains some function (see Table 10-4; see Fig. 10-7). An effective therapy of this type is used to manage **hereditary angioedema**, a rare but potentially fatal autosomal dominant condition due to mutations in the gene encoding the complement 1

(C1) esterase inhibitor. Affected individuals are subject to unpredictable episodes, of widely varying severity, of submucosal and subcutaneous edema. Attacks that involve the upper respiratory tract can be fatal. Because of the rapid and unpredictable nature of the attacks, long-term prophylaxis with attenuated androgens, particularly danazol, is often employed. Danazol significantly increases the abundance of the C1 esterase inhibitor mRNA by modulating transcription of the gene, presumably from both the normal and mutant loci. In the great majority of patients, the frequency of serious attacks is dramatically reduced, although long-term androgen administration is not free of side effects.

Table 10-4   Treatment by Modification of the Genome or its Expression

Type of Modification	Example	Status
Pharmacological modulation of gene expression	Decitabine therapy to stimulate γ-globin (and thus Hb F) synthesis in sickle cell disease	Effective in increasing Hb F levels; concerns about cytotoxicity drive the search for safer but effective cytidine analogues
RNA interference (RNAi) to reduce the abundance of a toxic or dominant negative protein	RNAi for transthyretinamyloidosis	Successful Phase I clinical trial completed
Induction of exon skipping	Use of antisense oligonucleotides to induce skipping of exon 51 in Duchenne muscular dystrophy	Investigational; clinical trials offer cautious optimism
Gene editing	CRISPR/Cas9 inactivation of the *CCR5* gene in CD4 T cells of HIV-infected individuals	Investigational; Phase I trial successful
Partial modification of the somatic genotype	Bone marrow transplantation in β-thalassemia	Curative with HLA-matched donor; good results overall
By transplantation	Bone marrow transplantation in storage diseases (e.g., Hurler syndrome)	Excellent results in some diseases, even if the brain is affected, such as Hurler syndrome
	Cord blood stem cell transplantation for presymptomatic Krabbe disease; Hurler syndrome	Excellent results for these two disorders
	Liver transplantation in α1-antitrypsin deficiency	Up to 80% survival over 5 yr for genetic liver disease
By gene transfer into somatic tissues (see Table 10-5)	See Table 10-5	See Table 10-5

Note: cas, CRISPR-associated; CRISPR, clustered regularly interspaced short palindromic repeats; Hb F, fetal hemoglobin; HLA, human leukocyte antigen.

(2) Increasing Gene Expression From a Locus Not Affected by the Disease

A related therapeutic strategy is to increase the expression of a normal gene that compensates for the effect of mutation at another locus. This approach is extremely promising in the management of sickle cell disease and β-thalassemia, for which drugs that induce **DNA hypomethylation** are being used to increase the abundance of fetal hemoglobin (Hb F), which normally constitutes less than 1% of total hemoglobin in adults. Sickle cell disease causes illness because of both the anemia and the sickling of red blood cells. The increase in the level of Hb F (α2γ2) benefits these patients because Hb F is a perfectly adequate oxygen carrier in postnatal life and because the polymerization of deoxyhemoglobin S is inhibited by Hb F. In β-thalassemia, Hb F restores the imbalance between α and non-α-globin chains, substituting Hb F (α2γ2) for Hb A (α2β2).

The normal postnatal decrease in the expression of the γ-globin gene is at least partly due to methylation of CpG residues in the promoter region of the gene. Methylation of the promoter is inhibited if a cytidine analogue such as decitabine (5-aza-2-deoxycytidine) is incorporated into DNA instead of cytidine. The inhibition of methylation is associated with substantial increases in γ-globin gene expression and, accordingly, in the proportion of Hb F in blood. Both patients with sickle cell anemia and patients with some forms of β-thalassemia treated with decitabine uniformly display increases in Hb F to levels that are likely to have a significant positive impact on morbidity and mortality (see Fig. 10-12). The use of inhibitors of γ-globin gene methylation is evolving rapidly, and more effective inhibitors of methylation, with fewer side effects, are likely to be developed.

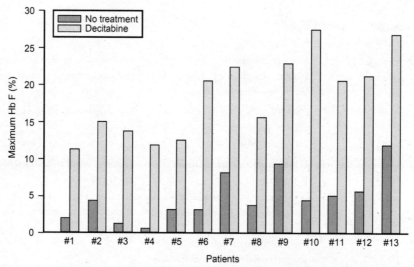

Figure 10-12   The effect of the cytosine analogue decitabine, a DNA hypomethylating agent, on the percentage of fetal hemoglobin (Hb F) in 13 patients with sickle cell disease, compared with their level of Hb F without any treatment

Note the wide variation between patients in the levels of Hb F without treatment. Every patient shown had a significant increase in Hb F during decitabine therapy.
(From SAUNTHARARAJAH Y, LAVELLE D, DESIMONE J. DNA hypo-methylating agents and sickle cell disease[J]. British journal of haematology, 2004,126(5):629−636.)

As described earlier, any approach that allows a patient with β-thalassemia or sickle cell anemia to retain Hb F expression is likely to be very beneficial to the patient. The BCL11A protein is a trans-acting effector of hemoglobin switching that turns off γ-globin production postnatally but nevertheless allows β-globin gene expression. Genome editing in hematopoietic stem cells (HSCs) is currently being explored as a method to delete an erythroid enhancer of the *BCL11A* gene, thereby blocking its expression in the erythroid cell lineage. As a result, hemoglobin switching from Hb F to Hb A would not occur, and patients would retain Hb F instead of a hemoglobin containing a mutant β-thalassemia or sickle cell allele.

(3) Reducing the Expression of a Dominant Mutant Gene Product: Small Interfering RNAs

The pathology of some inherited diseases results from the presence of a mutant protein that is toxic to the cell, as seen with proteins with expanded polyglutamine tracts, as in **Huntington disease**, or with disorders such as the inherited amyloidoses. The autosomal dominant disorder **transthyretin amyloidosis** is the result of any of more than 100 missense mutations in transthyretin, a protein produced mainly in liver, that transports retinol (one form of vitamin A) and thyroxine in body fluids. The major phenotypes are amyloidotic polyneuropathy, due to deposition of the amyloid in peripheral nerves (causing intractable peripheral sensory neuropathy and autonomic neuropathy), and amyloidotic cardiomyopathy, due to its deposition in the heart. Both disorders greatly shorten the life span, and the only current treatment is hepatic transplantation.

A promising therapy, however, is provided by a technology called **RNA interference** (**RNAi**), which can mediate the degradation of a specific target RNA, such as that encoding transthyretin. Briefly, short RNAs that correspond to specific sequences of the targeted RNA (see Fig. 10-7)—termed **small interfering RNAs** (**siRNAs**)—are introduced into cells by, for example, lipid nanoparticles or viral vectors. Strands of the interfering RNA, approximately 21 nucleotides long, bind to the target RNA and initiate its cleavage. A Phase I clinical trial using an siRNA (encapsulated in injected lipid nanoparticles) directed against transthyretin, led to a 56% to 67% reduction in transthyretin levels by the 28th day of study, with no significant toxicity. This trial established proof of concept for RNAi treatment of an inherited disease, an approach that will undoubtedly be applied to other diseases where elimination of the mutant gene product is the goal.

(4) Induction of Exon Skipping

Exon skipping refers to the use of molecular interventions to exclude an exon from a pre-mRNA that encodes a reading frame-disrupting mutation, thereby rescuing expression of the mutant gene. If the number of nucleotides in the excluded exon is a multiple of three, no frame shift will occur and, if the resulting polypeptide with the deleted amino acids retains sufficient function, a therapeutic benefit will result. The most widely studied method of inducing exon skipping is through the use of **antisense oligonucleotides** (**ASOs**), which are synthetic 15- to 35-nucleotide single-stranded molecules that can hybridize to specific corresponding sequences in a pre-mRNA (see Fig. 10-7). The clearest example of the potential of this strategy is provided by Duchenne muscular dystrophy (DMD).

The goal of exon skipping in DMD is to convert a DMD mutation into an in-frame counterpart that generates a functional dystrophin, just as the deletions that allow the production of a partially functioning dystrophin are associated with the milder phenotype of Becker muscular dystrophy. The distribution of DMD mutations is nonrandomly distributed in the gene, and thus, remarkably, the skipping of just exon 51 alone would restore the dystrophin reading frame of an estimated 13% of all DMD patients (see Fig. 10-13). This exon has therefore been the major focus of exon-skipping drug development. Several clinical trials have established that ASOs that cause skipping of exon 51 can produce significant increases in the number of dystrophin-positive muscle fibers of DMD patients. Moreover, one trial demonstrated stabilization of patient walking ability, but the treatment group was small and must be studied in a larger number of subjects. Irrespective of the specific challenges posed by DMD, it will be surprising if exon-skipping strategies do not ultimately play a significant role in the therapy of some inherited disorders.

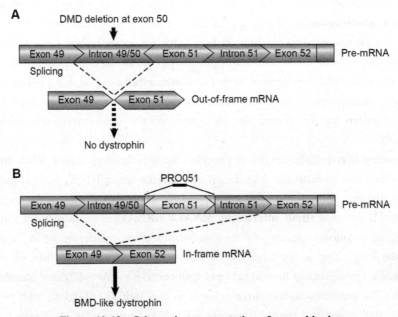

Figure 10-13 Schematic representation of exon skipping

(A) In a patient with Duchenne muscular dystrophy (DMD) who has a deletion of exon 50, an out-of-frame transcript is generated in which exon 49 is spliced to exon 51. (B) As a result, a stop codon is generated in exon 51, which prematurely aborts dystrophin synthesis. The sequence-specific binding of the exon-internal antisense oligonucleotide PRO051 interferes with the correct inclusion of exon 51 during splicing, so that the exon is actually skipped. This restores the open reading frame of the transcript and allows the synthesis of a dystrophin similar to that in patients with Becker muscular dystrophy (BMD). mRNA, Messenger RNA.

(From VAN DEUTEKOM J C, JANSON A A, GINJAAR I B, et al. Local dystrophin restoration with antisense oligonucleotide PRO051[J]. The new england journal of medicine, 2007,357(26): 2677-2686.)

(5) Gene Editing

Over the last decade, molecular biologists have developed methods to introduce site-specific genomic sequence changes into the DNA of intact organisms, including primates. The correction of a mutant gene sequence in its natural DNA context, in a sufficient number of target cells, would be an ideal treatment. This new technology, termed **genome editing**, uses engineered endonucleases containing a DNA-binding domain that will recognize a specific sequence in the genome, such as the sequence in which a missense mutation is embedded. Subsequently, a nuclease domain creates a double-stranded break, and cellular mechanisms for homology-directed repair (HDR) then repair the break, introducing the wild-type nucleotide to replace the mutant one. The template for the HDR must be based on a matching homologous wild-type DNA template that is introduced into the target cells before editing. The most widely used editing approach at present is the clustered regularly interspaced short palindromic repeats (CRISPR)/CRISPR-associated (Cas) 9 system, commonly referred to as CRISPR/Cas9.

In humans, genome editing offers possibilities for the correction of genetic defects in their natural genomic landscape, without the risks associated with the semirandom vector integration of some viral vectors used in gene therapy. The first clinical use of this technology was a Phase I (safety) clinical trial reported in 2014. This study took advantage of the knowledge that a naturally occurring deletion in CCR5, the gene that encodes the cell membrane coreceptor for human immunodeficiency virus (HIV), renders homozygous carriers resistant to HIV infection but does not impair CD4 T-cell function. When CD4 T-cells taken from HIV-infected patients were treated with an adenoviral vector expressing a nuclease designed to generate a null allele of the CCR5 gene, and then reinfused into the patient, the CCR5 gene was "knocked out" in 11% to 28% of the CD4 T-cells in these patients. The modified cells had a half-life of almost 1 year, and HIV RNA became undetectable in one of four patients who could be evaluated. This study demonstrates the great clinical potential of gene editing.

A major concern whose real dimensions are presently unknown is that the endonucleases can have off-target effects, which could cause mutations elsewhere in the genome. Nevertheless, considerable optimism is justified in thinking that this technology can be extended to the correction of mutations in the cells of individuals with genetic diseases in the future, including, for example, bone marrow stem cells for the treatment of inherited blood and immune system disorders.

10.4.3 Modification of the Somatic Genome by Transplantation

Transplanted cells retain the genotype of the donor, and consequently transplantation can be regarded as a form of gene transfer therapy because it leads to a modification of the somatic genome. There are two general indications for the use of transplantation in the treatment of genetic disease. First, cells or organs may be transplanted to introduce wild-type copies of a gene into a patient with mutations in that gene. This is the case, for example, in homozygous familial hypercholesterolemia, for which liver transplantation is an effective but high-risk procedure. The second and more common indication is for cell replacement, to compensate for an organ damaged by genetic disease (for example, a liver that has become cirrhotic in α1-antitrypsin deficiency). Some examples of the uses of transplantation in genetic disease are provided in Table 10-4.

(1) Stem Cell Transplantation

Stem cells are defined by two properties: (1) their ability to proliferate to form the differentiated cell types of a tissue in vivo; and (2) their ability to self-renew—that is, to form another stem cell.

Only three types of stem cells are in clinical use at present: hematopoietic stem cells (HSCs), which can reconstitute the blood system after bone marrow transplantation; **corneal stem cells**, which are used to regenerate the corneal epithelium, and **skin stem cells**. These cells are derived from immunologically compatible donors. The possibility that other types of stem cells will be used clinically in the future is enormous because stem cell research is one of the most active and promising areas of biomedical investigation. Although it is easy to overstate the potential of such treatment, optimism about the long-term future of stem cell therapy is justified.

① Hematopoietic Stem Cell Transplantation in Nonstorage Diseases

In addition to its extensive application in the management of cancer, HSC transplantation using bone marrow stem cells is the treatment of choice for a selected group of monogenic immune deficiency disorders, including SCID of any type. Its role in the management of genetic disease in general, however, is less certain and under careful evaluation. For example, excellent outcomes have been obtained with allogenic HSC transplantation in the treatment of children with β-thalassemia and sickle cell disease. Nevertheless, for each disease that bone marrow transplantation might benefit, its outcomes must be evaluated for many years and weighed against the results obtained with other therapies.

② Hematopoietic Stem Cell Transplantation for Lysosomal Storage Diseases

Transplantation of Hematopoietic Stem Cells from Bone Marrow

Bone marrow stem cell transplants are effective in correcting lysosomal storage in many tissues including, in some diseases, the brain, through the two mechanisms depicted in Figure 10-14. Firstly, the transplanted cells are a source of lysosomal enzymes that can be transferred to other cells through the extracellular fluid for Ⅰ-cell disease. Because bone marrow-derived cells constitute approximately 10% of the total cell mass of the body, the quantitative impact of enzymes transferred from them may be significant. Secondly, the mononuclear phagocyte system in tissues is derived from bone marrow stem cells so that, after bone marrow transplantation, this system is of donor origin throughout the body. Of special note are the brain perivascular microglial cells, whose bone marrow origin may partially account for the correction of nervous system abnormalities by bone marrow transplantation in some storage disorders, as we will see next in the case of **Hurler syndrome**, a lysosomal storage disease due to α-l-Iduronidase deficiency.

Bone marrow transplantation corrects or reduces the visceral abnormalities of many storage diseases. For example, a normalization or reduction in the size of the enlarged liver, spleen, and heart seen in Hurler syndrome can be achieved, and improvements in upper airway obstruction, joint mobility, and corneal clouding are also obtained. Most rewarding, however, has been the impact of transplantation on the neurological component of this disease. Patients who have good developmental indices before transplantation, and who receive transplants before 24 months of age, continue to develop cognitively after transplantation, in contrast to the inexorable loss of intellectual function that otherwise occurs. Interestingly, a gene dosage effect is manifested in the donor marrow. Children who receive cells from homozygous normal donors appear to be more likely to retain fully normal intelligence than do the recipients of heterozygous donor cells.

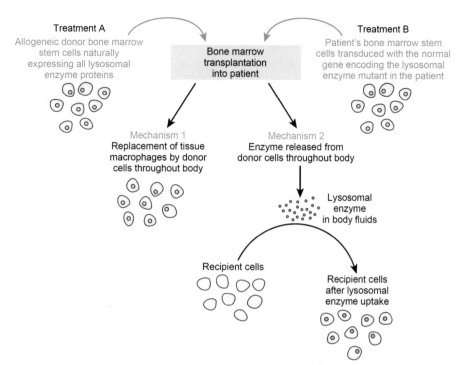

Figure 10-14   The two major mechanisms by which bone marrow transplantation or gene transfer into bone marrow may reduce the substrate accumulation in lysosomal storage diseases

In the case of either treatment, bone marrow transplantation from an allogeneic donor (A) or genetic correction of the patient's own bone marrow stem cells by gene transfer (B), the bone marrow stem cell progeny, now expressing the relevant lysosomal enzyme, expand to repopulate the monocyte-macrophage system of the patient (mechanism 1). In addition, lysosomal enzymes are released from the bone marrow cells derived from the donor or from the genetically modified marrow cells of the patient and taken up by enzyme-deficient cells from the extracellular fluid (mechanism 2).

Transplantation of Hematopoietic Stem Cells from Placental Cord Blood

The discovery that placental cord blood is a rich source of HSCs is beginning to make a substantial impact on the treatment of genetic disease. The use of placental cord blood has three great advantages over bone marrow as a source of transplantable HSCs. Firstly, recipients are more tolerant of histoincompatible placental blood than of other allogeneic donor cells. Thus engraftment occurs even if as many as three HLA antigens, cell surface markers encoded by the major histocompatibility complex, are mismatched between the donor and the recipient. Secondly, the wide availability of placental cord blood, together with the increased tolerance of histoincompatible donor cells, greatly expands the number of potential donors for any recipient. This feature is of particular significance to patients from minority ethnic groups, for whom the pool of potential donors is relatively small. Thirdly, the risk for graft-versus-host disease is substantially reduced with use of placental cord blood cells. Cord blood transplantation from unrelated donors appears to be as effective as bone marrow transplantation from a matched donor for the treatment of Hurler syndrome (see Fig. 10-15).

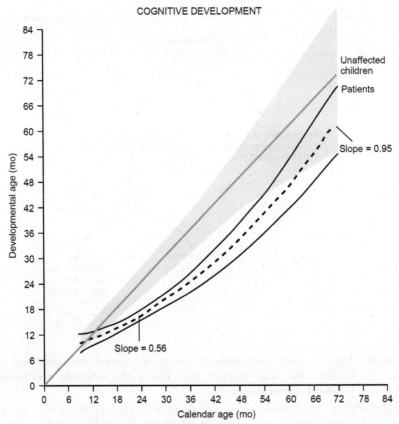

COGNITIVE DEVELOPMENT

Figure 10-15　Preservation of neurocognitive development in children with Hurler syndrome treated by cord blood transplantation

The figure displays the mean cognitive growth curve for transplanted patients compared with unaffected children. The *thin black lines* represent the 95% confidence interval for transplanted patients. (From STABA S L, ESCOLAR M L, POE M, et al. Cord-blood transplants from unrelated donors in patients with Hurler's syndrome[J]. The new england journal of medicine, 2004,350(19):1960−1969.)

(2) Liver Transplantation

For some metabolic liver diseases, liver transplantation is the only treatment of known benefit. For example, the chronic liver disease associated with CF or α1AT deficiency can be treated only by liver transplantation, and together these two disorders account for a large fraction of all the liver transplants performed in the pediatric population. Liver transplantation has now been undertaken for more than two dozen genetic diseases. At present, the 5-year survival rate of all children who receive liver transplants is in the range of 70% to 85%. For almost all of these patients, the quality of life is generally much improved, the specific metabolic abnormality necessitating the transplant is corrected, and in those conditions in which hepatic damage has occurred (such as α1AT deficiency), the provision of healthy hepatic tissue restores growth and normal pubertal development.

(3) The Problems and the Future of Transplantation

Two major problems limit the wider use of transplantation for the treatment of genetic disease. First, the mortality after transplantation is still significant, and the morbidity from superimposed infection due to the requirement for immunosuppression and graft-versus-host disease is substantial. Nevertheless, the ultimate goal of transplantation research—transplantation without immunosuppression—comes incrementally closer. The increased tolerance of the recipient to cord blood transplants, compared with bone marrow-derived donor cells, exemplifies the advances in this area.

The second problem with transplantation is the finite supply of organs, cord blood being a singular exception. For example, for all indications, including genetic disease, more than 6,000 liver transplants are performed annually in the United States alone, but more than double that number are added to the waiting list each year. In addition, it remains to be demonstrated that transplanted organs are generally capable of functioning normally for a lifetime.

One solution to these difficulties involves the combination of stem cell and either genome editing or gene therapy. Here, a patient's own stem cells would be cultured in vitro and either transfected by gene therapy with the gene of interest or corrected by CRISPR/Cas9 editing and returned to the patient to repopulate the affected tissue with genetically restored cells. The identification of stem cells in a variety of adult human tissues and recent advances in gene transfer therapy offer great hope for this strategy.

Induced Pluripotent Stem Cells

The recently developed ability to induce the formation of pluripotent stem cells (**iPSCs**) from somatic cells has the potential to provide the optimal solution to both of the challenges of transplantation posed earlier. In this approach somatic cells, such as skin fibroblasts, would be taken from a patient in need of a transplant, and induced to form differentiated cells of the organ of interest. For example, the loss-of-function mutation in the α1-antitrypsin gene in the fibroblasts cultured from a patient with α1AT deficiency could be corrected, either by gene editing or gene therapy. The corrected cells could then be induced to form liver-specific iPSCs, which could then be transplanted into the liver of the patient to differentiate into hepatocytes. Alternatively, mature hepatocytes derived in vitro from the genetically corrected iPSCs could be transplanted. The great merit of this approach is that the genetically corrected liver cells are derived from the patient's own genome, thus evading immunological rejection of the transplanted cells as well as graft-versus-host disease. Experimental work in animal models has established that this strategy is capable of correcting inherited disorders. Substantial hurdles with iPSCs must first be overcome, however, including establishing the safety of transplanting cells derived by iPSC methodology and preventing epigenetic modifications in the derived cell type that are not characteristic of wild-type cells of the tissue of interest.

10.5 Gene Therapy

Gene therapy is the introduction of a biologically active gene into a cell to achieve a therapeutic benefit. In 2012, the first gene therapy product was licensed in the United States and Europe for the treatment of lipoprotein lipase deficiency, and gene therapy has now been shown to be effective or extremely promising in clinical trials for almost a dozen inherited diseases, some of which are outlined in Table 10-5. These recent successes firmly establish that the treatment of genetic disease at its most fundamental level—the gene—will be increasingly feasible. The goal of gene therapy is to transfer the therapeutic gene early enough in the life of the patient to prevent the pathogenetic events that damage cells. Moreover, correction of the reversible features of genetic diseases should also be possible for many conditions.

Table 10-5 Examples of Inherited Diseases Treated by Gene Therapy of Somatic Tissues

Disease	Affected Protein (Gene)	Vector, Cell Transduced	Outcome
X-linked SCID	γc-cytokine receptor subunit of several interleukin receptors (*IL2RG*)	Retroviral vector Allogenic hematopoietic stem cells	Significant clinical improvement in 27 of 32 patients, 5 of whom developed a leukemia-like disorder that was treatable in 4
SCID due to ADA deficiency	Adenosine deaminase (*ADA*)	Retroviral vector Allogenic hematopoietic stem cells	29 of 40 treated patients are off PEG-ADA enzyme replacement therapy
X-linked adrenoleukodystrophy	A peroxisomal adenosine triphosphate-binding cassette transporter (*ABCD1*)	Lentiviral vector Autologous hematopoietic stem cells	Apparent arrest of cerebral demyelination in the two boys studied
Lipoprotein lipase deficiency	Lipoprotein lipase (*LPL*)	Adeno-associated virus vector injected intramuscularly	Decreased frequency of pancreatitis in affected individuals
Metachromatic leukodystrophy	Arylsulfatase A (*ARSA*)	Lentiviral vector expressing supraphysiological levels of ARSA Autologous hematopoietic stem cells	Apparent arrest of neurodegeneration in three patients, with no genotoxic effects. Long-term follow-up is required to know the true safety and efficacy of the treatment
Wiskott-Aldrich syndrome	WAS protein, a regulator of actin polymerization in hematopoietic cells (*WAS*)	Lentiviral vector Autologous hematopoietic stem cells	Marked immunological, hematological, and clinical improvement in the first three patients treated
Hemophilia B	Factor IX (*F9*)	Adeno-associated virus vector Patients received a single IV injection	Stable expression of factor IX at 1%～7% of normal levels up to 3 years post-treatment; 4 of 6 patients able to stop prophylactic factor IX treatment
β-Thalassemia	β-Globin (*HBA1*)	Lentiviral vector Autologous hematopoietic stem cells	A single patient, with compound βE/β0-thalassemia. Stable Hb levels of 9～10 g/dL, but only a third of the total Hb originated from the vector (see text)
Leber congenital amaurosis (one form)	RPE65, a protein required for the cycling of retinoids (vitamin A metabolites) to photoreceptors (*RPE65*)	Adeno-associated virus vector Retinal pigment epithelial cells	Initially improved vision in many patients in the first trials, but the evidence now suggests, unexpectedly, that the photoreceptor (PR) degeneration continues nevertheless. The cause of this PR death is unknown

Note: ADA, Adenosine deaminase; Hb, hemoglobin; IV, intravenous; PEG, polyethylene glycol; SCID, severe combined immunodeficiency; WAS, Wiskott-Aldrich syndrome.

In this section, we outline the potential, methods, and probable limitations of gene transfer for the treatment of human genetic disease. The minimal requirements that must be met before the use of gene transfer can be considered for the treatment of a genetic disorder are presented in the Table.

10.5.1   General Considerations for Gene Therapy

In the treatment of inherited disease, the most common use of gene therapy will be the introduction of functional copies of the relevant gene into the appropriate target cells of a patient with a loss-of-function mutation (because most genetic diseases result from such mutations).

In these instances, precisely where the transferred gene inserts into the genome of a cell would, in principle, generally not be important. If gene editing (see earlier discussion and Table 10-4) to treat inherited disease becomes possible, then correction of the defect in the mutant gene in its normal genomic context would be ideal and would alleviate concerns such as the activation of a nearby oncogene by the regulatory activity of a viral vector, or the inactivation of a tumor suppressor due to insertional mutagenesis by the vector. In some long-lived types of cells, stable, long-term expression may not require integration of the introduced gene into the host genome. For example, if the transferred gene is stabilized in the form of an episome (a stable nuclear but nonchromosomal DNA molecule, such as that formed by an adeno-associated viral vector, discussed later), and if the target cell is long-lived (e.g., T cells, neurons, myocytes, hepatocytes), then long-term expression can occur without integration.

Gene therapy may also be undertaken to inactivate the product of a dominant mutant allele whose abnormal product causes the disease. For example, vectors carrying siRNAs (see earlier section) could, in principle, be used to mediate the selective degradation of a mutant mRNA encoding a dominant negative $pro\alpha1(I)$ collagen that causes osteogenesis imperfecta.

10.5.2   Gene Transfer Strategies

An appropriately engineered gene may be transferred into target cells by one of two general strategies (see Fig. 10-16). The first involves introduction of the gene into cells that have been cultured from the patient ex vivo (that is, outside the body) and then reintroduction of the cells to the patient after the gene transfer. In the second approach, the gene is injected directly in vivo into the tissue or extracellular fluid of interest (from which it is taken up by the target cells). In some cases, it may be desirable to target the vector to a specific cell type. This is usually achieved by modifying the coat of a viral vector so that only the designated cells bind the viral particles.

10.5.3   The Target Cell

The ideal target cells are stem cells (which are self-replicating) or progenitor cells taken from the patient (thereby eliminating the risk for graft-versus-host disease). Both cell types have substantial replication potential. Introduction of the gene into stem cells can result in the expression of the transferred gene in a large population of daughter cells. At present, bone marrow is the only tissue whose stem cells have been successfully targeted as recipients of transferred genes. Genetically modified bone marrow stem cells have been used to cure two forms of SCID, as discussed later. Gene transfer therapy into blood stem cells is also likely to be effective for the treatment of hemoglobinopathies and storage diseases for which bone marrow transplantation has been effective, as discussed earlier.

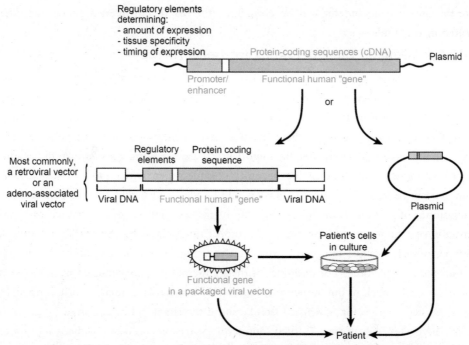

Figure 10-16　The two major strategies used to transfer a gene to a patient

For patients with a genetic disease, the most common approach is to construct a viral vector containing the human complementary DNA (cDNA) of interest and to introduce it directly into the patient or into cells cultured from the patient that are then returned to the patient. The viral components at the ends of the molecule are required for the integration of the vector into the host genome. In some instances, the gene of interest is placed in a plasmid, which is then used for the gene transfer.

An important logistical consideration is the number of cells into which the gene must be introduced in order to have a significant therapeutic effect. To treat PKU, for example, the approximate number of liver cells into which the phenylalanine hydroxylase gene would have to be transferred is approximately 5% of the hepatocyte mass, or approximately 1, 010 cells, although this number could be much less if the level of expression of the transferred gene is higher than wild type. A much greater challenge is gene therapy for muscular dystrophies, for which the gene must be inserted into a significant fraction of the huge number of myocytes in the body in order to have therapeutic efficacy.

10.5.4　DNA Transfer Into Cells: Viral Vectors

The ideal vector for gene therapy would be safe, readily made, and easily introduced into the appropriate target tissue, and it would express the gene of interest for life. Indeed, no single vector is likely to be satisfactory in all respects for all types of gene therapy, and a repertoire of vectors will probably be required. Here, we briefly review three of the most widely used classes of viral vectors, those derived from **retroviruses**, **adeno-associated viruses** (AAVs), and **adenoviruses**.

One of the most widely used classes of vectors is derived from retroviruses, simple RNA viruses that can integrate into the host genome. They contain only three structural genes, which can be removed and replaced with the gene to be transferred (see Fig. 10-16). The current generation of retroviral vectors has been engineered to render them incapable of replication. In addition, they are nontoxic to the cell, and only a low number of copies of the viral DNA (with the transferred gene) integrate into the host genome.

Moreover, the integrated DNA is stable and can accommodate up to 8 kb of added DNA, commodious enough for many genes that might be transferred. A major limitation of many retroviral vectors, however, is that the target cell must undergo division for integration of the virus into the host DNA, limiting the use of such vectors in nondividing cells such as neurons. In contrast, lentiviruses, the class of retroviruses that includes HIV, are capable of DNA integration in nondividing cells, including neurons.

Lentiviruses have the additional advantage of not showing preferential integration into any specific gene locus, thus reducing the chances of activating an oncogene in a large number of cells.

AAVs do not elicit strong immunological responses, a great advantage that enhances the longevity of their expression. Moreover, they infect dividing or nondividing cells to remain in a predominantly episomal form that is stable and confers long-term expression of the transduced gene. A disadvantage is that the current AAV vectors can accommodate inserts of up to only 5 kb, which is smaller than many genes in their natural context.

The third group of viral vectors, adenovirus-derived vectors, can be obtained at high titer, will infect a wide variety of dividing or nondividing cell types, and can accommodate inserts of 30 to 35 kb. However, in addition to other limitations, they have been associated with at least one death in a gene therapy trial through the elicitation of a strong immune response. At present their use is restricted to gene therapy for cancer.

10.5.5 Risks of Gene Therapy

Gene therapy for the treatment of human disease has risks of three general types:

- **Adverse response to the vector or vector-disease combination.** Principal among the concerns is that the patient will have an adverse reaction to the vector or the transferred gene. Such problems should be largely anticipated with appropriate animal and preliminary human studies.
- **Insertional mutagenesis causing malignancy.** The second concern is insertional mutagenesis, that is, that the transferred gene will integrate into the patient's DNA and activate a proto-oncogene or disrupt a tumor suppressor gene, leading possibly to cancer. The illicit expression of an oncogene is less likely to occur with the current generation of viral vectors, which have been altered to minimize the ability of their promoters to activate the expression of adjacent host genes. Insertional inactivation of a tumor suppressor gene is likely to be infrequent and, as such, is an acceptable risk in diseases for which there is no therapeutic alternative.
- **Insertional inactivation of an essential gene.** A third risk—that insertional inactivation could disrupt a gene essential for viability—will be without significant effect because such lethal mutations are expected to be rare and will kill only single cells. Although vectors appear to somewhat favor insertion into transcribed genes, the chance that the same gene will be disrupted in more than a few cells is extremely low. The one exception to this statement applies to the germline. An insertion into a gene in the

germline could create a dominant disease-causing mutation that might manifest in the treated patient's offspring. Such events, however, are likely to be rare and the risk acceptable because it would be difficult to justify withholding, on this basis, carefully planned and reviewed trials of gene therapy from patients who have no other recourse. Moreover, the problem of germline modification by disease treatment is not confined to gene therapy. For example, most chemotherapy used in the treatment of malignant disease is mutagenic, but this risk is accepted because of the therapeutic benefits.

10.5.6　Diseases That Have Been Amenable to Gene Therapy

Although nearly a dozen single-gene diseases have been shown to improve with gene therapy, a large number of other monogenic disorders are potential candidates for this strategy, including retinal degenerations; hematopoietic conditions, such as sickle cell anemia and thalassemia; and disorders affecting liver proteins, such as PKU, urea cycle disorders, familial hypercholesterolemia, and α1AT deficiency. Here we discuss several disorders in which gene therapy has been clearly effective, but which also highlight some of the challenges associated with this therapeutic approach.

(1) Severe X-Linked Combined Immunodeficiency

The SCIDs are due to mutations in genes required for lymphocyte maturation. Affected individuals fail to thrive and die early in life of infection because they lack functional B and T lymphocytes. The most common form of the disease, X-linked SCID, results from mutations in the X-linked gene (IL2RG) encoding the γc-cytokine receptor subunit of several interleukin receptors. The receptor deficiency causes an early block in T lymphocy and natural killer-lymphocyte growth, survival, and differentiation and is associated with severe infections, failure to thrive, and death in infancy or early childhood if left untreated. This condition was chosen for a gene therapy trial for two principal reasons. Firstly, bone marrow transplantation cures the disease, indicating that the restoration of lymphocyte expression of IL2RG can reverse the pathophysiological changes. Secondly, it was believed that so-called transduced cells carrying the transferred gene would have a selective survival advantage over untransduced cells.

The outcome of trials of X-linked SCID has been dramatic and resulted, in 2000, in the first gene therapy cure of a patient with a genetic disease. Subsequent confirmation has been obtained in most patients in subsequent clinical trials (see Table 10-5). Bone marrow stem cells from the patients were infected in culture (ex vivo) with a retroviral vector that expressed the γc cytokine subunit cDNA. A selective advantage was conferred on the transduced cells by the gene transfer. Transduced T cells and natural killer cells populated the blood of treated patients, and the T cells appeared to behave normally. Although the frequency of transduced B cells was low, adequate levels of serum immunoglobulin and antibody levels were obtained. Dramatic clinical improvement occurred, with resolution of protracted diarrhea and skin lesions and restoration of normal growth and development. These initial trials demonstrated the great potential of gene therapy for the correction of inherited disease.

This highly promising outcome, however, came at the cost of induction of a leukemia-like disorder in 5 of the 20 treated patients, who developed an extreme lymphocytosis resembling T-cell acute lymphocytic leukemia. 4 of them are now well after treatment of the leukemia. The malignancy was due to insertional mutagenesis: the retroviral vector inserted into the LMO2 locus, causing aberrant expression of the LMO2 mRNA, which encodes a component of a transcription factor complex that mediates hematopoietic development. Consequently, trials using integrating vectors in hematopoietic cells must now monitor insertion sites and survey for clonal proliferation. Current-generation vectors are designed to avoid this mutagenic effect by using strategies such as including a self-inactivating or "suicide" gene cassette in the vector to eliminate clones of malignant cells. At this point, bone marrow stem cell transplantation remains the treatment of choice for those children with SCID fortunate enough to have a donor with an HLA-identical match. For patients without such a match, autologous transplantation of hematopoietic stem and progenitor cells, in which the genetic defect has been corrected by gene therapy, offers a lifesaving alternative, but one that may not be without risk.

(2) Metachromatic Leukodystrophy

Metachromatic leukodystrophy (MLD) is an autosomal recessive neurodegenerative disorder that, in the late infantile form, is generally fatal by 5 years of age. It results from mutations in the gene, ARSA, that encodes arylsulfatase A, a lysosomal enzyme that degrades sulfatides that are neurotoxic, leading to demyelination in the central and peripheral nervous system. As described earlier, HSC transplantation is an effective treatment of some lysosomal storage diseases because some of the donor-derived macrophages and microglia can enter the central nervous system, scavenge the stored material (such as sulfatide in MLD), and release lysosomal enzymes that are taken up by the mutant cells of the patient. HSC transplants have not been successful for MLD, however, a failure thought to be due to a level of ARSA expression from the transplanted cells that is too low to have a therapeutic effect.

In an apparently successful treatment, the autologous HSCs of three patients with MLD were transduced with a lentiviral vector that was engineered to produce above-normal levels of arylsulfatase A from a functional ARSA gene, and the genetically corrected HSCs were then engrafted (see Fig. 10-17). Although more than 36,000 different lentiviral integration sites were examined, no evidence of genotoxicity was observed, suggesting that lentiviral vectors can be effective in the gene therapy of HSCs. Dramatically, disease progression was arrested, at least up to 24 months after treatment, but long-term follow-up will be required to establish that the effect of the gene therapy is benign and enduring.

(3) Hemophilia B

Hemophilia B is an X-linked disorder of coagulation caused by mutations in the F9 gene, leading to a deficiency or dysfunction of clotting factor IX. The disease is characterized by bleeding into soft tissues, muscles, and weight-bearing joints, and occurs within hours to days after trauma. Severely affected subjects, with less than 1% of normal levels of factor IX, have frequent bleeding that causes crippling joint disease and early death. Prophylactic—but not curative—treatment with intravenous factor IX concentrate several times a week is expensive and leads to the generation of inhibitory antibodies.

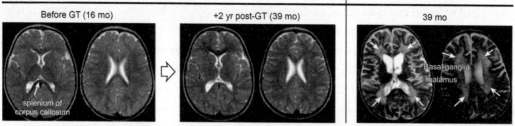

| MLD01 | | UT LI MLD |
| Before GT (16 mo) | +2 yr post-GT (39 mo) | 39 mo |

Figure 10-17　Clinical follow-up of a metachromatic leukodystrophy（MLD）patient after hematopoietic stem cell gene therapy（GT）with the arylsulfatase A gene

Magnetic resonance images from patient MLD01 before gene therapy and 2 years after treatment. The brain of this patient appeared largely normal 2 years after treatment. In contrast, the brain of an untreated, age matched late infantile MLD patient（UT LI MLD）showed severe demyelination associated with diffuse atrophy. In MLD01 images, a small area of hyperintensity is present within the splenium of the corpus callosum（ *white arrow* ）. This area appeared at the 12-month follow-up and remained stable thereafter. In UT LI MLD images, extensive, diffuse symmetrical hyperintensities with typical striped "tigroid pattern"（ *white arrows* ）are seen within periventricular white matter, corpus callosum, external and internal capsules, and cerebellar deep white matter. Severe diffuse brain atrophy involving basal ganglia and thalamus, which show a T2 hypointense signal, is also present.
（From BIFFI A, MONTINI E, LORIOLI L, et al. Lentiviral hematopoietic stem cell gene therapy benefits metachromatic leukodystrophy[J]. Science, 2013,341（6148）:1233158.）

In 2011, the first successful gene therapy treatment of hemophilia B was reported in six patients using an AAV8 vector that is tropic for hepatocytes, where factor IX is normally produced. After a single infusion of the AAV8-F9 vector, four patients were able to discontinue prophylactic factor IX infusions, whereas the other two tolerated longer intervals between infusions. The two patients who received the highest dose of the vector had transient asymptomatic increases in liver enzyme levels—which resolved with steroid treatment— indicating that immune-related side effects must remain a concern in future studies. Unfortunately, the AAV vectors cannot accommodate the gene for factor VIII, so that other vectors will have to be developed for hemophilia A patients. Apart from this limitation of cargo size, however, AAV-mediated gene therapy targeted to hepatocytes may be applicable to any genetic disease in which production of the protein in the liver is the desired goal.

（4）β-Thalassemia

The hemoglobinopathies are the most common genetic defects in the world, but at present they are incurable except by HSC transplantation from a matched donor. Consequently, the development of effective, safe, and affordable gene therapy for these disorders, the most common being sickle cell disease and the α-and β-thalassemias, would be a medical triumph.

In 2010, the first successful gene therapy trial for a hemoglobinopathy was reported, in a single patient with β-thalassemia who was transfusion-dependent, with hemoglobin levels of only 4 to 6 g/dL. This individual was a genetic compound of β^E and β^0 alleles, the β^E allele generating a mutant β-globin of decreased abundance, with the β^0 allele being a null. The patient's HSCs were transduced with a lentiviral vector containing a β-globin gene. The patient became transfusion-independent, with hemoglobin levels ranging from 9 to 10 g/dL, although the vector-encoded hemoglobin accounted for only approximately one third of the total, the remainder being the mutant Hb E and Hb F. Unexpectedly, the increase in normal β-globin expression was largely attributable to one bone marrow cell clone, in which the lentiviral vector integrated into a gene encoding a transcriptional regulator called HMGA2. This integration activated expression in erythroid cells of a truncated form of HMGA2, an event that confounded the interpretation of the result, because the extent to which the clonal dominance of cells expressing the truncated HMGA2 accounted for the therapeutic benefits of the gene therapy is unclear.

This study offers great promise but highlights the potential risks associated with the random insertion of viral vectors in the genome. Much current research is therefore devoted to the development of safer gene delivery vectors, including modified lentiviral vectors.

10.5.7 The Prospects for Gene Therapy

To date, almost 2,000 clinical gene therapy trials (approximately two thirds of which are for cancer) have been undertaken worldwide to evaluate both the safety and efficacy of this long-promised and conceptually promising technology. Approximately 180 of these trials were for the treatment of monogenic diseases. The exciting results obtained with gene therapy to date, albeit with small numbers of patients and only a few diseases, validates the optimism behind this immense effort. Although the breadth of applications remains uncertain, it is to be hoped that over the next few decades, gene therapy for both monogenic and genetically complex diseases will contribute to the management of many disorders, both common and rare.

10.6 Precision Medicine: the Present and Future of the Treatment of Mendelian Disease

The treatment of single-gene diseases embodies the concept of precision medicine tailored to the individual patient as deeply as any other area of medical treatment. Knowledge of the specific mutant sequence in an individual is central to many of the targeted therapies described in this chapter. The promise of gene therapy for an individual with a mendelian disorder must be based on the identification of the mutant gene in each affected individual and on the design of a vector that will deliver the therapeutic gene to the targeted tissue. Similarly, approaches based on gene editing require knowledge of the specific mutation to be corrected.

Beyond this, however, precision medicine will frequently require knowledge of the precise mutant allele and of its specific effect on the mRNA and protein. In many cases, the exact nature of the mutation will define the drug that will bind to a specific regulatory sequence to enhance or reduce the expression of a gene. In other cases, the mutation will dictate the sequence of an allele-specific oligonucleotide to mediate the skipping of an exon with a premature termination codon, or of an siRNA to suppress a dominant negative allele. A compendium of small molecules will gradually become available to suppress particular stop codons, to act as chaperones that will rescue mutant proteins from misfolding and proteosomal degradation, or to potentiate the activity of mutant proteins.

Genetic treatment is not only becoming more and more creative, it is becoming more and more precise. The future promises not only a longer life for many patients, but a life of vastly better quality.

Study Questions:

1. Identify some of the limitations on the types of proteins that can be considered for extracellular replacement therapy, as exemplified by polyethylene glycol-adenosine deaminase (PEG-ADA). What makes this approach inappropriate for phenylalanine hydroxylase deficiency? If Tay-Sachs disease caused only liver disease, would this strategy succeed? If not, why?

2. A 3-year-old girl, Rhonda, has familial hypercholesterolemia due to a deletion of the 5'end of each of her low density lipoprotein (LDL) receptor genes that removed the promoter and the first two exons. (Rhonda's parents are second cousins.) You explain to the parents that she will require plasmapheresis every 1 to 2 weeks for years. At the clinic, however, they meet another family with a 5-year-old boy with the same disease. The boy has been treated with drugs with some success. Rhonda's parents want to know why she has not been offered similar pharmacological therapy. Please explain.

3. Both alleles of an autosomal gene that is mutant in your patient produce a protein that is decreased in abundance but has residual function. What therapeutic strategies might you consider in such a situation?

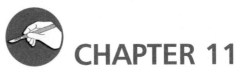

CHAPTER 11
Genetic Counseling and Risk Assessment

Purpose and Requirement:

In this chapter students should understand genetic counseling is the process by which the patients or relatives at risk of an inherited disorder are advised of the consequences and nature of the disorder, the probability of developing or transmitting it, and the options open to them in management and family planning. This complex process can be separated into diagnostic (the actual estimation of risk) and supportive aspects.

In this chapter, we present the fundamentals of the practice of genetic counseling as applied to families in which an individual is known or suspected to have a hereditary condition. Genetic counseling includes a discussion of the natural history of the disease as well as determination of the risk for disease in other family members based on the inheritance pattern, empirical risk figures, and medical testing, especially molecular genetic and genomic testing. Counseling includes a discussion of approaches available to mitigate or reduce the risk for heritable disease. Finally, the counselor carries out a careful assessment of the psychological and social impact of the diagnosis on the patient and family and works to help the family cope with the presence of a heritable condition.

11.1 Family History in Risk Assessment

Family history is clearly of great importance in diagnosis and risk assessment. Applying the known rules of mendelian inheritance, as introduced in Chapter 3, allows the geneticist to provide accurate evaluations of risk for disease in relatives of affected individuals. Family history is also important when a geneticist assesses the risk for complex disorders, as discussed in Chapter 6. Because a person's genes are shared with his or her relatives, family history provides the clinician with information on the impact that an individual's genetic makeup might have on one's health, using the medical history of relatives as an indicator of one's own genetic susceptibilities. Furthermore, family members often share environmental factors, such as diet and behavior, and thus relatives provide information about both shared genes and shared environmental factors that may interact to cause the common, genetically complex diseases. Having a first-degree relative with a common disease of adulthood—such as cardiovascular disease, cancer of the breast, cancer of the colon or prostate, type 2 diabetes, osteoporosis, or asthma—raises an individual's risk for the disease approximately 2-fold to 3-fold relative to the general population, a moderate increase compared with the average population risk. The more first-degree relatives one has with a complex trait and the earlier in life the disease occurs in a family member, the greater the load of susceptibility genes and environmental exposures likely to be present in the patient's family. Thus consideration of family history can lead to the designation of a patient as being at high risk for a particular disease on the basis of family history. For example, a male with three male first-degree relatives with prostate cancer has an 11-fold greater relative risk for development of the disease than does a man with no such family history.

Determining that an individual is at increased risk on the basis of family history can have an impact on individual medical care. For example, two individuals with deep venous thrombosis—one with a family history of unexplained deep venous thrombosis in a relative younger than 50 years and another with no family history of any coagulation disorder—should receive different management with respect to testing for factor V Leiden or prothrombin 20210G>A and anticoagulation therapy. Similarly, having a first-degree relative with colon cancer is sufficient to trigger the initiation of colon cancer screening by colonoscopy at the age of 40 years, 10 years earlier than for the general population. This is because the cumulative incidence for development of the disease for someone 40 years old with a positive family history equals the risk for someone at the age of 50 years with no family history. The increase in risk is even more pronounced if two or more relatives have had the disease, an empirical observation that has driven standards of clinical care for screening in this condition.

Family history is admittedly an indirect method of assessing the contribution of an individual's own genetic variants to health and disease susceptibility. Direct detection of genetic risk factors and demonstrating that they are valid for guiding health care is a major challenge in applying genomics to medicine.

11.2 Genetic Counseling in Clinical Practice

Clinical genetics is concerned with the diagnosis and management of the medical, social, and psychological aspects of hereditary disease. As in all other areas of medicine, it is essential in clinical genetics to do the following:

- Make a correct diagnosis, which often involves laboratory testing, including genetic testing to find the mutations responsible.
- Help the affected person and family members understand and come to terms with the nature and consequences of the disorder.
- Provide appropriate treatment and management, including referrals to other specialist providers as needed.

Just as the unique feature of genetic disease is its tendency to recur within families, the unique aspect of genetic counseling is its focus on both the original patient and also on members of his or her family, both present and future. Genetic counselors have a responsibility to do the following:

- Work with the patient to inform other family members of their potential risk.
- Offer mutation or other testing to provide the most precise risk assessments possible for other family members.
- Explain what approaches are available to the patient and family members to modify these risks.

Finally, genetic counseling is not limited to the provision of information and identification of individuals at risk for disease. Rather, it is a process of exploration and communication. Genetic counselors define and address the complex psychosocial issues associated with a genetic disorder in a family and provide psychologically oriented counseling to help individuals adapt and adjust to the impact and implications of the disorder in the family. For this reason, genetic counseling may be most effectively accomplished through periodic contact with the family as the medical or social issues become relevant to the lives of those involved.

11.2.1 Genetic Counseling Providers

Clinical genetics is particularly time-consuming in comparison with other clinical fields because it requires extensive preparation and follow-up in addition to time for direct contact with patients. In many countries, genetic counseling is provided by physicians. However, in the United States, Canada, the United Kingdom, and a few other countries, genetic counseling services are often provided by **genetic counselors** or **nurse geneticists**, professionals specially trained in genetics and counseling, who serve as members of a health care team with physicians. Genetic counseling in the United States and Canada is a self-regulating health profession with its own board (the American and Canadian Boards of Genetic Counselors) for accreditation of training programs and certification of practitioners. Some states in the United States are also licensing genetic counselors. Nurses with genetics expertise are accredited through a separate credentialing commission. In China, genetic counseling is steered by the Chinese Board of Genetic Counseling (CBGC).

Genetic counselors and nurse geneticists play an essential role in clinical genetics, participating in many aspects of the investigation and management of genetic problems. A genetic counselor is often the first point of contact that a patient has with clinical genetic services, provides genetic counseling directly to individuals, helps patients and families deal with the many psychological and social issues that arise during genetic counseling, and continues in a supportive role and as a source of information after the clinical investigation and formal counseling have been completed. Genetic counselors are also active in the field of genetic testing. They provide close liaison among the referring physicians, the diagnostic laboratories, and the families themselves. Their special expertise is invaluable to clinical laboratories because explaining and interpreting genetic testing to patients and referring physicians often requires a sophisticated knowledge of genetics and genomics, as well as excellent communication skills.

11.2.2 Common Indications for Genetic Counseling

Table 11-1 lists some of the most common situations that lead people to pursue genetic counseling. Individuals seeking genetic counseling (referred to as the consultands) may themselves be the probands in the family, or they may be the parents of an affected child or have relatives with a potential or known genetic condition. Genetic counseling is also an integral part of prenatal testing and of genetic testing and screening programs.

Established standards of medical care require that providers of genetic services obtain a history that includes family and ethnic information, inquire as to possible consanguinity, advise patients of the genetic risks to them and other family members, offer genetic testing or prenatal diagnosis when indicated, and outline the various treatment or management options for reducing the risk for disease. Although genetic counseling case management must be individualized for each patient's needs and situation, a generic approach can be summarized (see Table 11-2). In general, patients are not told what decisions to make with regard to the various testing and management options but are instead provided with information and support in coming to a decision that seems most appropriate for the patients, the consultands, and their families. This approach to counseling, referred to as **nondirective counseling**, has its origins in the setting of prenatal counseling, where the guiding principle is respect for an individual couple's autonomy, that is, their right to make reproductive choices free of coercion.

Table 11-1 Common Indications for Genetic Counseling

- Previous child with multiple congenital anomalies, intellectual disability, or an isolated birth defect such as neural tube defect or cleft lip and palate
- Personal history or family history of a hereditary condition, such as cystic fibrosis, fragile X syndrome, congenital heart defect, hereditary cancer, or diabetes
- Pregnancy at risk for a chromosomal or hereditary disorder
- Consanguinity
- Teratogen exposure, such as to occupational chemicals, medications, alcohol
- Repeated pregnancy loss or infertility
- Newly diagnosed abnormality or geneticcondition
- Before undertaking genetic testing and after receiving results, particularly in testing for susceptibility to late-onset disorders, such as hereditary cancer syndromes or neurological disease
- As follow-up for a positive result of a newborn test, as with phenylketonuria; a heterozygote (preconception carrier) screening test, such as Tay-Sachs; or a positive first- or second-trimester maternal serum screen, a noninvasive prenatal screen by free fetal DNA analysis or abnormal fetal ultrasound examination results

Table 11-2 Genetic Counseling Case Management

• Collection of information Family history (questionnaire) Medical history Tests or additional assessments • Assessment Physical examination Laboratory and radiological testing Validation or establishment of diagnosis—if possible	• Counseling Nature and consequence of disorder • Recurrence risk Availability of further or future testing • Decision making Referral to other specialists, health agencies, support groups • Continuing clinical assessment, especially if no diagnosis • Psychosocial support

11.2.3 Managing the Risk for Recurrence in Families

Many families seek genetic counseling to ascertain the risk for heritable disease in their children and to learn what options are available to reduce the risk for recurrence of the particular genetic disorder in question. Genetic laboratory tests for carrier testing (karyotyping, biochemical analysis, or genome analysis) are frequently used to determine the actual risk to couples with a family history of a genetic disorder. Genetic counseling is recommended both before and after such testing, to assist consultands in making an informed decision to undergo testing, as well as to understand and to use the information gained through testing.

When family history or laboratory testing indicate an increased risk for a hereditary condition in a future pregnancy, prenatal diagnosis is one approach that can often be offered to families. Prenatal diagnosis is, however, by no means a universal solution to the risk for genetic problems in offspring. There are disorders for which prenatal diagnosis is not available and, for many parents, pregnancy termination is not an acceptable option, even if prenatal diagnosis is available. Preimplantation diagnosis by blastocyst or blastomere biopsy avoids the problems of pregnancy termination but requires in vitro fertilization.

Other measures besides prenatal diagnosis are available for the management of recurrence and include the following:

- Genetic laboratory tests for carrier testing can sometimes reassure couples with a family history of a genetic disorder that they themselves are not at increased risk for having a child with a specific genetic disease. In other cases, such tests indicate that the couple is at increased risk. Genetic counseling is recommended both before and after such testing, to assist consultands in making an informed decision to undergo testing, as well as understanding and using the information gained through testing.

- If the parents plan to have no more children or no children at all, contraception or sterilization may be their choice, and they may need information about the possible procedures or an appropriate referral.

- **Adoption** is a possibility for parents who want a child or more children.

- **Artificial insemination** may be appropriate if the father has a gene for an autosomal dominant or X-linked defect or has a heritable chromosome defect, but it is obviously not indicated if it is the mother who has such a defect. Artificial insemination is also useful if both parents are carriers of an autosomal recessive disorder. In vitro fertilization with a **donated egg** may be appropriate if the mother has an autosomal dominant defect or carries an X-linked disease. In either case, genetic counseling and appropriate genetic tests of the sperm or egg donor should be part of the process.

If the parents decide to terminate a pregnancy, provision of relevant information and support is an appropriate part of genetic counseling. Periodic follow-up through additional visits or by telephone is often arranged for a few months or more after a pregnancy termination.

11.2.4   Psychological Aspects

Patients and families dealing with a risk for a genetic disorder or coping with the illness itself are subject to varying degrees of emotional and social stress. Although this is also true of nongenetic disorders, the concern generated by knowledge that the condition might recur, the guilt or censure felt by some individuals, and the need for reproductive decisions can give rise to severe distress. Many persons have the strength to deal personally with such problems. They prefer receiving even bad news to remaining uninformed, and they make their own decisions on the basis of the most complete and accurate information they can obtain. Other persons require much more support and may need referral for psychotherapy.

Genetic counselors often refer a patient and family with a genetic disorder or birth defect to family and patient **support groups**. These organizations, which can be focused either on a single disease or on a group of diseases, can help those concerned to share their experience, to learn how to deal with the day-to-day problems caused by the disorder, to hear of new developments in therapy or prevention, and to promote research into the condition. Many support groups have Internet sites and electronic chat rooms, through which patients and families give and receive information and advice, ask and answer questions, and obtain much needed emotional support. Similar disease-specific, self-help organizations are active in many nations around the world.

11.3　Determining Recurrence Risks

The estimation of recurrence risks is a central concern in genetic counseling. Ideally, it is based on knowledge of the genetic nature of the disorder in question and on the pedigree of the particular family being counseled. The family member whose risk for a genetic disorder is to be determined is usually a relative of a proband, such as a sibling of an affected child or a living or future child of an affected adult. In some families, especially for some autosomal dominant and X-linked traits, it may also be necessary to estimate the risk for more remote relatives.

When a disorder is known to have single-gene inheritance, the recurrence risk for specific family members can usually be determined from basic mendelian principles (see Fig. 11-1). On the other hand, risk calculations may be less than straightforward if there is reduced penetrance or variability of expression, or if the disease is frequently the result of new mutation, as in many X-linked and autosomal dominant disorders. Laboratory tests that give equivocal results can add further complications. Under these circumstances, mendelian risk estimates can sometimes be modified by means of applying conditional probability to the pedigree, which takes into account information about the family that may increase or decrease the underlying mendelian risk.

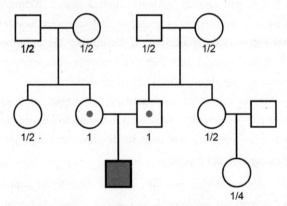

Figure 11-1　Pedigree of a family with an autosomal recessive condition
The probability of being a carrier is shown beneath each individual symbol in the pedigree.

In contrast to single-gene disorders, the underlying mechanisms of inheritance for most chromosomal or genomic disorders and complex traits are unknown, and estimates of recurrence risk are based on previous experience (see Fig. 11-2). This approach to risk assessment is valuable if there are reliable data on the frequency of recurrence of the disorder in families and if the phenotype is not heterogeneous. However, when a particular phenotype has an undetermined risk or can result from a variety of causes with different frequencies and with widely different risks, estimation of the recurrence risk is hazardous at best. In a later section, the estimation of recurrence risk in some typical clinical situations, both straightforward and more complicated, is considered.

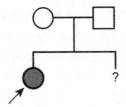

Figure 11-2   Empirical risk estimates in genetic counseling

A family with no other positive family history has one child affected with a disorder known to be multifactorial or chromosomal. What is the recurrence risk? If the child is affected with spina bifida, the empirical risk to a subsequent child is approximately 4%. If the child has Down syndrome, the empirical risk for recurrence would be approximately 1% if the karyotype is trisomy 21, but it might be substantially higher if one of the parents is a carrier of a Robertsonian translocation involving chromosome 21.

11.3.1   Risk Estimation by Use of Mendel's Laws When Genotypes are Fully Known

The simplest risk estimates apply to families in which the relevant genotypes of all family members are known or can be inferred. For example, if both members of a couple are known to be heterozygous carriers of an autosomal recessive condition because they have a child with the disorder or because of carrier testing, the risk (probability) is one in four with each pregnancy that the child will inherit two mutant alleles and inherit the disease (see Fig. 11-3A). Even if the couple were to have six unaffected children subsequent to the affected child (see Fig. 11-3B), the risk in the eighth, ninth, or tenth pregnancy would still be one in four for each pregnancy (assuming there is no misattributed paternity for the first affected child).

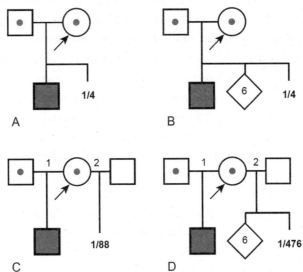

Figure 11-3   Series of pedigrees showing autosomal recessive inheritance with contrasting recurrence risks

(A) and (B) The genotypes of the parents are known. (C) The genotype of the consultand's second partner is inferred from the carrier frequency in the population. (D) The inferred genotype is modified by additional pedigree information. *Arrows* indicate the consultand. Numbers indicate recurrence risk in the consultand's next pregnancy.

11. 3. 2　Risk Estimation by Use of Conditional Probability When Alternative Genotypes are Possible

In contrast to the simple case just described, situations arise in which the genotypes of the relevant individuals in the family are not definitively known. The risk for recurrence will be very different, depending on whether or not the consultand is a carrier of an abnormal allele of a disease gene. For example, the chance that a woman, who is known from her first marriage to be a carrier of cystic fibrosis (CF), might have an affected child depends on the chance that her husband by her second marriage is a carrier (see Fig. 11-3C). The risk for the partner's being a carrier depends on his ethnic background. For the general non-Hispanic white population, this chance is approximately 1 in 22. Therefore the chance that a known carrier and her unrelated partner would have an affected first child is the product of these probabilities, or $1/22 \times 1/4 = 1/88$ (approximately 1.1%).

Of course, if the husband really were a carrier, the chance that the child of two carriers would be a homozygote or a compound heterozygote for mutant CF alleles is one in four. If the husband were not a carrier, then the chance of having an affected child is zero. Suppose, however, that one cannot test his carrier status directly. A carrier risk of 1 in 22 is the best estimate one can make for individuals of his ethnic background and no family history of CF without direct carrier testing; in fact, however, a person either is a carrier or is not. The problem is that we do not know. In this situation, the more opportunities the male in Figure 11-3C (who may or may not be a carrier of a mutant gene) has to pass on the mutant gene and fails to do so, the less likely it would be that he is indeed a carrier. Thus, if the couple were to come for counseling already with six children, none of whom is affected (see Fig. 11-3D), it would seem reasonable, intuitively, that the husband's chance of being a carrier should be less than the 1 in 22 risk that the childless male partner in Figure 11-3C was assigned on the basis of the population carrier frequency. In this situation, we apply conditional probability (also known as **Bayesian analysis**, based on Bayes's theorem on probability published in 1763), a method that takes advantage of phenotypic information in a pedigree to assess the relative probability of two or more alternative genotypic possibilities and to condition the risk on the basis of that information. In Figure 11-3D, the chance that the second husband is a carrier is actually 1 in 119, and the chance that this couple would have a child with CF is therefore 1 in 476, not 1 in 88, as calculated in Fig. 11-3C. Some examples of the use of Bayesian analysis for risk assessment in pedigrees are examined in the following section.

(1) Conditional Probability

To illustrate the application of Bayesian analysis, consider the pedigrees shown in Figure 11-4. In Family A, the mother II-1 is an **obligate carrier** for the X-linked bleeding disorder hemophilia A because her father was affected. Her risk for transmitting the mutant factor VIII (F8) allele responsible for hemophilia A is 1 in 2, and the fact that she has already had four unaffected sons does not reduce this risk. Thus the risk that the consultand (III-5) is a carrier of a mutant F8 allele is 1 in 2 because she is the daughter of a known carrier.

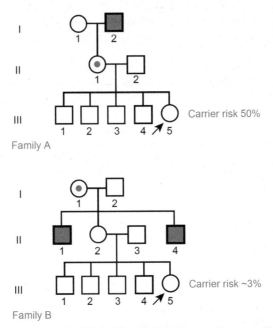

Figure 11-4 Modified risk estimates in genetic counseling

The consultands in the two families are at risk for having a son with hemophilia A. In Family A, the consultand's mother is an obligate heterozygote; in Family B, the consultand's mother may or may not be a carrier. Application of Bayesian analysis reduces the risk for being a carrier to only approximately 3% for the consultand in Family B but not the consultand in Family A. See text for derivation of the modified risk.

In Family B, however, the consultand's mother (individual II-2) may or may not be a carrier, depending on whether she has inherited a mutant *F8* allele from her mother, I-1. If III-5 were the only child of her mother, III-5's risk for being a carrier would be 1 in 4, calculated as 1/2 (her mother's risk for being a carrier) ×1/2 (her risk for inheriting the mutant allele from her mother). Short of testing III-5 directly for the mutant allele, we cannot tell whether she is a carrier. In this case, however, the fact that III-5 has four unaffected brothers is relevant because every time II-2 had a son, the chance that the son would be unaffected is only 1 in 2 if II-2 were a carrier, whereas it is a near certainty (probability=1) that the son would be unaffected if II-2 were, in fact, not a carrier at all. With each son, II-2 has, in effect, tested her carrier status by placing herself at a 50% risk for having an affected son. To have four unaffected sons might suggest that maybe her mother is not a carrier. Bayesian analysis allows one to take this kind of indirect information into account in calculating whether II-2 is a carrier, thus modifying the consultand's risk for being a carrier. In fact, as we show in the next section, her carrier risk is far lower than 50%.

(2) Identify the Possible Scenarios

To translate this intuition into actual risk calculation, we use a Bayesian probability calculation. First, we list all possible alternative genotypes that may be present in the relevant individuals in the pedigree (see Fig. 11-5). In this case, there are three scenarios, each reflecting a different combination of alternative genotypes:

A. II-2 is a carrier, but the consultand is not.

B. II -2 and the consultand are both carriers.

C. II -2 is not a carrier, which implies that the consultand could not be one either because there is no mutant allele to inherit.

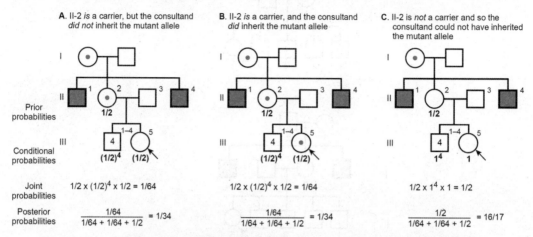

Figure 11-5 Conditional probability used to estimate carrier risk for a consultand in a family with hemophilia in which the prior probability of the carrier state is determined by mendelian inheritance from a known carrier at the top of the pedigree

These risk estimates, based on genetic principles, can be further modified by considering information obtained from family history, carrier detection testing, or molecular genetic methods for direct detection of the mutation in the affected boy, with use of Bayesian calculations. (A) to (C) The three mutually exclusive situations that could explain the pedigree.

Why do we not consider the possibility that the consultand is a carrier even though II -2 is not? We do not list this scenario because it would require that two mutations in the same gene occur independently in the same family, one inherited by the probands and one new mutation in the consultand, a scenario so vanishingly unlikely that it can be dismissed out of hand.

First, we draw the three possible scenarios as pedigrees (as in Fig. 11-5) and write down the probability of individual II -2's being a carrier or not. This is referred to as her **prior probability** because it depends simply on her risk for carrying a mutant allele inherited from her known carrier mother, I -1, and it has not been modified ("conditioned") at all by her own reproductive history.

Next, we write down the probabilities that individuals III -1 through III -4 would be unaffected under each scenario. These probabilities are different, depending on whether II -2 is a carrier or not. If she is a carrier (situations A and B), then the chance that individuals III -1 through III -4 would all be unaffected is the chance that each did not inherit II -2's mutant $F8$ allele, which is 1 in 2 for each of her sons or $(1/2)^4$ for all four. In situation C, however, II -2 is not a carrier, so the chance that her four sons would all be unaffected is 1 because II -2 does not have a mutant $F8$ to pass on to any of them. These are called **conditional probabilities** because they are probabilities affected by the condition of whether II -2 is a carrier.

Similarly, we can write down the probability that the consultand (III -5) is a carrier. In A, she did not inherit the mutant allele from her carrier mother, with a probability of 1 in 2. In B, she did inherit the mutant allele (probability $=1/2$). In C, her mother is not a carrier, and so

III-5 has essentially a 100% chance of not being a carrier. Multiply the prior and conditional probabilities together to form the **joint probabilities** for each situation, A, B, and C.

Finally, we determine what fraction of the total joint probability is represented by any scenario of interest; this is called the **posterior probability** of each of the three situations. Because III-5 is the consultand and wants to know her risk for being a carrier, we need the posterior probability of situation B, which is:

$$\frac{1/64}{1/64+1/64+1/2}=1/34\approx3\%$$

If we wish to know the chance that II-2 is a carrier, we add the posterior probabilities of the two situations in which she is a carrier, A and B, to get a carrier risk of 1 in 17, or approximately 6%.

If III-5 were also to have unaffected sons, her carrier risk could also be modified downward by a Bayesian calculation. However, if II-2 were to have an affected child, then she would have proved herself a carrier, and III-5's risk would thus become 1 in 2. Similarly, if III-5 were to have an affected child, then she must be a carrier, and Bayesian analysis would no longer be necessary.

Bayesian analysis may seem to some like mere statistical maneuvering. However, the analysis allows genetic counselors to quantify what seemed to be intuitively likely from inspection of the pedigree: the fact that the consultand had four unaffected brothers provides support for the hypothesis that her mother is not a carrier. The analysis having been performed, the final risk that III-5 is a carrier can be used in genetic counseling. The risk that her first child will have hemophilia A is $1/34\times1/4$, or less than 1%. This risk is appreciably below the prior probability estimated without taking into account the genetic evidence provided by her brothers.

11.4   Empirical Recurrence Risks

11.4.1   Counseling for Complex Disorders

Genetic counselors deal with many conditions that are not single-gene disorders. Instead, counselors may be called on to provide risk estimates for complex trait disorders with a strong genetic component and familial clustering, such as cleft lip and palate, congenital heart disease, meningomyelocele, psychiatric illness, and coronary artery disease. In these situations, the risk for recurrence in first-degree relatives of affected individuals may be increased over the background incidence of the disease in the population. For the vast majority of these disorders, however, we do not know the relevant underlying genetic variants or how they interact with each other or with the environment to cause disease.

As the information gained through the Human Genome Project is applied to the problem of diseases with complex inheritance, physicians and genetic counselors and other health professionals in the years ahead will have more of the information they need to provide accurate molecular diagnosis and risk assessment and to develop rational preventive and therapeutic measures. In the meantime, however, geneticists must rely on **empirically derived risk figures** to give patients and their relatives some answers to their questions about disease risk and how to manage that risk. Recurrence risks are estimated empirically by studying as many families with the disorder as possible and observing how frequently the disorder recurs. The observed frequency of a recurrence is taken as an **empirical recurrence risk**. With time, research should make empirical recurrence risks obsolete, replacing them with individualized assessments of risk based on knowledge of a person's genotype and environmental exposures.

Another area in which empirical recurrence risks must be applied is for chromosomal abnormalities. When one member of a couple is carrying a chromosomal or genome abnormality, such as a balanced translocation or a chromosomal inversion, the risk for a liveborn, chromosomally unbalanced child depends on a number of factors. These include the following:

- Whether the couple was ascertained through a previous liveborn, chromosomally abnormal child, in which case a viable offspring with the chromosome abnormality is clearly possible, or the ascertainment was through chromosome or genome studies for infertility or recurrent miscarriage.
- The chromosomes involved, which region of the chromosome was affected, and the size of the regions that could be potentially trisomic or monosomic in the fetus.
- Whether the mother or father is the carrier of the balanced translocation or inversion.

These factors must all be considered when empirical recurrence risks are determined for a couple in which one member is carrying a balanced translocation or a seemingly "normal" genomic copy number variant.

Empirical recurrence risks are also applied when both parents are chromosomally normal but have a child with, for example, trisomy 21. In this case, the age of the mother plays a major role in that, in a young woman younger than 30 years, recurrence risk for trisomy 21 is approximately 5 per 1,000 and the risk for any chromosome abnormality is approximately 10 per 1,000 as opposed to the population risk of approximately 1.6 per 1,000 live births. Over age 30, however, the age-specific risk becomes the dominant factor, and the fact of a previously affected child with trisomy 21 plays much less of a role in determining recurrence risk.

Genetic counselors must use caution in applying empirical risk figures to a particular family. Firstly, empirical estimates are an average over what is undoubtedly a group of heterogeneous disorders with different mechanisms of inheritance. In any one family, the real recurrence risk may actually be higher or lower than the average. Secondly, empirical risk estimates use history to make predictions about future occurrences. If the underlying biological causes are changing through time, data from the past may not be accurate for the future.

For example, neural tube defects (myelomeningocele and anencephaly) occur in approximately 3.3 per 1,000 live births in the U.S. white population. If, however, a couple has a child with a neural tube defect, the risk in the next pregnancy has been shown to be 40 per 1,000 (13 times higher). The risks remained elevated compared with the general population risk for more distantly related individuals; a second-degree relative (e.g., a nephew or niece) of an individual with a neural tube defect was found to have a 1.7% chance of a similar birth defect. Thus neural tube defects manifest many of the features typical of multifactorial inheritance. However, these empirical recurrence risks were calculated before widespread folic acid supplementation. With folate supplementation before conception and during early pregnancy, these recurrence risk figures have fallen dramatically. This is not because the allelic variants in the families have changed, but rather because a critical environmental factor has changed.

Finally, it is important to emphasize that empirical figures are derived from a particular population, and so the data from one ethnic group, socioeconomic class, or geographical location may not be accurate for an individual from a different background. Nonetheless, such figures are useful when patients ask genetic counselors to give a best estimate for recurrence risk for disorders with complex inheritance.

11.4.2　Genetic Counseling for Consanguinity

Consanguineous couples sometimes request genetic counseling before they have children because an increased risk for birth defects in their offspring is widely appreciated. In the absence of a family history for a known autosomal recessive condition, we use empirical risk figures for the offspring of consanguineous couples, based on population surveys of birth defects in children born to first-cousin couples compared with nonconsanguineous couples (see Table 11-3).

Table 11-3　Incidence of Birth Defects in Children Born to Nonconsanguineous and First-Cousin Couples

First-Cousin Marriage or not	Incidence of First Birth Defect in Sibship (per 1,000)	Incidence of Recurrence of Any Birth Defect in Subsequent Children in Sibship (per 1,000)
First-cousin marriage	36	68
Nonconsanguineous marriage	15	30

(Data from STOLTENBERG C, MAGNUS P, SKRONDAL A, LIE R T. Consanguinity and recurrence risk of birth defects: a population-based study[J]. American journal of medical genetics, 1999, 82 (5):423-428.)

These results provide empirical risk figures in the counseling of first cousins. Although the relative risk for abnormal offspring is higher for related than for unrelated parents, it is still quite low: approximately double in the offspring of first cousins, compared with baseline risk figures for any abnormality of 15 to 20 per 1,000 for any child, regardless of consanguinity. This increased risk is not exclusively for single-gene autosomal recessive diseases but includes the entire spectrum of single-gene and complex trait disorders. However, any couple, consanguineous or not, who has a child with a birth defect is at greater risk for having another child with a birth defect in a subsequent pregnancy.

These risk estimates for consanguinity may be slightly inflated given they are derived from communities in which first-cousin marriages are widespread and encouraged. These are societies in which the degree of relationship (coefficient of inbreeding) between two first cousins may actually be greater than the theoretical due to multiple other lines of relatedness. Furthermore, these same societies may also limit marriages to individuals from the same clan, leading to substantial population stratification, which also increases the rate of autosomal recessive disease beyond what might be expected based on mutant allele frequency alone.

Review Points:

1. Genetic counselors.

A genetic counselor is an expert with a Master of Science degree in genetic counseling. In the United States, they are certified by the American Board of Genetic Counseling. In Canada, genetic counselors are certified by the Canadian Association of Genetic Counsellors. In China, genetic counseling is steered by the Chinese Board of Genetic Counseling (CBGC). Most enter the field from a variety of disciplines, including biology, genetics, nursing, psychology, public health and social work. Genetic counselors should be expert educators, skilled in translating the complex language of genomic medicine into terms that are easy to understand.

2. Patients.

Any person may seek out genetic counseling for a condition they may have inherited from their biological parents.

3. Families or individuals may choose to attend counseling or undergo prenatal testing for a number of reasons.

(1) Family history of a genetic condition or chromosome abnormality.

(2) Molecular test for single gene disorder.

(3) Increased maternal age (35 years and older).

(4) Increased paternal age (40 years and older).

(5) Abnormal maternal serum screening results or ultrasound findings.

(6) Increased nuchal translucency measurements on ultrasound.

(7) Strong family history of cancer.

(8) Predictive testing for adult-onset conditions.

4. Determining recurrence risks. The estimation or recurrence risk is a central concern in genetic counseling.

(1) When a disorder is known to have single-gene inheritance, the recurrence risk for specific family members can usually be determined from basic Mendelian principles.

(2) Risk estimation by use of conditional probability when alternative genotypes are possible.

Study Questions:

1. In a village in Wales in 1984, 13 boys were born in succession before a girl was born. What is the probability of 13 successive male births? What is the probability of 13 successive births of a single sex? What is the probability that after 13 male births, the 14th child will be a boy?
2. Ira and Margie each have a sibling affected with cystic fibrosis.
   a. What are their prior risks for being carriers?
   b. What is the risk for their having an affected child in their first pregnancy?
   c. They have had three unaffected children and now wish to know their risk for having an affected child. Using Bayesian analysis to take into consideration that they have already had three unaffected children, calculate the chance that their next child will be affected.

REFERENCES

[1] FEERO W G, GUTTMACHER A E, COLLINS F S. Genomic medicine—an updated primer[J]. The new england journal of medicine, 2010,362(20):2001−2011.

[2] GINSBURG G, WILLARD H F. Genomic and personalized medicine (vols 1 & 2) [M]. 2nd ed. New York: Elsevier, 2012.

[3] FRAZER K A. Decoding the human genome[J]. Genome research. 2012,22(9): 1599−1601.

[4] VENTER J, ADAMS M, MYERS E, et al. The sequence of the human genome [J]. Science, 2001,291(5507):1304−1351.

[5] BENNETT R L, FRENCH K S, RESTA R G, DOYLE D L. Standardized human pedigree nomenclature: update and assessment of the recommendations of the National Society of Genetic Counselors[J]. Journal of genetic counseling, 2008,17(5):424−433.

[6] SCRIVER C R, BEAUDET A L, SLY W S, et al. The metabolic and molecular bases of inherited disease 8th edition 2001[J]. Journal of inherited metabolic disease, 2001,24: 519−520.

[7] BALDWIN E L, MAY L F, JUSTICE A N, et al. Mechanisms and consequences of small supernumerary marker chromosomes[J]. The american journal of human genetics, 2008, 82(2):398−410.

[8] COULTER M E, MILLER D T, HARRIS D J, et al. Chromosomal microarray testing influences medical management[J]. Genetics in medicine, 2011,13(9):770−776.

[9] FIRTH H V, RICHARDS S M, BEVAN A P, et al. DECIPHER: database of chromosomal imbalance and phenotype in humans using ensembl resources[J]. The american journal of human genetics, 2009,84(4):524−533.

[10] HIGGINS A W, ALKURAYA F S, BOSCO A F, et al. Characterization of apparently balanced chromosomal rearrangements from the Developmental Genome Anatomy Project[J]. The american journal of human genetics, 2008,82(3):712−722.

[11] NAGAOKA S I, HASSOLD T J, HUNT P A. Human aneuploidy: mechanisms

and new insights into an age-old problem[J]. Nature reviews genetics, 2012,13(7):493-504.

[12] REDDY U M, PAGE G P, SAADE G R, et al. Karyotype versus microarray testing for genetic abnormalities after stillbirth[J]. The new england journal of medicine, 2012, 367(23):2185-2193.

[13] TALKOWSKI M E, ERNST C, HEILBUT A, et al. Next-generation sequencing strategies enable routine detection of balanced chromosome rearrangements for clinical diagnostics and genetic research[J]. The american journal of human genetics, 2011,88(4): 469-481.

[14] BAXTER R M, VILAIN E. Translational genetics for diagnosis of human disorders of sex development[J]. Annual review of genomics and human genetics, 2013, 14:371-392.

[15] COOPER G M, COE B P, GIRIRAJAN S, et al. A copy number variation morbidity map of developmental delay[J]. Nature genetics, 2011,43(9):838-846.

[16] HUGHES I A, DAVIES J D, BUNCH T I, et al. Androgen insensitivity syndrome [J]. The lancet, 2012,380(9851):1419-1428.

[17] KAMINSKY E B, KAUL V, PASCHALL J, et al. An evidence-based approach to establish the functional and clinical significance of copy number variants in intellectual and developmental disabilities[J]. Genetics in medicine, 2011,13(9):777-784.

[18] KORBEL J O, TIROSH-WAGNER T, URBAN A E, et al. The genetic architecture of Down syndrome phenotypes revealed by high-resolution analysis of human segmental trisomies[J]. Proceedings of the national academy of sciences of the united states of america, 2009,106(29):12031-12036.

[19] NAJMABADI H, HU H, GARSHASBI M, et al. Deep sequencing reveals 50 novel genes for recessive cognitive disorders[J]. Nature, 2011,478(7367):57-63.

[20] TALKOWSKI M E, ROSENFELD J A, BLUMENTHAL I, et al. Sequencing chromosomal abnormalities reveals neurodevelopmental loci that confer risk across diagnostic boundaries[J]. Cell, 2012,149(3):525-537.

[21] WEISCHENFELDT J, SYMMONS O, SPITZ F, et al. Phenotypic impact of genomic structural variation: insights from and for human disease[J]. Nature reviews genetics, 2013,14(2):125-138.

[22] AMIEL J, SPROAT-EMISON E, GARCIA-BARCELO M, et al. Hirschsprung disease, associated syndromes, and genetics: a review[J]. Journal of medical genetics, 2008,45 (1):1-14.

[23] MALHOTRA D, MCCARTHY S, MICHAELSON J J, et al. High frequencies of de novo CNVs in bipolar disorder and schizophrenia[J]. Neuron, 2011,72(6):951-963.

[24] TROWSDALE J, KNIGHT J C. Major histocompatibility complex genomics and

human disease[J]. Annual review of genomics and human genetics, 2013,14:301−323.

[25] BECK C R, GARCIA-PEREZ J L, BADGE R M, et al. LINE-1 elements in structural variation and disease[J]. Annual review of genomics and human genetics, 2011,12: 187−215.

[26] CHESS A. Mechanisms and consequences of widespread random monoallelic expression[J]. Nature reviews genetics, 2012,13(6):421−428.

[27] DEKKER J. Gene regulation in the third dimension [J]. Science, 2008, 319 (5871):1793−1794.

[28] DJEBALI S, DAVIS C A, MERKEL A, et al. Landscape of transcription in human cells[J]. Nature, 2012,489(7414):101−108.

[29] HEYN H, ESTELLER M. DNA methylation profiling in the clinic: applications and challenges[J]. Nature reviews genetics, 2012,13(10):679−692.

[30] HÜBNER M R, SPECTOR D L. Chromatin dynamics [J]. Annual review of biophysics, 2010, 39:471−489.

[31] ZHOU V W, GOREN A, BERNSTEIN B E. Charting histone modifications and the functional organization of mammalian genomes[J]. Nature reviews genetics, 2011,12(1): 7−18.

[32] CHIN L, ANDERSEN J N, FUTREAL P A. Cancer genomics, from discovery science to personalized medicine[J]. Nature medicine, 2011,17(3):297−303.

[33] KILPLIVARA O, AALTONEN L A. Diagnostic cancer genome sequencing and the contribution of germline variants[J]. Science, 2013,339(6127):1559−1562.

[34] LAL A, PANOS R, MARJANOVIC M, et al. A gene expression profile test to resolve head & neck squamous versus lung squamous cancers[J]. Diagnostic pathology, 2013,8 (1):44.

[35] WATSON I R, TAKAHASHI K, FUTREAL P A, et al. Emerging patterns of somatic mutations in cancer[J]. Nature reviews genetics, 2013,14(10):703−718.

[36] ALKAN C, COE B P, EICHLER E E. Genome structural variation discovery and genotyping[J]. Nature reviews genetics, 2011,12(5):363−376.

[37] KONG A, FRIGGE M L, MASSON G, et al. Rate of de novo mutations and the importance of father's age to disease risk[J]. Nature, 2012,488(7412):471−475.

[38] LAPPALAINEN T, SAMMETH M, FRIEDLÄNDER M R, et al. Transcriptome and genome sequencing uncovers functional variation in humans [J]. Nature, 2013, 501 (7468):506−511.

[39] MACARTHUR D G, BALASUBRAMANIAN S, FRANKISH A, et al. A systematic survey of loss-of function variants in human protein-coding genes[J]. Science, 2012,

335(6070):823-828.

[40] SUN J X, HELGASON A, MASSON G, et al. A direct characterization of human mutation based on microsatellites[J]. Nature genetics, 2012,44(10):1161-1165.

[41] BIFFI A, MONTINI E, LORIOLI L, et al. Lentiviral hematopoietic stem cell gene therapy benefits metachromatic leukodystrophy[J]. Science, 2013,341(6148):1233158.

[42] CATHOMEN T, EHL S. Translating the genomic revolution—targeted genome editing in primates[J]. The new england journal of medicine, 2014,370(24):2342-2345.

[43] COELHO T, ADAMS D, SILVA A, et al. Safety and efficacy of RNAi therapy for transthyretin amyloidosis[J]. The new england journal of medicine, 2013,369(9):819-829.

[44] DALEY G Q. The promise and perils of stem cell therapeutics[J]. Cell stem cell, 2012,10(6):740-749.

[45] DONG A, RIVELLA S, BREDA L. Gene therapy for hemoglobinopathies: progress and challenges[J]. Translational research, 2013,161(4):293-306.

[46] GAZIEV J, LUCARELLI G. Hematopoietic stem cell transplantation for thalassemia [J]. Current stem cell research & therapy, 2011,6(2):162-169.

[47] HANNA J H, SAHA K, JAENISCH R. Pluripotency and cellular reprogramming: facts, hypotheses, unresolved issues[J]. Cell, 2010,143(4):508-525.

[48] LI M, SUZUKI K, KIM N Y, et al. A cut above the rest: targeted genome editing technologies in human pluripotent stem cells[J]. The journal of biological chemistry, 2014,289 (8):4594-4599.

[49] ROBINTON D A, DALEY G Q. The promise of induced pluripotent stem cells in research and therapy[J]. Nature, 2012,481(7381):295-305.

[50] SANDER J D, JOUNG J K. CRISPR-Cas systems for editing, regulating and targeting genomes[J]. Nature biotechnology, 2014,32(4):347-355.

[51] BIESECKER L G, GREEN R C. Diagnostic clinical genome and exome sequencing[J]. The new england journal of medicine, 2014,370(25):2418-2425.

[52] GUTTMACHER A E, COLLINS F S, CARMONA R H. The family history: More important than ever[J]. The new england journal of medicine, 2004,351(22):2333-2336.

[53] SHERIDAN E, WRIGHT J, SMALL N, et al. Risk factors for congenital anomaly in a multiethnic birth cohort: an analysis of the Born in Bradford study[J]. The lancet, 2013, 382(9901):1350-1359.

[54] YANG Y P, MUZNY D M, REID J G, et al. Clinical whole-exome sequencing for the diagnosis of mendelian disorders[J]. The new england journal of medicine, 2013,369 (16):1502-1511.